Theory and Treatment Planning in Counseling and Psychotherapy

DIANE R. GEHART, Ph.D.

California State University, Northridge

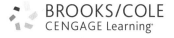

BROOKS/COLE
CENGAGE Learning

Australia • Brazil • Japan • Korea • Mexico • Singapore • Spain • United Kingdom • United States

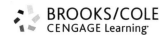

Theory and Treatment Planning in Counseling and Psychotherapy
Diane R. Gehart, Ph.D.

Publisher/Executive Editor: Jon-David Hague

Acquisitions Editor: Seth Dobrin

Assistant Editor: Naomi Dreyer

Editorial Assistant/Associate: Suzanna Kincaid

Media Editor: Elizabeth Momb

Marketing Program Manager: Tami Strang

Manufacturing Planner: Judy Inouye

Rights Acquisitions Specialist: Tom McDonough

Design Direction, Production Management, and Composition: PreMediaGlobal

Cover Designer: Norman Baugher

Cover Image: © szefei/Shutterstock, © Adrian Chinery/Shutterstock, © dmiskv/Shutterstock, © karam Miri/Shutterstock

Library of Congress Control Number: 2012930177

ISBN-13: 978-0-8400-2860-0

ISBN-10: 0-8400-2860-1

Brooks/Cole
20 Davis Drive
Belmont, CA 94002-3098
USA

Cengage Learning is a leading provider of customized learning solutions with office locations around the globe, including Singapore, the United Kingdom, Australia, Mexico, Brazil, and Japan. Locate your local office at **www.cengage.com/global**.

Cengage Learning products are represented in Canada by Nelson Education, Ltd.

To learn more about Brooks/Cole, visit **www.cengage.com/brookscole**

Purchase any of our products at your local college store or at our preferred online store **www.cengagebrain.com**.

Printed in the United States of America
1 2 3 4 5 6 7 16 15 14 13 12

Dedication

This book is dedicated to my son, Michael,
whose first two years of life have brought inspiration and joy
to the writing of this book—while the many printed rough drafts
became the canvas for his first creative projects.

Brief Table of Contents

Detailed Table of Contents

Preface

Using state-of-the-art pedagogical methods, *Theory and Treatment Planning in Counseling and Psychotherapy* is a new generation textbook specifically designed to enable faculty to easily and consistently measure student learning outcomes and competency, a task now required by all regional and professional accrediting bodies. Using a learning-centered, outcome-based pedagogy, the text engages students in an *active learning process* rather than deliver content in a traditional narrative style. More specifically, the text introduces counseling and psychotherapy theories using a) *theory-informed case conceptualization* and b) *treatment planning*. These assignments empower students to apply theoretical concepts and develop real-world skills as early as possible in their training, resulting in greater mastery of the material. Furthermore, the author uses a friendly and fun style to explain concepts in clear and practical language that contemporary students appreciate. Instructors will enjoy the simplicity of having the text and assignments work seamlessly together, thus requiring less time in class preparation and grading. The extensive set of instructor materials—which include syllabi templates, detailed PowerPoints, test banks, online lectures, and scoring rubrics designed for accreditation assessment—further reduce educators' workloads. In summary, the book employs the most efficient and effective pedagogical methods available to teach counseling and psychotherapy theories, resulting in a win/win for instructors and students alike.

Appropriate Courses

A versatile book that serves as a reference across the curriculum, this text is specifically designed for use as a primary or secondary textbook in the following courses:

- Introductory or advanced counseling and psychotherapy theories courses
- Pre-practicum skills classes
- Practicum or fieldwork classes

Assessing Student Learning and Competence

The learning assignments in the text are designed to simplify the process of measuring student learning for regional and national accreditation. The case conceptualization and treatment plans in the book come with scoring rubrics, which are available on the student and instructor websites for the book at www.cengagebrain.com. Scoring rubrics are available for all major mental health disciplines using the following sets of competencies:

- *Counseling:* 2009 Council on the Accreditation of Counseling and Related Educational Programs (CACREP) standards for each of the six areas of specialization
- *Marriage and Family Therapy:* MFT core competencies
- *Psychology:* Psychology competency benchmarks (2011 revision)
- *Social work:* Council for Social Work Education (CSWE) accreditation standards

Each scoring rubric is linked to competencies identified in these disciplinary standards, and discipline-specific sample syllabi on the website include lists of the competencies covered on the treatment plan and case conceptualization assignments.

Organization

This book is organized into three parts:

- **Part I: Introduction to Counseling Theories and Treatment Planning** provides an introduction to counseling, competencies, research, and treatment planning.
- **Part II: Counseling Theories** covers the major schools of counseling and psychotherapy theory.
  - **Analytic Theories**
    - Psychoanalytic and psychodynamic theories
    - Jungian Analysis
    - Adler's Individual Psychology
  - **Humanistic-Existential Theories**
    - Person-Centered
    - Existential
    - Gestalt
  - **Action-Oriented Theories**
    - Behavioral and Cognitive-Behavioral
    - Family systems
  - **Postmodern Theories**
    - Solution-focused
    - Narrative
    - Collaborative
    - Feminist
- **Part III: Integration and Case Conceptualization** describes current trends towards integration and includes a comprehensive integrative case conceptualization approach to help solidify your understanding of theories.

The theory chapters in Part II are organized in a user-friendly way to maximize students' ability to use the book when developing case conceptualizations, writing treatment plans, and designing interventions with clients. The theory chapters follow this outline consistently through the book:

- **In a Nutshell**: The Least You Need to Know
- **The Juice**: Significant Contributions to the Field: If there is one thing to remember from this chapter it should be…
- **Rumor Has It**: The People and Their Stories
- **The Big Picture**: Overview of the Counseling Process
- **Making Connection**: The Counseling Relationship
- **The Viewing**: Case Conceptualization
- **Targeting Change**: Goal Setting
- **The Doing**: Interventions
- **Snapshot**: Research and Evidence Base
- **Snapshot**: Working with Diverse Populations
- Online Resources
- Reference List
- **Case Example**: Vignette with Case Conceptualization and Treatment Plan

Student Supplements

At www.cengagebrain.com students will find the following resources to help them in the learning process:

- **Online lectures**: video files with PowerPoints and the author lecturing on selected chapters in the book
- Blank treatment plan and integrated case conceptualization templates to use when completing assignments

- Per-chapter **online quizzes** to check understanding
- **Scoring rubric** correlated to each discipline's required core competencies that may be used by their instructors for grading the assignment.
- **Glossary** of key terms with definitions to assist students while studying

Instructor's Supplements

An online instructor's manual and test bank is available for download at www.cengage.com/login. The manual includes:

- Detailed **PowerPoint slides** for each chapter
- Sample **syllabi** templates for faculty, with discipline-specific lists of competencies covered on all assignments:
    ○ Counseling and psychotherapy theory courses: counseling, family therapy, social work, and psychology
    ○ Practicum/fieldwork courses: counseling, family therapy, social work, and psychology
- **Online lectures:** video files with PowerPoints and the author lecturing on selected chapters in the book
- Extensive multiple-choice **test bank,** with answer key and page references
- **Treatment plan** and integrated case conceptualization templates for student assignment
- **Scoring rubrics** pre-correlated for national accreditation bodies
    ○ *Counseling:* 2009 Council on the Accreditation of Counseling and Related Educational Programs (CACREP) standards for each of the six areas of specialization
    ○ *Marriage and Family Therapy:* MFT core competencies
    ○ *Psychology:* 2011 Psychology Competency Benchmarks
    ○ *Social work:* Council for Social Work Education competencies

Instructors can access these materials through their "Instructor Bookshelf" at Cengage Learning (www.cengage.com/login) which they can create by completing a brief online registration form. Instructors can add the ancillaries for this title, and others, to their virtual bookshelves at any time.

Acknowledgments

I would like to thank the following content experts who gave their time and energy to ensure that the information in this textbook was accurate and current:

Rie Rogers Mitchell: Jungian sand play, psychodynamic theories
Luis Rubalcava: psychodynamic theories
Stan Charnofsky: humanistic, person centered, Gestalt, existential
Wendel Ray and his doctoral students, Todd Gunter and Allison Lux: systemic theories
Marion Lindblad-Goldberg: systemic theories
Scott Woolley: emotionally focused therapy
Bill O'Hanlon: solution-based therapies
Harlene Anderson: collaborative therapy
Gerald Monk: narrative therapy
Ron Chenail: Competencies Assessment System
Thorana Nelson: Competencies Assessment System
William Northey: Competencies Assessment System

I would also like to thank the following people for their assistance:

Alejandra Trujillo: My volunteer research assistant who helped me locate hundreds of original sources cited in this text and one of the most competent women I have had the pleasure to work with.
Eric Garcia: The amazing CSUN librarian assigned to my department who helped locate many of resources used in this book.
Seth Dobrin: The book's fabulous and supportive editor at Cengage who helped make this book a success. Thank you for always being a joy to work with.
Joseph McNicholas: My incredible husband, whose encouragement, support, and understanding made the process fun; I hope he enjoyed the dinner conversations about counseling theories along the way.
Michael McNicholas: My son, whose magical first two years of life provided inspiration and joy while writing this book—you add so much light to my life!

Finally, I would like to thank the following reviewers and survey respondents who provided invaluable feedback on making this book work for faculty:

Reviewers:

Gregg Allinson, Beaufort County Community College
Samantha Anders, University of Minnesota
Kathleen Arveson, Regent University
Nancy Baily, University of West Alabama
Jayne Barnes, Nashua Community College
Eric Burns, Campbellsville University

Tamara Clingerman, Syracuse University

Paul DeSena, Loyola Marymount University

Annmarie Early, Eastner Mennonite University

Bengu Erguner-Tekinalp, Drake University, Des Moines

Yvonne Garza, Sam Houston State University

Helene Halvorson, East Tennessee State University

Glenda Hufnagel, University of Oklahoma, Norman

Donna Huger, South Carolina State University

Nithya Karuppaswamy, University of Illinois, Springfield

Mary Livingston, Louisiana Technical University

Krista Medina, University of Cincinnati

Paula Nelson, Saint Leo University

Jenny Savage, Jacksonville State University

Cheryl Warner, Clemson University

Kelly Wester, University of North Carolina, Greensboro

Survey Respondents:

Ernestine C. Brittingham, Delaware State University

Charmaine D. Caldwell, Valdosta State University

Mathilda Catarina, William Paterson University

Dibya Choudhuri, Eastern Michigan University

Nancy DeCesare, Chestnut Hill College

Faith Drew, Pfeiffer University

Kevin R. Galey, Dallas Baptist University

Amy Ginsberg, Long Island University

Nicholas Greco, Adler School of Professional Psychology

Kathleen Hathaway, Clover Park Technical College

James M. Hepburn, Waynesburg University

Mary Kay Houston-Vega, University of Texas at San Antonio

Stuart G. Itzkowitz, Wayne State University

Kelly James, Brigham Young University

Randi Kim, Rhode Island College

Cynthia N. Lepley, Thomas College

David Lutz, Missouri State University

Don Lynch, Unity College

Jeanie McCarville Kerber, Des Moines Area Community College

Polly McMahon, Spokane Falls Community College

Richard McWhorter, Prairie View A&M University

C. Michael Nina, William Paterson University

Gwen Newsom, North Carolina Central University

Kate Pandolpho, Kean University

Lois Pasapane, Palm Beach State College

Kim-Anne Perkins, University of Maine at Presque Isle

David Rentler, Northwestern Connecticut Community College

Barbara Roland, Grayson County College

Allen R. Stata, Judson College

Jenny Warren, Liberty University

About the Author

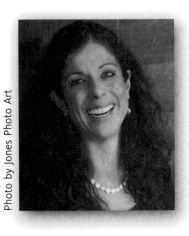

DR. DIANE R. GEHART is a professor in the Marriage and Family Therapy and Counseling Programs at California State University, Northridge. Having practiced, taught, and supervised for nearly 20 years, she has authored/edited the following:

- *Mastering Competencies in Family Therapy*
- *Mindfulness and Acceptance in Couple and Family Therapy*
- *The Complete MFT Core Competency Assessment System*
- *The Complete Counseling Assessment System*
- *Collaborative Therapy: Relationships and Conversations That Make a Difference* (coedited)
- *Theory-Based Treatment Planning for Marriage and Family Therapists* (coauthored)

She has also written extensively on postmodern therapies, mindfulness, mental health recovery, sexual abuse treatment, gender issues, children and adolescents, client advocacy, qualitative research, and counselor and marriage and family therapy education. She speaks internationally, having given workshops to professional and general audiences in the United States, Canada, Europe, and Mexico. Her work has been featured in newspapers, radio shows, and television worldwide, including the BBC, National Public Radio, Oprah Winfrey's O magazine, and *Ladies' Home Journal*. She is an associate faculty member at three international postgraduate training institutes: the Houston Galveston Institute, the Taos Institute, and the Marburg Institute for Collaborative Studies in Germany. Additionally, she is an active leader in state and national professional organizations. She maintains a private practice in Thousand Oaks, California, specializing in couples, families, women's issues, trauma, life transitions, and difficult-to-treat cases. For fun, she enjoys spending time with her family, hiking, swimming, yoga, salsa dancing, meditating, and savoring all forms of dark chocolate. You can learn more about her work at www.dianegehart.com.

Author's Introduction

Bridge Across the Grand Canyon

Known for making its visitors audibly gasp in awe, the Grand Canyon is so wide at points that it is hard to see the other side. Having inspired reverence for generations, this great natural wonder provides many with a palpable experience of the divine. However, these qualities are not what I believe students over the years were referring to when they told me that the gap between their university course work and fieldwork experiences was like the Grand Canyon. In marked contrast, my students were referring to the canyon's gaping and seemingly impassable chasms that appear impossible to traverse, at least not without hiring a personal jet, helicopter, or the starship *Enterprise*. Clearly, my students were feeling as though they were not able to connect their classroom experiences to their internships with the tools they had been given. Thus, I am writing this book to create a bridge across the Grand Canyon of Counseling—or at least a zip line—to help new counselors and therapists gracefully traverse two worlds that have been far too distant for too long: the worlds of academic theory and real-world practice.

You might be thinking, "That is a bold claim. How is she going to achieve this lofty goal?" As often happens in life, the answer lies in the question. In this case, the key is the term *goal*. As you learn about counseling and psychotherapy theories in this book, you are also going to learn how these theories are used to generate meaningful clinical goals to help clients and their counselors skillfully address the concerns brought to counseling. Thus, you will be introduced to counseling theories from the perspective of a practitioner rather than an academic. You will get less history and more information about how these ideas inform action in the counseling room. Furthermore, you will be given two vehicles for translating theory into practice: case conceptualizations and treatment plans. These tools are what counselors in the field use to help them do their job—and the versions in this book are specifically designed to integrate theoretical knowledge.

This introduction continues in Chapter 1; once you get there, you'll see why. If you happen to have read this first, congratulations. You are way ahead of me!

Diane R. Gehart, PhD
Westlake Village, CA
July 2011

Section I

Introduction to Theories, Competencies, and Treatment Planning

1

Start Here: Introduction and Instructions for Using This Book

Start Here

Similar to many people reading this book, I was one of those students in school who always worked hard and went the extra mile. Perhaps I was simply a nerd (ironically, the last four digits of my family's childhood phone number was 4335, or G-E-E-K). Perhaps it was my immigrant father's constant reminder that without a good education one becomes a ditch digger. Regardless of the reasons, I have always loved the whole "school thing" far more than playing soccer or watching television (okay, confession: being bad at sports may have also played a role). This love of education may have also started with those toddler activity books. I cannot wait for my now 2-year-old son to have homework because few things are more exciting than filling out elementary workbooks—pictures, colors, dots, lines, puzzles, and mazes—much more engaging than dull, dry, black-and-white textbooks (present text excluded).

In graduate school, this overdo-it tendency took another form: never leaving the library. When it came time to write the doctoral dissertation, which some consider the crowning academic assignment in Western civilization, it only seemed natural that one *had* to write an exhaustive literature review. It took me 2 years to write that review. Toward the end, my professor offhandedly mentioned that the review did not have to include every last study related to my topic. After a wave of now-you-tell-me thoughts washed over me, I returned to my personal brand of "sanity" (i.e., overdo-it logic), looked at him, and said, "But I want to," and just kept searching for everything ever written on the subject (please note: my dissertation was written at a time in history when this was possible—the library had a "card catalogue" and only the earliest forms of digital databases).

Given this tendency, it is amazing to look back and realize—and now confess to you—that I never once read the introduction to any of the hundreds of books I "read" in graduate school. Professors never listed them as "required reading," the publisher never cared enough to give a formal chapter or real page number, and they were short, seemingly too short to possibly be of value. Now, sitting here writing to you, I realize that it was foolhardy to skip the introduction. In most cases, authors reveal the most important information, summarize the really big idea behind the book, and tell you how to read and learn from it. In short: it's where the secrets are.

Thus, although anyone reading this book is likely to lean toward the industrious end of the spectrum (but not necessarily a geek and failed athlete like me), I am concerned that they may miss reading the information in the introduction, as I had for decades. So, to avoid that error—easily made by even the most devout learners—the introduction has been placed in Chapter 1. It is also labeled "Start Here" just in case it wasn't clear. Hopefully, you will find that it greatly enhances your ability to get the most out of this book. Also, you may want to take a quick glace at introductions for your future reads.

How This Book Is Different and What It Means to You

Theory and Treatment Planning in Counseling and Psychotherapy is a different kind of textbook. Based on a new pedagogical model, learning-centered teaching (Killen, 2004; Weimer, 2002), this book is designed to help you *actively learn* the content rather than simply deliver the content and hope that you will memorize it. Thus, learning activities are woven into the text so that you have opportunities to apply and use the information in ways that facilitate learning (not unlike my son's elementary school activity books). The specific learning activities in this book are (a) case conceptualization and (b) treatment plans that translate the theory learned in each chapter to client situations. This book teaches real-world skills that you can immediately use to better serve your clients.

Also, this book is different in another way: it is organized by key concepts rather than general headings with long narratives sections. This organization—which evolved from my personal study notes for my doctoral and licensing exams back before I had email (and, no, dinosaurs were not roaming the planet then)—facilitates the retention of vocabulary and terms because of the visual layout. Each year, I receive numerous emails from enthusiastic newly licensed counselors and therapists thanking me for helping them to pass their licensing exams—they all say that the organization of the book made the difference. So, spending some time with this text should better prepare you for the big exams in your future (and if you have already passed these, you should be all the more impressed with yourself for doing it the hard way).

Lay of the Land

This book is organized into three parts:

- **Part I: Introduction to Counseling Theories and Treatment Planning** provides an introduction to counseling, competencies, research, and treatment planning.
- **Part II: Counseling Theories** covers the major schools of counseling and psychotherapy theory.
  - **Analytic theories**
  - **Humanistic-existential theories**
  - **Action-oriented theories**
  - **Postmodern theories**
- **Part III: Integration and Case Conceptualization** describes current trends toward integration and includes a comprehensive integrative case conceptualization approach to help solidify your understanding of theories.

Anatomy of a Theory

The theory chapters in Part II are organized in a user-friendly way to maximize your ability to use this book to support you when developing case conceptualizations, writing treatment plans, and designing interventions with clients. The anatomy of each of the theory chapters in Part II (Chapters 4–13) follows this outline:

Anatomy of a Theory

- **In a Nutshell:** The Least You Need to Know
- **The Juice:** Significant Contributions to the Field

(continued)

- **Rumor Has It:** The People and Their Stories
- **The Big Picture:** Overview of the Counseling Process
- **Making Connection:** The Counseling Relationship
- **The Viewing:** Case Conceptualization
- **Targeting Change:** Goal Setting
- **The Doing:** Interventions
- **Putting It All Together:** Treatment Plan Template
- **Snapshot:** Research and Evidence Base
- **Snapshot:** Working With Diverse Populations
- **Online Resources**
- **Reference List**
- **Case Example:** Vignette With Case Conceptualization and Treatment Plan

- *In a Nutshell: The Least You Need to Know:* The chapters begin with a brief summary of the key features of the theory. Although it may not be the absolute least you need to know to get an A in a theory class or help a client, it is the basic information you should have memorized and be able to quickly articulate at any moment to help you keep your theories straight.
- *The Juice: Significant Contributions to the Field:* In the next section, I use the principle of primacy (first information introduced) to help you remember one of the most significant contributions of the theory to the field of counseling. In most cases, well-trained clinicians who generally use another approach to counseling are likely to be skilled and use this particular concept because it has shaped standard practice in the field. This section is your red flag to remember a seminal concept or practice for the theory. Feedback from students indicates this is often one of their favorite sections.
- *Rumor Has It: The People and Their Stories:* In this section, you can read about the developers of the theory and how their personal stories shaped the evolution of the ideas. And, yes, some of the rumors are juicier than others. As the focus of this text is how counseling theories are actually used in contemporary settings, I have de-emphasized the history and development of the theory, but you will find brief summaries of such history here.
- *The Big Picture: Overview of the Counseling Process:* The big picture provides an overview of the flow of the counseling process: what happens in the beginning, middle, and end and how change is facilitated across these phases.
- *Making Connection: The Counseling Relationship:* All approaches start by establishing a working relationship with clients, but each approach does it differently. In this section, you will read about the unique ways that counselors of various schools build relationships that provide the foundation for change.
- *The Viewing: Case Conceptualization:* The case conceptualization section will identify the signature theory concepts that counselors from each school use to identify and assess clients and their problems. This really is the heart of the theory and where the real differences emerge. *I encourage you to pay particularly close attention to these.* You can also read more about case conceptualization in Chapters 14 and 15.
- *Targeting Change: Goal Setting:* Based on the areas assessed in the case conceptualization and the overall counseling process, each approach has a unique strategy for identifying client goals that become the foundation for the treatment plan.
- *The Doing: Interventions:* Probably the most exciting part for most new counselors, this section outlines the common techniques and interventions for each theory. In some cases, a section for techniques used with special populations is included if these are notably different than those in standard practice.
- *Putting It All Together: Treatment Plan Template:* After graduation, you will probably thank me most for this section, which provides a template for a treatment plan that can

be used for addressing depression, anxiety, and similar concerns. This plan ties everything in the chapter together.

- *Snapshot: Research and Evidence Base:* A short review of the research and evidence base for each theory is provided to offer a general sense of empirical foundations for the theory. In some cases, influential evidence-based treatments (see Chapter 2 for a definition) are highlighted.
- *Snapshot: Working With Diverse Populations:* A second short review of the research related to working with diverse populations is also included to help you consider for whom this approach is best suited and/or not well suited.
- *Online Resources:* A list of Web pages and Web documents are included for those who want to pursue specialized training or conduct further research on the theory.
- *Reference List:* Many students pass right over reference lists and forget all about them. But if you have to do an academic paper or literature review on any of these theories, this should be your first stop. You might remember my historical difficulty with leaving the library. In this case, I had several hundred books go through my 12-by-12-foot office while writing this book over 2 years. Thus, you can certainly shorten the time it takes to locate key resources by pursuing these before you hit the library yourself (oh, I forgot, no one steps foot in these places any more; I meant "surf" the library's Web page while still in your bunny slippers).
- *Case Example: Vignette With Case Conceptualization and Treatment Plan:* Finally, each chapter ends with a case vignette, case conceptualization, and treatment plan to give you a sense of how the theory looks in action and how to put it down on paper. I use examples of adults presenting for individual counseling in this text; see my other text *Mastering Competencies in Family Therapy* (Gehart, 2010) for examples with couples, families, and children. Again, I think you will find this most useful once your instructor or supervisor asks you to write one yourself.

Theoretical Friends and Families

Although each theory presented is wholly unique and independent, like the rest of us, each has friends and families with whom they associate. These are generally referred to as "schools" of counseling or therapy, and these are increasingly important as more and more counselors move toward integrated approaches (see Chapters 14 and 15). Unfortunately, like virtually all systems of grouping individuals, these groupings do not capture the full complexity of their characters. For example, in this book, Adlerian individual psychology is in the "analytic approach" section because it includes analytic elements; however, it also has humanistic, cognitive-behavioral, and even systemic elements. Obviously, reprinting the chapter four times would not help you, so you will have to read each chapter to learn about the similarities and differences between approaches in the same school. The *rough* and *imperfect* classifications of theories in this book are as follows:

- **Analytic approaches**
    - Psychodynamic
    - Jungian analytic
    - Adlerian individual psychology
- **Humanistic-existential approaches**
    - Person centered
    - Existential
    - Gestalt
- **Action-based approaches**
    - Behavioral
    - Cognitive-behavioral
    - Systemic/family
- **Postmodern and multicultural approaches**
    - Solution based
    - Feminist
    - Narrative
    - Collaborative
    - Reflecting teams

Voice and Tone

Finally, I should mention that the voice and tone of this textbook is a bit different than your average college read. Hopefully, you have noticed by now that I am talking right at ya. I also like to add some humor and have some fun while I write. Why? Well, first I have more fun writing this way. But, more important, I want to engage you as if you were one of my students or supervisees learning about how to apply these ideas for the first time. Counseling and psychotherapy are relationship-based practices, one in which both the parties are fully present in their humanity (at least in most approaches). Thus, it is hard for me to write about how to be genuine and present to clients as a detached, faceless author. So, as I write, I am imagining you as a full and real person eager to learn about how to use these ideas to help others. I am going to try to reach out to you, answer questions I imagine you have, and periodically tap you on the shoulder to make sure you are still awake.

Suggested Uses

Suggestions for Thinking About Counseling Theories

As you read the chapters in this book, you are going to be tempted to identify which ones you like the best and de-emphasize the ones to which you are less attracted. This may seem like a great idea at first, but here are some points to consider:

- **Favorite Versus Useful:** The theories that the average counselor finds personally useful are probably not the same ones that the average client of new counselors is likely to find useful. Many counselors are psychologically minded, meaning that they enjoy thinking about the inner world and how it works. However, most new counselors begin working with diverse, multiproblem clients and families many (but not all) of whom are not psychologically minded because they are often struggling with issues of survival and/or come from cultural traditions that place less value on analysis and understanding of the inner world. So the theory you find most useful to you personally may not be a good fit for your first client.
- **Appreciation:** The theories in this book are not casually chosen. They have become part of the standard canon of theories because generations of counselors and therapists have found them helpful. Each has wisdom worthy of study. The one lesson I have learned over the years is that the more theories counselors understand, the better able they are to serve their clients because their understanding of the human condition and its concomitant problems is broader. Thus, I recommend approaching each theory with an attitude of searching for its essential and useful parts. I facilitate this for you in the "Juice" section of each chapter that identifies the one thing you should work hardest to remember from the chapter.
- **Common Threads:** Counseling theories are ironic: in one sense, they are very different and inform distinct and mutually exclusive behaviors and attitudes. However, the better you understand one, the better you understand them all. In fact, some counselors, the common factors proponents, argue that theories are generally equally effective because they are simply different modes for delivering the same factors (Miller, Duncan, & Hubble, 1997; you will read more in Chapter 2). So, it is quite possible that commonalities across theories are *more important* than their differences.

Suggestions for Using This Book to Learn Theories

First, I recommend that you set aside an hour or two to read about a single theory from beginning to end (from "In a Nutshell" to "Putting It All Together") to help get the full sense of the theory. Some chapters have a couple of theories in one, so for these it is fine to read the chapter in chunks. Additionally, some learners may find it helpful to scan the treatment plan (either the template or the example at the end of the chapter) or some other section first to provide a practical overview; that said, I have tried to organize the ideas in the way most people seem to prefer. But I encourage you to discover what works best for you, as different learners have different strategies that work best for them. When you are done with a chapter, you might want to try completing a case conceptualization and treatment plan for yourself (you may have to make up a problem if you are nearly perfect) or someone else to get a sense of how this would work.

Finally, I strongly recommend that either after reading the chapter or after going to class, you take good old-fashioned notes. Yes, I mean it. I recommend that you type up (or, if you prefer, handwrite) a complete outline of the key concepts in your own words. Why do I advocate for such painful torture? All of us, myself included, when we read long, dense books such as this one, fade in and out of alert attentiveness to what we are reading—often lapsing into more interesting fantasies or less interesting to do lists—and—gasp!—sometimes even skim large sections of the text (no, I am not surprised or offended). The only way to make sure that you really understand the concepts you read about is to put them in your own words and organize them in a way that makes sense to you. If you need to take culminating exams or plan to pursue licensure, you will have to log the concepts in this book into your long-term memory, which requires more than cramming for a final exam. If you are new to graduate and professional school, I am sorry to be the bearer of the sad news, unlike undergraduate study, where forgetting everything you learned the week after finals was generally not a problem. Being a mental health professional requires that you master and build on what you learn, and you will be expected to know what is in this book for the entire time you are active in the profession (seriously—and if you think that is bad, just wait until you get to a class on diagnosis—you'll have to memorize an even longer book). Thus, if your former study habits included all-night cramming, gallons of espresso (or other favorite caffeine delivery system), and little recall after the exam, you might want to try my note-taking tip or some other strategy as you move forward.

Suggestions for Using This Book to Write Treatment Plans

Because I know some of you might be tempted to skip ahead to the examples and avoid the boring theory, I feel it necessary to recommend taking a few minutes to read Chapter 3 on treatment planning before trying to quickly write one for class or your supervisor. There are some basic "rules" of good treatment planning that all counselors use and that are clearly spelled out in Chapter 3, and in the end, if you need to get a signature or grade on your treatment plan, it will save you lots of time to read the "how-tos" in Chapter 3 first.

I want to emphasize that the treatment plan format, templates, and examples in this book are just that: formats, templates, and examples. They do not represent the only approach or the only right approach but simply a solid approach based on the common standards and expectations. You most likely will work at a counseling agency or institution that uses another format, but the same general rules (the ones in Chapter 3) will still apply. That is why understanding the principles of how to write good goals and interventions is more important than memorizing the format.

Furthermore, don't use the templates and examples too rigidly. Feel free to modify the goal statements and techniques to fit the unique needs of your client. I have provided some relatively specific goals as an example of what might work and encourage you to tailor these for each client's unique needs.

Suggestions for Use in Internships and Clinical Practice

When working as an intern or licensed mental health professional, this book can be useful for teaching yourself theories and techniques in addition to learning how to write treatment plans. You will likely find that when you work with new populations and problems, you may be interested in considering how other therapy models might approach these situations. This book is designed to be a prime resource for quickly scanning to identify other possibilities. Alternatively, you might have a colleague or supervisor who uses a theory with which you are not familiar. You can use this book to quickly review that theory and keep from looking uneducated. In addition, this book is written to help you appreciate and find common ground across theories, which can be of particular benefit when working in a "mixed-theory" context. However, to actually learn to practice any of these theories well, I strongly urge you to take advanced training from experts in that approach.

Suggestions for Studying for Licensing Exams

Licensing exams are designed not to be unnecessarily tricky or scary but simply to ensure that you have knowledge necessary to practice counseling and psychotherapy without supervision *and not harm anybody*. And it is a vocabulary test. If you have honestly engaged your classes, done your homework, avoided cramming for tests and papers, and made it a priority to get decent supervision, you should have a strong foundation for taking your licensing exam. You should already have in your possession books (such as this) that cover all the content to be studied for the exam. If your exam is to be taken on finishing a lengthy post-master's internship, you should use the entire 2- to 4-year period to read as many books as possible on the theories and materials covered by the exam (no novels for a few years).

I do not recommend that all my students take long, expensive "review courses" because such courses are not necessary for those who are proactive in mastering the material on the exam long before they sign up to take it. If you start studying only after you are approved to take the test, you are starting about 2 to 4 years too late—and then, yes, you will need to take a crash course. My basic suggestion for studying for mental health licensing exam is this: read an original text on each major theory during your postdegree internship, use the *Diagnostic and Statistical Manual of Mental Disorders* (*DSM*), and keep up with laws and ethics, then buy the practice exams (without the study guides) and take them until you consistently get 5% above the required passing score (e.g., 75% if the passing score is 70%). If you find that you are weak in a particular area, such as theory or *DSM*, use a text such as this, which is designed with the license review in mind. Once you consistently get 75%, you are ready to take the test with the most learning and the least expense.

Suggestions for Faculty to Measure Competencies and Student Learning

This book is specifically designed to help faculty and supervisors simplify and streamline the onerous task of measuring student competencies as required by the various accreditation bodies. The forms and scoring rubrics for assessing student learning using counseling, psychology, social work, and family therapy competencies are available on this book's Web page for instructors (see **www.cengage.com** or **www.masteringcompetencies.com**). On this website, instructors will also find free online lectures, PowerPoints, sample syllabi, and a test bank (test banks are available only from your Cengage sales representative to maintain security of the questions). This text may be used as the primary or secondary text in a counseling theories class or as the primary text in a pre-practicum or practicum/ fieldwork class. Because of its combination of solid theory and practical skills, it can easily be used across more than one class to develop students' abilities to conceptualize theory and write treatment plans, skills that are not likely to be mastered in a single class.

When designing a class to measure competencies and student learning using these treatment plans and case conceptualizations, I recommend initially going over the scoring rubrics with students so that they understand how these are used to clearly define what needs to be done and the expectations for the final product. I have found that it is most helpful to provide two or three opportunities to practice case conceptualization and treatment planning over a semester to provide feedback and enable students to improve and build on these skills in a systematic fashion. The online instructor resources includes several example syllabi for the different mental health disciplines. Specifically, I have a small group present a case conceptualization and treatment plan with each theory studied based on a video the class watches on the theory; that way, they have enough information to actually conceptualize the client dynamics and treatment. Then the entire class can see an example and discuss the thought process of developing the plan. A later or final assignment for the class can be to independently develop a treatment plan for a case (either one assigned by the instructor or one from a popular movie, personal life, or actual client). By the end of a semester with these activities, students will have developed not only competence but also confidence in their case conceptualization and treatment planning abilities.

Student Resources

Students will find numerous useful resources for this text on the Cengage website (**www .cengage.com**) and the author's websites (**www.dianegehart.com** and **www.mastering competencies.com**). These include the following:

- Online lectures: mp4 recordings of yours truly discussing content of the various chapters
- Digital forms for the treatment plan and integrative case conceptualization
- Scoring rubrics
- Links to related websites and readings
- Glossary of key concepts and terms

Instructor Resources

Instructors will find numerous resources for the book online on the Cengage website (**www.cengage.com**) or the author's websites (**www.masteringcompetencies.com** and **www.dianegehart.com**):

- Online lectures by the author
- Sample syllabi for how to use this book in a theory class or practicum class in counseling, family therapy, psychology, or social work. These syllabi include detailed lists of the competencies covered for each discipline to meet accreditation requirements
- Detailed PowerPoints for all of the chapters
- Downloadable versions of the integrative case conceptualization, treatment plan, and scoring rubrics (rubrics are correlated to competencies for each of the CACREP specialities as well as the core competencies/benchmarks for family therapy, psychology, and social work)
- Test bank and Web quizzes (available only from your Cengage representative)

Next Steps

Now that you are acquainted with the lay of the land, it is time to get down to business. In the chapters that follow, you will learn more about competencies in the field of counseling and psychotherapy and what they mean for you and your future as a professional. Part of this tour includes a review of what it means to be a professional and the ethical duties that come with the job. We will also explore the purpose of counseling theories and consider two streams of research that inform the use and development of these theories: the common factors research and evidence-based treatment studies. Then you will learn about the nuts and bolts of treatment planning in Chapter 3. This one may be a bit dry, but I promise that once you are assigned to write your first one, you will find it to be one of the most exciting in this book—nothing like the pressure of having to write your first plan to alter your perspective of what is fascinating. The remainder of this book will take you on a grand tour of some of the most exciting ideas from the 20th and 21st centuries. I have confidence that it will be the trip of a lifetime.

   Bon voyage!

   And congratulations on reading your first (secretly disguised) book introduction! I hope you can see the value now.

ONLINE RESOURCES

Webpage for this book: www.cengagebrain.com

Student Resource Page:

- Treatment plan and case conceptualization forms
- Scoring rubrics
- Online lectures (also at www.masteringcompentencies.com)
- Glossary of key concepts and terms

Instructor Resource Page:

- Sample syllabi with detailed list of competencies covered in the class
- PowerPoints for each chapter
- Treatment plan and case conceptualization forms
- Scoring rubrics correlated to accreditation competencies for counseling, family therapy, psychology, and social work.
- Test bank and Web quizzes

My Web page that has resources for clients but will always contain a link to the site for this page. www.dianegehart.com

My Web page that contains many of the resources also available on the Cengage page as well as live links and other resources on this and my other textbooks. www.masteringcompetencies.com

References

Gehart, D. (2010). *Mastering competencies in family therapy: A practical approach to theory and clinical case documentation.* Pacific Grove, CA: Brooks/Cole.

Killen, R. (2004). *Teaching strategies for outcome-based education.* Cape Town: Juta Academic.

Miller, S. D., Duncan, B. L., & Hubble, M. (1997). *Escape from Babel: Toward a unifying language for psychotherapy practice.* New York: Norton.

Weimer, M. (2002). *Learner-centered teaching: Five key changes to practice.* New York: Jossey-Bass.

2

Counseling Theory, Competency, Research, and You: Connecting the Dots

What Distinguishes a Counselor From a Bartender?

What makes a counselor or therapist different from a good bartender, hairdresser, or friend? In many cases, the latter are excellent listeners, can be empathetic, and help solve problems. Aside from the obvious fact that bartenders and friends are cheaper than counselors, and hairdressers are more expensive, counselors go beyond these basic helping skills and do something more. Counselors use counseling *theory* to (a) develop a specific form of helping relationship, (b) articulate more useful understandings of clients' situations, and (c) identify effective means to resolve clients' presenting problems. In the end, it is the ability to skillfully translate theory into action that makes counselors different from those helpful others. Counseling theories provide powerful lenses through which to view clients' situations and identify the most expedient means to resolve their concerns. This book will show you how counselors do it—and perhaps one day you will use this skill to make nearly as much as your stylist.

Why Theory Matters

Although much has changed in the past decade in mental health care—better research to guide us, new knowledge about the brain, more details about mental health disorders, and increased use of psychotropic medication—the primary tool that counselors and psychotherapists use to help people has not: *theory*. Counseling theory provides a means for quickly sifting through the tremendous amount of information clients bring; then targeting specific thoughts, behaviors, or emotional processes for change; and finally helping clients to effectively make these changes to resolve their initial concerns. Even with fancy functional magnetic resonance imaging, neurofeedback machines, and hundreds of available medications, no other technology has taken the place of theory. However, the changing landscape of mental health care has changed how counseling theories are understood and used.

Do I Have to Choose?

Over the years, the role of theory in counseling and psychotherapy has become less rather than more clear. Initially, the general recommendation was to select and train in one theory, which became a counselor's primary identity and style of working; it was a personal choice, and the story ended there. Textbooks such as this one are grounded around this honorable tradition, a tradition in which I was "raised." However, many counselors like to "mix it up," integrating theories, which has been an increasingly popular and justified practice in the field (see the "Common Factors Research: Reframing Theory" section; Miller, Duncan, & Hubble, 2004).

Similarly, many of my students, on reading their first theory textbook, enthusiastically exclaim, "I like them all; do I have to choose?" It's one of those questions that they quickly regret asking. Because rather than give a simple yes-or-no answer (anyone who asks is hoping for "no"), I must instead go into a long lecture on epistemological foundations, developmental stages of becoming a counselor, research on outcomes, evidence-based treatment, and so on. Within 15 minutes, the class gets very quiet. After half an hour, most are scrunching their faces with stress. By the end of the first hour, all have given up hope for a simple answer to their question. So now it's your turn to listen to the answer to this question, and out of compassion, I will provide you with a quick overview and road map.

Counseling theory and how it is being used and understood has been recontextualized by two major movements in recent years: (a) the competency movement, which includes multicultural competency, and (b) expanding research base and the evidence-based treatment movement. These movements have not ended the need for theory but have instead changed how we conceptualize, adapt, and apply theory.

Counseling and Psychotherapy Theory Recontextualized: A Road Map

- **Competency: Common Threads in Competent Use of Theory**
  - ◦ Diversity and multicultural competence
  - ◦ Research competence
  - ◦ Law and ethics
  - ◦ Person-of-the-counselor
- **Research and the Evidence Base: Reframing and Redesigning Theory**
  - ◦ Common factors (across theories) research
  - ◦ Evidence-based practice and treatments

Competency in Counseling and Psychotherapy

Stereotypes are dangerous and typically inaccurate. Nonetheless, I am going to risk stating such a generalization, namely, that counselors and therapists care about others. Most counselors feel called to the profession to help others and to make a difference in the world. Few report being motivated by fame and riches, as there are easier and more expedient means to these ends (you may need to chat with a career counselor if this comes as a surprise). Many find inspiration from the work of Carl Rogers (1951, 1961), who radically claimed that accurate empathy, unconditional positive regard, and genuineness are not only necessary but also *sufficient* conditions for promoting change in clients. At the grassroots level, clients often describe effective counselors as "nice," good-hearted people. Research indicates that this human connection is one of the strongest predictors of change in the counseling process (Miller, Duncan, & Hubble, 1997). But the counseling relationship does not account for all the change; in fact, many argue that it is not enough.

Regardless of whether you side with Rogers or those who claim that more is needed, competent counseling in the 21st century demands that counselors do more than care, that they are more than nice, and that they demonstrate more than the core conditions that Rogers advocated. The standard of practice in today's treatment environments involves several key elements that counselors must master to be considered *competent*: having the necessary skills for the job. All mental health professionals who provide counseling and psychotherapy services must master a core set of competencies, including counselors, family therapists, clinical and counseling psychologists, clinical social workers, psychiatric nurses, and psychiatrists. The core elements of competent counseling are consistent across disciplines, but the specifics of how they are enacted can vary by training and discipline.

Competency and (Not) You

Although at first it may seem insensitive, the vernacular expression commonly used by my teen clients sums up the mind-set of competency best: "It's not about you." It's not about *your* theoretical preference, what worked for *you* in your personal counseling, what *you* are good at, what *you* find interesting, or even what *you* believe will be most helpful. Competent counseling requires that *you* get outside your comfort zone, stretch, and learn how to interact with clients in a way that works for *them*. In short, you need to be competent in a wide range of theories and techniques to be helpful to all the clients with whom you work. If you allow me to go on, you might even begin to see how this makes some sense and might even be in your best interest.

Perhaps it is best to explain with an example: you will likely either have a natural propensity for generating a broad-view case conceptualization using counseling theories, or you will have a disposition that favors a detail-focused mental health assessment and diagnosis; humans tend to be good either with the big picture or with details. However, to be competent, a counselor needs to get good at doing both, even if one is easier, preferred, and philosophically favored. Similarly, you may prefer theories that promote insight and personal reflection; after all, that may be what works for *you* in *your* life. However, that may not work for your client, and/or research may indicate that such an approach is not the most effective approach for your client's situation or background. Thus, you will need to master theories of counseling that may not particularly interest you or even fit with your theory of counseling. Although at first you may not like this idea, I think that by the time you are done with this book, you might just warm up to it.

I first learned this competency lesson when working with families in which the parents had difficulty managing the behaviors of their young children. I was never a huge fan of behaviorism, but it did not take too many hysterically screaming, clawing, and biting 2-year-olds before I was preaching the value of reinforcement schedules and consistency. Given my strong—admittedly zealous—attachment to my postmodern approach at the time, I have every faith that you will be driven either by principle (ideally) or by desperation (more likely) to move beyond your comfort zone to become a well-rounded, competent counselor.

Common Threads of Competency

Although each major mental health profession—such as counseling, marriage and family therapy, psychology, psychiatry, psychiatric nursing, and chemical dependency counseling—uses a different set of competencies, there are many similarities across them. They agree that competent use of theory entails attending four key areas:

- *Diversity and multicultural competence:* The use of counseling theory is always contextualized by diversity issues, which means that the application and applicability varies—sometimes dramatically—on the basis of diversity issues, such as age, ethnicity, sexual orientation, ability, socioeconomic status, immigration status, and so on.
- *Research and the evidence base:* To be competent, counselors must be aware of the research and the evidence base related to their theory, client populations, and presenting problem.
- *Ethics:* Perhaps the most obvious commonality across sets of competencies is law and ethics; without a firm grasp of the laws and ethical standards that relate to professional mental health practice, well, let's just say you won't be practicing very long. A solid understanding of ethical principles such as confidentiality is a prerequisite for applying theory well.

- *Person-of-the-counselor/person-of-the-therapist:* Finally, unlike most other professions, specific personal qualities are identified as competencies for mental health professionals.

Diversity and Competency

Over the past couple of decades, counselors have begun to take seriously the role of diversity in the counseling process, including factors such as age, gender, ethnicity, race, socioeconomic status, immigration, sexual orientation, ability, language, and religion. These factors inform the selection of theory, development of the counseling relationship, assessment and diagnosis process, and choice of interventions (Monk, Winslade, & Sinclair, 2008). In short, everything you think, do, or say as a professional is contextualized and should be informed by diversity issues. If you think that effectively responding to diversity is easy or can be easily learned or that perhaps your instructors, supervisors, or some famous author has magic answers to make it easy, you are going to be in for an unpleasant surprise. Rather than a black-and-white still life, dealing with diversity issues is more like finger painting: there are few lines to follow, it is messy for everyone involved, and it requires enthusiasm and openheartedness to make it fun.

I have often heard new and experienced counselors alike claim that because they are from a diverse or marginalized group, they don't need to worry about diversity issues. Conversely, I have heard counselors from majority groups say things such as "I don't have any culture." Both parties have much to learn on the diversity front. First of all, we are all part of numerous sociological groups that exert cultural norms on us, with the more common and powerful ones stemming from gender, ethnicity, socioeconomic class, religion, and age. Many if not most Americans belong to some groups that align more with dominant culture and some that are marginalized. However, it is important to realize that some groups experience far more traumatic and painful forms of marginalization than others, and to further complicate matters, each individual responds to these pressures differently.

To illustrate, some people experienced the process of coming out as gay as highly traumatic and want counselors to address these issues gingerly, while others find it insulting when counselors *assume* that they feel oppressed due to sexual orientation because they live in communities that are largely supportive. Furthermore, many Americans seem unaware that there is a very strong and distinct "American culture" of which they are a part; in fact, the various regions of America have very unique characteristics of which counselors need to be aware. As another example, midwestern men typically express their emotions far differently than men in California, and counselors who expect the two types of men to handle emotions in a similar way are going to unfairly pathologize one or the other.

Suffice it to say that competently handling diversity issues requires great attention to the unique needs of each person, and it is a career-long struggle and journey that adds great depth and humanity to the person of the counselor. In this book, you will begin this journey by examining diversity issues related to each of the theories covered and start integrating these issues into treatment planning. Although these issues are briefly summarized at the end of each theory chapter, you will find that more detailed and practical discussions are included throughout the chapter as they relate to specific concepts in each theory.

Research and Competency

Another common thread found in mental health competencies is understanding and, more important, *using* research to inform treatment and to measure one's effectiveness and client progress. In recent years, there has been powerful movement within the field to become more evidence based in mental health care, which involves two key practices: (a) using existing research to inform clinical decisions and treatment planning and (b) learning to use evidence-based treatments, which are specific and structured approaches for working with distinct populations and issues (Sprenkle, 2002). These movements are discussed in detail later in this chapter (perhaps too much detail for some), and issues related to the evidence base for each counseling theory are also discussed at the end of each theory chapter, with related evidence-based treatment highlighted. If you were hoping to escape discussion of research in your theory text, you will be initially disappointed, but I hope that by the end you find the integration an invigorating addition.

Law, Ethics, and Competency

I often quip with students entering the field that if they think counselors can cut corners with legal or ethical issues, they should transfer to a business program so that they can make some money without worrying about such details and avoid a felony prison sentence after working as an unpaid intern for 4 or more years. Okay, that might be a bit of an exaggeration, but not much. Counselors who fail to develop competence in legal and ethical issues will not last long. Although this book does not directly cover these issues, they are so central to the profession that even before you begin reading about theories and treatment planning, you need a brief introduction because you might just be tempted to run off and start applying the concepts in this book to identify the underlying causes of problems in your clients, friends, family, neighbors, pets, and self. All mental health professional organizations—such as the American Counseling Association, the American Association for Marriage and Family Therapy, the American Psychological Association, and the National Association of Social Workers—have codes of ethics that their members must follow. Thankfully, there is significant agreement between the various organizations, resulting in general agreement on most key issues; federal and state laws also generally agree on the key principles. Although ethical and legal issues require their own textbook to adequately address, I will quickly review some of the more applicable guidelines here:

- *Confidentiality:* Client information is confidential, meaning that it cannot be shared with others unless written releases or state law permits; *if you are using real clients for the exercises in this book, you must take steps to remove any and all identifying information before turning in your work.*
- *Diversity:* Counselors adapt assessment and treatment approaches to be respectful of and appropriately adapted for client diversity, including ethnicity, age, gender, socioeconomic status, physical and mental ability, sexual orientation, religious beliefs, language, and so on.
- *Scopes of competence and practice:* Counselors practice only within their *scope of competence*, areas in which they have been adequately trained or obtain supervision in areas of growth; if you are using this book in a class setting, your instructor will serve as your supervisor in how to use the concepts in this book. The *scope of practice* refers to what one's specific license allows one to do (e.g., licensed counselors are not allowed to do personal training under the license).
- *Dual relationships:* Counselors avoid dual relationships with clients to avoid exploitation, meaning that counselors should avoid working with people they know from other contexts (although this varies from country to country). Thus, I recommend that you avoid trying to casually assess, treat, or otherwise make sense of your family and friends by trying to apply the ideas in this book (as tempting as it is sometimes).
- *Defining the client:* When initiating counseling with individuals, couples, or families, the counselor carefully identifies "who" the client is (the individual, couple, or family system) and discusses how confidential information will be handled between clients.
- *Children's rights to confidentiality:* A particularly difficult issue when working with children and families are children's rights to privacy and confidentiality versus the parents' right to information about their children. Each state has different laws pertaining to children's rights to privacy, with more progressive states allowing children or teens with serious disorders to seek treatment without the knowledge of their parents (counselors need to justify potential harm) and more conservative states allowing parents full access to children's treatment information.
- *Personal concerns:* When counselors become aware of personal concerns that may affect their ability to interact, assess, or intervene with a client, the counselor addresses these issues by seeking personal psychotherapy, supervision, or otherwise resolving the problem. Most training programs (and many state legislatures) strongly encourage counselors in training to seek their own personal counseling.

- *Mandated reporting:* Most states have detailed laws that require counselors to report suspected child abuse and neglect, elder abuse and neglect, dependent adult abuse, serious suicidal threats, homicidal threats, and threats to personal property. Additionally, ethical standards encourage counselors to take action to manage self-harming behaviors and domestic violence that involve serious life-threatening issues not typically addressed by state laws.

Person-of-the-Counselor and Competency

Finally, being a competent counselor or therapist requires particular personal characteristics that are often difficult to define. Some qualities are basically assumed to be prerequisites for a professional—integrity, honesty, and diligence—and take the form of following through on instructions the first time asked, raising concerns before they spiral into problems, staying true to one's word, and so on. It is hard to establish competency in anything without these basic life skills.

The more subtle issues of the person-of-the-counselor come out in building relationships with clients. To begin with, the research is clear that clients need to feel heard, understood, and accepted by counselors, which often takes the form of offering empathy and avoiding advice giving (Miller et al., 1997). Furthermore, counselors need to identify and work through their personal issues to avoid bias or what psychodynamic counselors call *countertransference* (see Chapter 4 for a full discussion). Although more difficult to quantify, these issues often become quickly apparent by strong emotions or unusual interactions in relationships with clients, supervisors, instructors, and peers. Managing these well is part of being a competent counselor.

Finally, a more difficult aspect to define is *therapeutic presence*, a quality of self considered to have intrapersonal, interpersonal, and transpersonal elements, including elements of empathy, compassion, charisma, spirituality, transpersonal communication, patient responsiveness, optimism, and expectancies, making it elusive and difficult to operationalize (McDonough-Means, Kreitzer, & Bell, 2004). Clients—rather than a professional—are the best judges of this subtle quality because in the end it comes down to how the client experiences the counselor as a human being in the room. Although these competencies are more difficult to measure, they are nonetheless some of the more important to develop.

Research and the Evidence Base

Research and the evidence base have presented the greatest challenge to how counselors have traditionally thought about theory: as a personal choice that each counselor makes on the basis of personal beliefs about the human condition and the best remedies for suffering. Instead, two seemingly disparate streams of research have upset the proverbial applecart and forced counselors and therapists to reexamine their assumptions about theory: the common factors research and the evidence-based treatment research. The common factors research draws on studies that indicate that it is the common elements across theories that account for the effectiveness of counseling, thus undermining the often vicious competition between models of therapy to determine who is king of the hill. From the other direction, evidence-based treatments focus on developing specifically designed treatments for particular populations to improve outcomes, thus promoting a paradigm of selecting theory on the basis of client needs rather than therapist preference. As you can imagine, these two streams of research have lead to impassioned debates in the field, deliberations you are sure to be part of in the years ahead.

Common Factors Research: Reframing Theory

Much of the questioning of the role of theory has been spurred by what is commonly referred to as the *common factors debate* (Blow, Sprenkle, & Davis, 2007; Duncan et al., 1997; Sprenkle & Blow, 2004; Sprenkle, Davis, & Lebow, 2009). In a nutshell, the common factors proponents contend that the effectiveness of counseling has more to do with key elements found in all theories rather than the unique components of a specific theory. To simplify the argument even further, *it is the similarities more than the differences across models that are the critical change element.* This position is supported by meta-analyses (research on several research studies) of the outcome studies in the field: when confounding variables are controlled for (e.g., counselor loyalty, comparison group, measures of outcome), there is little evidence to support the superiority of one theory over another (Lambert, 1992; Wampold, 2001).

Within the common factors community, there are differences in the valuing of theoretical models. Some (Duncan et al., 1997) lean toward emphasizing the common factors while minimizing the role of theory, while others take a more moderate approach (Sprenkle & Blow, 2004), maintaining that theories are still important because they are the *vehicles through which* counselors deliver the common factors and that specific models may have an added benefit in certain contexts. Sprenkle and Blow (2004) emphasize that the common factors approach requires counselors not to relinquish counseling models but rather to understand their purpose differently. Rather than the "answer" or "truth" that solves the client problems, common factor proponents propose that using a structured treatment allows counselors to coherently actualize common factors, inspiring confidence from clients in the counseling process. From this perspective, a counseling model is better understood as *a tool that increases counselor effectiveness* rather than the "one and only true path" that resolves the client's problem.

The most frequently cited common factor's model is grounded in the work of Michael Lambert (1992). After reviewing outcome studies in psychotherapy, he *estimated* that outcome variance (the degree to which change is attributed to a specific variable) could be attributed to the following factors:

Lambert's Common Factors Model

- *Client factors:* Approximately 40%. Includes client motivation, resources, and so on.
- *Therapeutic/Counseling relationship:* Approximately 30%. Quality of the counseling relationship as the *client* evaluates it.
- *Therapeutic/Counseling model:* Approximately 15%. Counselor's specific model and techniques used.
- *Hope/placebo effect:* Approximately 15%. Client's level of hope and belief that counseling will help.

Often these percentages are cited as "fact," and although they are well-informed estimates based on a careful analysis of existing research, the numbers were not generated through an actual research study. These should be considered general trends in the research that inspire counselors to critically reconsider how they can help clients rather than exact percentages that should dictate how counselors operate.

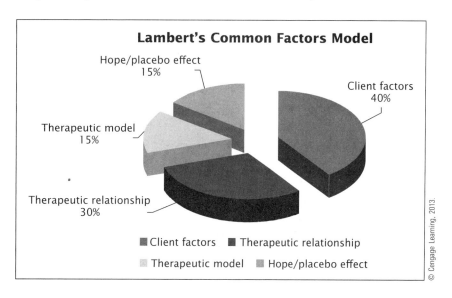

© Cengage Learning, 2013.

Wampold (2001), who conducted a meta-analysis similar to Lambert's but compared only studies that included two or more bona fide counseling models (rather than comparing a model to the generic "treatment as usual" or a no-treatment control group), presents evidence for the following:

Wampold's Common Factors Model

- *Therapeutic/Counseling models:* 8%. Unique contributions of specific theory (compare with 15% above).
- *General factors:* 70%. Counseling alliance, expectancy/hope, and so on.
- *Unknown factors:* 22%. Variance that is not related with known variables.

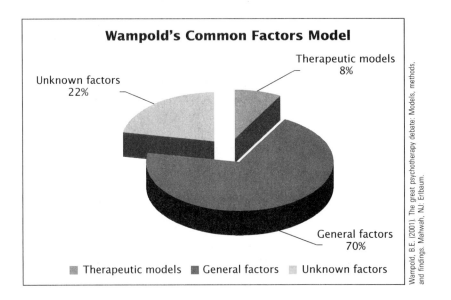

Wampold, B.E. (2001). The great psychotherapy debate: Models, methods, and findings. Mahwah, NJ: Erlbaum.

Wampold's research further underscores that common elements across theories may contribute to positive counseling outcome more than the unique elements of a specific theory. Thus, research across theories continually points to general or common factors having the greatest impact on outcome; of course, this may be due to the limits of our research (Sprenkle & Blow, 2004) or other factors, but for now, this is the best information we have on the subject.

Client Factors

Lambert's (1992) research, which has been made most accessible to clinicians in the work of Miller et al. (1997), emphasizes the importance of activating client resources, such as encouraging clients to create and use support networks and increasing client motivation and engagement in the process. Tallman and Bohart (1999) propose that the reason most theories work equally well is due to the client's ability to adapt and utilize whatever techniques and insights the counselor may offer, the counseling process effectively becoming a Rorschach-like inkblot that the client uses to create change. Miller et al. (1997) describe two general categories of client factors—client characteristics and extratherapeutic factors:

- *Client characteristics:* Client motivation to change, attitude about counseling/change, commitment to change, personal strengths and resources (e.g., cognitive, emotional, social, financial, spiritual), duration of complaints, and so on.
- *Extratherapeutic factors:* Social support, community involvement, fortuitous life events, and so on.

Counseling Relationship

A consistent finding in both Lambert's and Wampold's research, the quality of the counseling relationship appears to be more important than the specific model in predicting outcome; this finding is consistent with much of the traditional wisdom in the field. An effective counseling relationship is characterized by accommodating to the client's level of motivation, working toward the client's goals, and demonstrating a genuine, nonjudgmental attitude. A particularly interesting—and humbling—finding, the *client's evaluation* of the relationship is more strongly correlated with positive outcome than is the counselor's evaluation (Miller et al., 1997).

Despite the clear and consistent evidence regarding the importance of the counseling relationship, the majority of outcome studies in the field, especially studies on evidence-based therapies, try to control for and factor out the impact of the counselor on treatment, thereby obscuring the role of the counselor in effective treatment (Blow et al., 2007). Perhaps because it is difficult to fully operationalize and measure the quality of the counseling relationship or perhaps because researchers want a more scientific sounding explanation (the treatment did it, not the relationship), the research literature seems to undervalue and underestimate the importance of the counseling relationship. The common factors research redirects counselors' attention to the importance of the counseling relationship.

Theory-Specific Factors: Techniques

Theory-specific factors refer to the "doing" of counseling: what the counselor says and does to facilitate change. This typically is what counselors and third-party payers think of contributing most directly to change. Lambert's (1992) research and estimations indicate that technique may not be *as important* as typically assumed, as it may account for only *half* the outcome variance in comparison with the counseling relationship. However, it is still an influential factor over which counselors have significant control. Thus, new counselors still need to study books such as this.

Hope and Expectancy

Hope, expectancy, or the *placebo* effect, which refers to the client's belief that counseling will be helpful to them in resolving their problem, is a specific client factor emphasized in Lambert's (1992) research. Lambert's emphasis of this factor heightens counselors' awareness of an often neglected aspect of counseling process, at least in the research literature (Blow et al., 2007). Aware of the potential impact of hope, counselors can more consciously work to instill hope, which is particularly critical in the initial sessions.

Diversity and the Common Factors

Common factors can be particularly useful when working with diverse clients—whether culturally, sexually, linguistically, ability-wise, or otherwise—because diversity *always* implies unique client resources and challenges, particularly for the counseling relationship, choice of approach, and strategies for instilling hope. For example, when working with marginalized social groups such as gay/lesbian/bisexual/transgendered clients, although they are ostracized in the general community, many have extensive informal and formal social networks, creating a unique social support; the same is true of many ethnic groups as well as disabled or chronically ill people. Thus, the inherent societal challenge is partially offset with unique resources. Counselors can help clients leverage these resources to better manage the complementary and often daunting challenges of being different from the majority.

Similarly, creating an effective counseling relationship requires counselors to create a relationship where the client feels accepted rather than judged; with diverse clients, the task requires more mindfulness and thoughtfulness because there are often dynamics and traditions of which the counselor may not be aware. Education on local diverse communities is of course necessary, but humility and admitting that you do not know is often even more important because it cultivates respect and openness (Anderson, 1997). When counselors working with diverse clients proceed with curiosity and a willingness to learn, they often discover distinct and effective means for instilling hope in a way that is deeply meaningful from within the client's culture and primary community, further strengthening the counseling relationship.

Do We Still Need Theory?

The natural question that follows from the common factors debate, the one my students are quick to ask, is *do we still need theory?* As noted by Sprenkle and Blow (2004), some counselors lean toward the "dodo bird verdict," suggesting that theory matters very little. The more moderate stance of Sprenkle and Blow (2004) emphasizes that "the models are important because they are the vehicles through which the common factors do their work" (p. 126).

Following this moderate position, theory still plays a critical role for new and seasoned clinicians; the catch is that it is not the role one might initially expect it to play. It seems logical and reasonable to think that the role of theory is to provide a system to help clients alleviate their symptoms and resolve their problems. But that may not be it. It may be better to think of theory as a *tool* that helps the counselor help the client. *Thus, theory may be most relevant for the counselor—not the client.*

Theory gives counselors a system for making useful meaning of the information they get about clients so that they can say and do things that will be useful to clients. It also helps counselors know how best to relate and respond to clients. Without theory, it is easy to get lost in a sea of information, emotion, and challenging behaviors. Theory gives counselors a systematic way of dealing with the wide range of difficulties clients bring. Thus, choosing a theory involves identifying a theory that makes sense to the counselor and is useful to the counselor in navigating the "wild ride" that is counseling. That said, future research will perhaps more clearly identify specific circumstances when certain models work better for certain clients (Sprenkle & Blow, 2004).

Show Me Proof: Evidence-Based Treatments and Practice

If you are not confused enough, there is yet another thread in the theory debate that is pulling counselors in the apparent opposite direction of the common factors research: *empirically supported treatments*, generally referred to as *evidenced-based therapies*, counseling models that were developed through research and randomized clinical trials (frequently referred to as RCTs) (Sprenkle, 2002). These should not be confused with *evidence-based practice*, which, although sounding quite similar, refers to a different practice: *using* "evidence" and research to make clinical decisions (Patterson, Miller, Carnes, & Wilson, 2004).

When counselors, licensing boards, or funding institutions refer to counseling models as "evidence based," they are generally referring to a set of standards that a 1993 task force of the American Psychological Association (APA) established for what was initially called *empirically validated treatments* and later called *empirically supported treatments (ESTs)*, the change underscoring that a treatment is always in the process of being further studied and refined (APA, 1993; Chambless et al., 1996). The APA established several categories for describing empirically supported therapies, and similar categories have been developed by others, all of which are generally considered "evidence-based therapies."

ESTs and Their Kin

ESTs meet the following criteria (Chambless & Hollon, 1998):

- Subjects are randomly assigned to treatment groups.
- In addition to a group receiving the treatment being studied, there must also be
  - a no-treatment control (usually subjects are on a waiting list) or
  - an alternative treatment (for comparison; may be an unspecified approach: "treatment as usual") or
  - placebo treatment.
- Treatment is significantly better than no-treatment control and at least equally as effective as an established alternative.
- Treatment is based on a written treatment manual with specific criteria for including/excluding clients.
- A specific population with a specific problem is identified.
- Researchers use reliable and valid outcome measures with appropriate statistical measures.

Efficacious Treatments: Meet the above requirements plus the following (Chambless & Hollon, 1998):

- Two independent investigations (studies conducted by someone who is not closely involved in the development of the treatment or invested in the outcome of treatment)

Efficacious and Specific Treatments: Meet the above criteria for Efficacious Treatments plus the following (Chambless & Hollon, 1998):

- *Superior* to alternative treatments in *at least two* independent studies

Advantages of ESTs and Efficacious Treatments

- Greater scientific support
- Written manuals to guide treatment; highly structured
- Target a specific population with a specific problem

Disadvantages of ESTs and Efficacious Treatments

- Limited applicability: targets a specific and therefore limited population
- Expensive: counselors need highly specific training in the model *and* need to be trained in a number of models to function effectively in most work environments

Real-World Applications of ESTs

The findings of the APA's 2005 follow-up report on ESTs highlight the necessity for more broadly defined standards of evidence-based treatments (Woody, Weisz, & McLean, 2005). This survey indicated that although a higher percentage of ESTs were taught in the classroom, there was a *significant drop in clinical training* in ESTs from 1993 to 2003. When asked to identify the obstacles to clinical training in ESTs, supervisors cited "uncertainty about how to conceptualize training in ESTs, lack of time, shortage of trained supervisors, inappropriateness of established ESTs for a given population, and philosophical opposition" (Woody et al., 2005, p. 9). Arguably, all but perhaps the last of these obstacles are clearly linked to the exact things that make ESTs unique: written treatment manuals and narrowly defined population. Thus, although promising, ESTs have significant practical limitations at this time.

Evidence-Based Practice

More commonly used in the medical field, *evidence-based practice (EBP)* refers to using research findings to inform clinical decisions for the care of individual clients. Patterson et al. (2004) describe five steps in employing EBPs:

Step 1. Develop an answerable question to focus the search for information (e.g., What treatments are most effective for teens who cut to relieve emotional pain?)

Step 2. Search the literature for the best empirical evidence to answer the question (e.g., search digital databases such as PsycINFO and **scholar.google.com** using key words: "adolescents," "self harm," "treatment")

Step 3. Evaluate the validity, impact, and applicability of the research to determine its usefulness in this case (e.g., Is the study randomized? Were there comparison groups? What was the treatment effect size? Were the findings clinically relevant?)

Step 4. Determine whether the research findings are applicable to the current client's situation (e.g., What are the potential benefits and risks to applying these findings with this current client? Are there age, ethnicity, class, family system, or other diversity factors that I need to consider?)

Step 5. After implementing the EBP, evaluate the effectiveness in this client's individual case (e.g., How did the client respond? Were there signs of improvement, no change, or worsening?)

In comparison to ESTs, EBP is a practical and practice-friendly approach for using research to enhance the practice of counseling.

Research in Perspective

Counselors need to keep the evidence-based counseling movement in perspective. Almost all research indicates that any counseling is better than no treatment at all: that is one of the major motivation factors behind the common factors movement (Miller et al., 1997; Sprenkle & Blow, 2004). The evidence-based counseling approach refines what we know and aims to develop better and more specific theories; however, this should not be misinterpreted as though *nothing* in the field has ever been researched or studied before. A more fair and realistic assessment is that mental health theories have an established history of meaningful research, and our ability to do so more precisely continually increases. Research courses have been part of mental health curricula from the beginning and are increasingly valued and expanded. A research orientation is not new; however, our ability to conduct more meticulous and useful studies is improving.

Rock-Paper-Scissors and Other Strategies for Choosing a Theory

Regardless of challenges from the competency and research movements, for most, choosing a counseling theory to work from still compares to the search for love: some preferring the "one and only" and others preferring to "play the field." Those yearning for the perfect mate engage in a focused and passionate pursuit: scanning the Web, reading books, going to seminars, or searching for that *one* theory that shares your beliefs, style, and chemistry, leaving you with a "meant to be" feeling. Others set out with a preference for dating, not wanting to commit to any one theory but instead preferring the "string-free" freedom of being eclectic. Before you rush to join one of these two camps, I am going to caution that neither approach is likely to lead to counseling theory nirvana, immediate competence, or similar form of bliss. You need to begin by carefully examining research on the role of theory in counseling before declaring your intent. I expect that you will be convinced to proceed with a bit more caution, just as you did after your heart was broken the first time (sorry in advance to those romantic and free-love readers for being a killjoy).

To Be Continued ...

"To be continued ...": the most dreaded end-of-season conclusion to a favorite television show. Now, I'm doing it to you in a textbook. Sorry. For now, I encourage you to neither be on the prowl for your "match-made-in-heaven" theory nor assume that you can do it all by being wildly "eclectic." Instead, simply focus on understanding the intricacies of each theory—one by one—in the chapters that follow (Chapters 4 to 13). Try to keep an open and curious mind and enjoy getting to learn more about the foundational schools of counseling and psychotherapy.

P.S. For those of you who can't wait to know how this ends, you can sneak a peek at Chapters 14 and 15 to learn more about what responsible integration looks like.

ONLINE RESOURCES

American Counseling Association Code of Ethics
www.counseling.org

American Association for Marriage and Family Therapy Code of Ethics
www.aamft.org

American Psychological Association Code of Ethics
www.apa.org

American Psychological Association Competency Assessment Resources
www.apa.org/ed/graduate/competency.aspx

CACREP: Council on Accreditation of Counseling and Related Educational Programs: Competency-Based Standards for Counselors
www.cacrep.org

Center for Clinical Excellence: Common Factors
www.centerforclinicalexcellence.com

Empirically Supported Treatment Documents: Links to APA documents on ESTs
www.apa.org/divisions/div12/journals.html

Heart and Soul of Change: Common Factors
http://heartandsoulofchange.com

National Association of Social Workers Code of Ethics
www.socialworkers.org

National Association of Social Workers Practice Standards for Specialties and Special Populations
www.socialworkers.org/practice/default.asp

SAMHSA Registry of Evidence-Based Programs and Practices
www.nrepp.samhsa.gov

References

American Psychological Association. (1993, October). *Task force on promotion and dissemination of psychological procedures: A report adopted by the Division 12 Board.* Available: http://www.apa.org/divisions/div12/journals.html

Anderson, H. (1997). *Conversations, language, and possibilities: A postmodern approach to therapy.* New York: Basic Books.

Blow, A. J., Sprenkle, D. H., & Davis, S. D. (2007). Is who delivers the treatment more important than the treatment itself? *Journal of Marital and Family Therapy, 33,* 298–317.

Chambless, D. L., & Hollon, S. D. (1998). Defining empirically supported therapies. *Journal of Consulting and Clinical Psychology, 66,* 7–18.

Chambless, D. L., Sanderson, W. C., Shoham, V., Johnson, S. B., Pope, K. S., Crits-Christoph, P., et al. (1996.). An update on empirically validated treatments. *The Clinical Psychologist, 49*(2), 5–18. Available: http://www.apa.org/divisions/div12/journals.html

Lambert, M. (1992). Psychotherapy outcome research: Implications for integrative and eclectic counselors. In J. C. Norcross & M. R. Goldfried (Eds.), *Handbook of psychotherapy integration* (pp. 94–129). New York: Wiley.

McDonough-Means, S. I., Kreitzer, M. J., & Bell, I. R. (2004). Fostering a healing presence and investigating its mediators. *Journal of Alternative and Complementary Medicine, 10,* S25–S41.

Miller, S. D., Duncan, B. L., & Hubble, M. (1997). *Escape from Babel: Toward a unifying language for psychotherapy practice.* New York: Norton.

Miller, S. D., Duncan, B. L., & Hubble, M. A. (2004). Beyond integration: The triumph of outcome over process in clinical practice. *Psychotherapy in Australia, 10*(2), 2–19.

Monk, G., Winslade, J., & Sinclair, S. (2008). *New horizons in multicultural counseling.* Thousand Oaks, CA: Sage.

Patterson, J. E., Miller, R. B., Carnes, S., & Wilson, S. (2004). Evidence-based practice for marriage and family therapies. *Journal of Marital and Family Therapy, 30,* 183–195.

Rogers, C. (1951). *Client-centered therapy.* Boston: Houghton Mifflin.

Rogers, C. (1961). *On becoming a person: A counselor's view of psychocounseling.* London: Constable.

Sprenkle, D. H. (Ed.). (2002). Editor's introduction. In *Effectiveness research in marriage and family therapy* (pp. 9–25). Alexandria, VA: American Association for Marriage and Family Therapy.

Sprenkle, D. H., & Blow, A. J. (2004). Common factors and our sacred models. *Journal of Marital and Family Therapy, 30,* 113–129.

Sprenkle, D. H., Davis, S. D., & Lebow, J. L. (2009). *Common factors in couple and family therapy: The overlooked foundation for effective practice.* New York: Guilford.

Tallman, K., & Bohart, A. C. (1999). The client as a common factor: Clients as self-healers. In M. A. Hubble, B. L. Duncan, & S. D. Miller (Eds.), *The heart and soul of change: What works in therapy* (pp. 91–131). Washington, DC: American Psychological Association.

Wampold, B. E. (2001). *The great psychotherapy debate: Models, methods, and findings.* Mahwah, NJ: Lawrence Erlbaum Associates.

Woody, S. R., Weisz, J., & McLean, C. (2005). Empirically supported treatments: 10 years later. *The Clinical Psychologists, 58,* 5–11.

3

Treatment Planning

Treatment Planning

Shanna was 12 when I met her. She was alone in witnessing her mother die of a stroke 3 years before. Her aunt tried to take care of her the first year but had to give her up to social services because she did not want the trouble. To be fair, Shanna was trouble. She frequently ran away, talked back, and didn't do her homework. Her foster parents—there were several in the past 2 years—had similar experiences. So, when I submitted by treatment plan to county mental health, I included the following in my goals:

1. Reduce episodes of running away to none; sustain for 3 months.
2. Reduce arguing with foster parents to no more than one mild episode per week.
3. Increase completion of homework to 90% every week; sustain for 3 months.
4. Work through grief related to loss of mother.

My treatment plan was rejected. So, I called the county mental health department to ask how best to revise the plan. The assessor on the other end of the phone said, "You just need to make the last goal measurable." In trying to get her to lighten up, I jokingly said, "Something like count how many tears she cries each week?" To my shock and horror, without skipping a beat, she said, "Yes, that would be perfect." That's when I realized I was dealing with an out-of-control bureaucracy rather than a system that promotes client welfare. Rather than demean my client's loss, I told her to strike the fourth goal from the plan and approve it with the first three. She agreed. I then documented in my notes how I worked on grief to help her let go of the guilt that held her back from building a relationship with her foster parents and kept her from investing herself in school so she could make a life for herself.

However, the anger I felt over the dehumanizing practice of reducing a child's grief to a simple matter of counting tears did not dissipate. So, in an act of rebellion and classic sublimation (if you are curious, see Chapter 4 for definition), I did all that an academic could do to make a difference in the world: I wrote a book (we are a wimpy lot when it comes to revolution). Over the following year, I spent my weekends writing a book that would provide justification for writing goals like "resolve grief related to loss of mother." I figured if it was in the literature, I could argue my case much better the next time a client needed me. In this book, *Theory-Based Treatment Planning for Marriage and Family Therapists*, I developed a *theory-based* approach to treatment planning, a model I developed for helping students conceptualize their cases. It's been almost 10 years since then, and my treatment plan approach has had to evolve to keep up with new demands from third-party payers and revised federal guidelines. In this chapter, you are going to learn a more comprehensive model for treatment planning that should enable you to get yours approved for payment the first time you submit—without counting tears.

Creative Planning

Treatments plans are fun and perhaps one of the most creative acts of a counselor. However, they also come with the burden of professional responsibility. As numerous good plans can be developed for any one client, counselors are free to choose—as well as responsible for choosing—a theory and techniques that are the best fit for *this client*, the specific *problem*, and the particular counselor–client relationship. In developing a treatment plan, counselors need to consider the evidence base related to the client issue, client demographics, and theory chosen. Ultimately, a counselor's job is to shepherd an effective intervention process that addresses the client's concerns, and coherent, thoughtful treatment plans are a primary vehicle for demonstrating the ability to do so.

The Brief History of Mental Health Treatment Planning

This section is brief because the history of mental health treatment planning is quite short. The original theorists did not talk or write about treatment planning, and, in fact, if you search the literature, you will not find any published in a form that a managed care company would approve for payment. If the approved approach to treatment planning isn't found in mental health literature, where did it come from? The short answer: the medical field.

The type of treatment planning that the vast majority of counselors must complete in order to receive third-party payment and, arguably, to maintain standard practice of care in the 21st century is derived from the medical model: it's what medical doctors use for medical treatment. Within the field of mental health, Jongsma and his colleagues (Dattilio & Jongsma, 2000; Jongsma, Peterson, & Bruce, 2006; Jongsma, Peterson, McInnis, & Bruce, 2006; O'Leary, Heyman, & Jongsma, 1998) have developed the most extensive models for this form of treatment planning, which is focused solely on clients' medical symptoms and referred to as *symptom-based treatment plans*. Most publications on mental health treatment planning use a similar symptom-based model (Johnson, 2004; Wiger, 2005). The strength of these plans is that they are relevant to those in the medical community; the weakness is that they do not sufficiently help counselors to conceptualize their treatment in useful ways.

For example, if a parent brings a child to counseling who is having tantrums and the counselor develops a plan around the presenting problem (e.g., "reduce child's tantrums to less than once per week") and follows that plan without thoroughly conceptualizing the case from a theoretical perspective, treatment is less likely to be successful. In this particular situation, a systemic assessment will typically reveal that there are marital and/or parenting issues that contribute to the presenting problem. In many cases, I find that doing couples counseling that targets tension in the marriage is the best way to reduce the child's tantrums. The danger of symptom-based treatment planning is that the counselor will *under*utilize counseling theories to conceptualize and overfocus on symptoms. Or, to borrow from the cliché, they are likely to miss the forest because they are focusing on the trees. Arguably, a "good" counselor would not do this; however, today's workplace realities include (a) heavy caseloads, (b) pressure to complete diagnosis and treatment plans by the end of the first session, and (c) highly structured paperwork and payment systems, all of which make it hard for a good counselor to do a good job. Thus, symptom-based treatment planning, although convenient, may not be the best choice for today's practice environments.

In Gehart and Tuttle (2003), we promoted theory-based treatment planning, which involved using theory to generate more clinically relevant treatment plans than the symptom model offers. Berman (1997) developed a similar approach for traditional psychotherapies. The strength of these models was that they include goals that are informed by clinical theories. However, after using theory-based plans with new trainees, I discovered that theory-based goals and interventions are easily confused because they use the same theory-based language. Furthermore, it was difficult for most students to address diagnostic issues and clinical symptoms in these theory-based plans because the language of these two systems is radically different. So, I have developed a new, "both/and" model that draws from the best of theory-based and symptom-based treatment plans and adds more recent elements of measurability.

Treatment Plans in a Nutshell

The treatment plans in this book provide a straightforward yet comprehensive overview of treatment. They are the "Hummers" of the treatment plan world: luxury meets invincibility. If you can do these, you can go anywhere and do just about any other treatment plan out there.

Clinical treatment plans include the following elements:

- *Counseling tasks:* Counseling tasks are "standard practice" tasks that the counselor should perform at each stage of counseling, namely, the initial, working, and closing phases of counseling. These tasks are informed by theory as well as ethical and legal requirements. These are rarely included in other plans but spell out standards of practice that are important to consider and document.
- *Client goals:* The key element of all treatment plans, client goals are unique to each client and describe what behaviors, thoughts, feelings, or interactions will be either increased or decreased as a result of treatment. Client goals are derived from the assessment of the presenting problem and are in theory-specific language.
- *Interventions:* Each goal includes two or three interventions that describe how the counselor plans to achieve these goals using the counselor's chosen theory. Interventions may or may not be included in other types of treatment plans.

Treatment Plan Format

Treatment Plan

Initial Phase of Treatment (First One to Three Sessions)
Initial Phase Counseling Tasks

1. Develop working counseling relationship. *Diversity note:* _____

   Relationship-building approach/intervention:

   a. _____

2. Assess individual, systemic, and broader cultural dynamics. *Diversity note:* _____

   Assessment strategies:

   a. _____

   b. _____

Initial Phase Client Goals *(One to Two Goals):* Manage crisis issues, increase hope, and/or reduce most distressing symptoms

1. ❐ Increase   ❐ Decrease _____ (personal/relational dynamic using

   terms from theory) to reduce _____ (symptom).

   Interventions:

   a. _____

   b. _____

(continued)

Working Phase of Treatment (Three or More Sessions)
Working Phase Counseling Task

1. Monitor quality of the working alliance. *Diversity note:* _____

    a. *Assessment Intervention:* _____

Working Client Goals *(Two to Three Goals).* Target individual and relational dynamics using theoretical language (e.g., decrease avoidance of intimacy, increase awareness of emotion, increase agency)

1. ❐ Increase   ❐ Decrease _____ (personal/relational dynamic using terms from theory) to reduce _____ (symptom).

    Interventions:

    a. _____

    b. _____

2. ❐ Increase   ❐ Decrease _____ (personal/relational dynamic using terms from theory) to reduce _____ (symptom).

    Interventions:

    a. _____

    b. _____

3. ❐ Increase   ❐ Decrease _____ (personal/relational dynamic using terms from theory) to reduce _____ (symptom).

    Interventions:

    a. _____

    b. _____

Closing Phase of Treatment (Last Four or More Sessions)
Closing Phase Counseling Task

1. Develop aftercare plan and maintain gains. *Diversity note:* _____

    Intervention:

    a. _____

Closing Phase Client Goals *(One to Two Goals):* Determined by theory's definition of health and normalcy

1. ❐ Increase   ❐ Decrease _____ (personal/relational dynamic using terms from theory) to reduce _____ (symptom).

    Interventions:

    a. _____

    b. _____

(continued)

2. ❑ Increase   ❑ Decrease _____ (personal/relational dynamic using

    terms from theory) to reduce _____ (symptom).

    Interventions:

    a. _____

    b. _____

Writing Useful Counseling Tasks

Counseling tasks are generally the easiest part of the treatment plan to develop because they are the most formulaic. Each theory has its own language and interventions for describing how to create a counseling relationship, and a good plan should reflect these differences. For example, a person-centered counselor uses empathy, unconditional positive regard, and genuineness in the relationship, while a systemic counselor focuses on joining each member of the family by adapting to their rhythm and style.

Initial Phase Counseling Tasks

Perhaps not surprisingly, counselors have the most tasks in the initial phase of treatment. This is when the counselor establishes the foundation for counseling. Virtually all theories include, in some form, these two initial counselor tasks early in counseling:

• Establish a counseling relationship
• Assess individual, family, and social dynamics

Although each theoretical approach has different ways to do these things, the cross-theory similarities make it easy for counselors to conceptualize this early phase of treatment. If ever problems arise in treatment, counselors can be sure that one of these initial tasks needs to be readdressed.

Working Phase Counseling Tasks

As counseling progresses, counselors need to continually monitor to ensure that they maintain a strong rapport with clients. As counseling progresses, the counseling relationship can be weakened by numerous obvious and not-so-obvious factors, including lack of progress, a necessary confrontation, a counselor's ill-timed self-disclosure, a misinterpreted comment, a random remark by a stranger, or the outcome of a Google search. Thus, counselors must continue to monitor the relationship to ensure that there is a solid working foundation for the treatment plan. Monitoring of the relationship should always be done by observation and verbally "checking in" every few weeks.

Closing Phase Counseling Tasks

Simply put, the primary task of the closing phase is for counselors to make themselves unnecessary in clients' lives. During this phase of counseling, counselors work with clients to develop aftercare plans that include identifying (a) what they did to make the changes they have made, (b) how they will maintain their success, and (c) how they will handle the next set of challenges in their lives. Each counseling model has different ways of doing this, but there is a cross-theoretical consistency as well as a consistent logic to this task that is useful in most counseling situations. When done well, clients leave counseling feeling better able to handle the inevitable problems that will continue to arise in their lives. As systemic practitioner John Weakland reportedly stated, "Clients come in experiencing the same damn problem over and over. Therapy is successful when life is one damn problem after another" (Gehart & McCollum, 2007, p. 214).

Diversity in Counseling Tasks

Each counseling task requires specifying how the task will be adapted for working with diversity factors, such as age, gender, ethnicity, sexual orientation, education level, socio-economic class, and so on. Forming a working counseling relationship—a key counseling task—demands careful attention to these issues. For example, when working with a teenager or men clients, I often use more humor and direct communication. Certain ethnic groups place a high value on saving face, which should also be reflected in how counselors relate to them. These types of diversity issues should be noted when specifying counseling tasks.

Writing Useful Client Goals

I am going to tell you the truth: writing good client goals is hard. Writing excellent ones is even harder. Writing goals reveals the clarity of your thinking, namely, your ability to conceptualize and understand the complex interplay between your client's presenting problem, personal dynamics, relational dynamics, and manifest psychiatric symptoms. Meaningful client goals strategically target two to three key threads that link these seemingly unrelated dynamics and issues. If you ever tried to open a large bag of flour (sugar, cat litter, bird seed, etc.) sealed with a braided thread, you know how this works. When you find the right thread to pull on, you achieve your goal effortlessly and quickly. If you can't find the right thread, nothing moves, you get wildly frustrated, and you end up cursing when you finally use scissors to get the job done (at this point, the flour explodes in your face to further your humiliation—if you are laughing, I know you've been there too). Similarly in counseling, when you know which threads to pull on, things go smoothly. When you don't, things don't move, and frustration ensues. To help you find the right thread, you can use the following goal writing worksheet.

Goal Writing Worksheet

When you are ready to write client goals for your treatment plan, begin by completing the goal writing worksheet. It combines (a) the client's description of the problem and (b) findings from the case conceptualization to help you quickly identify the key personal and relational dynamics that should be targeted for change. These become the foundation for the treatment plan.

Goal Writing Worksheet

Presenting Problem: These are used to help identify problem *dynamics*

What does the client say is the problem(s)? Use the client's words and phrases as much as possible.

1. _____

2. _____

3. _____

4. _____

Dynamics: These are used to write your *goals*

Develop a case conceptualization based on "The Viewing: Case Conceptualization" section of each theory chapter or use the integrative case conceptualization in Chapter 15. Identify two to four of the most salient problematic psychological or relational dynamics from the case conceptualization; these are the dynamics that are most likely to be contributing to the client's presenting problem. In some cases, you will see that certain dynamics overlap or are related; in these situations, try to summarize these overlapping dynamics into one point below.

(continued)

1. _____

2. _____

3. _____

Symptoms

Identify two to four of the most salient psychological symptoms or issues (e.g., depression, anxiety, substance use, conflict with loved ones, isolation, loss of interest, hallucinations). List these below.

1. _____

2. _____

3. _____

Put It All Together

This keeps you honest: Do all the pieces fit together?

Dynamic: *List the salient psychological and relational dynamics below.*	Problem: *Identify which of the client's presenting problems this dynamic relates to.*	Symptom: *Identify which symptom(s) is(are) likely to improve if the dynamic improves.*
1.		
2.		
3.		

Diversity note: If for any reason you have symptoms that don't seem to be related to the dynamics you chose, review your case conceptualization again.

Evidence-Based Practice (Optional): *Helps you determine theory and technique*

Use PsycINFO or a similar search engine to do a review of the research literature related to (a) the client's presenting problem, (b) diagnosis, (c) personal demographics/ diversity factors, and/or (d) your intended counseling approach. Describe the key interventions, techniques, or guidelines below.

1. _____

2. _____

3. _____

4. _____

Based on the most salient dynamics and evidence base as well as your client's needs, which theory and/or techniques do you plan to use with this case?

_____

Once you have identified the key dynamics, you should review the research literature to identify treatments that may have particular relevance for your client. For example, if you are working with a teen struggling with substance abuse issues, a quick PsycINFO or Google Scholar search will reveal that there are numerous studies showing that systemic family treatments are most effective with this population. In this case, you will want to include some family sessions in your plan.

The Goal Writing Process

The hardest part is always writing the goal. There are not any clear rules that work for every situation because each client is unique. However, there are some guidelines that can be useful.

Guidelines for Writing Useful Goals

- **Start With a Key Concept/Assessment Area From Theory of Choice:** Begin the goal with "increase" or "decrease" followed by a description using language from your chosen theory as to what is going to change.
- **Link to Symptoms:** Describe what symptoms will be addressed by changing the personal/relational dynamic.
- **Use Client's Name:** When you use the client's name (or equivalent confidential notation), you ensure that it is a unique goal rather than a formulaic one.

Anatomy of a Client Goal

"Increase/Decrease" + [theoretical concept/assessment area] + "to reduce" + [symptom]

Part A   Part B

Sample Goals:

- *Increase* positive self-talk about body *to reduce* binging and body image distortion. (cognitive-behavioral)
- *Reduce* compliance to socially imposed "shoulds" related to making others happy *to reduce* AF sense of hopelessness and depression. (person-centered)
- *Increase* frequency of social interaction and reengagement in music and sports hobbies *to reduce* severity of depressed mood. (solution focused)

Each part has a different function:

Function of Part A and Part B of Goal Statement

Part A: Gives the counselor a clear focus of treatment that fits with the theory of choice.

Part B: Provides third-party payers with a clear description of how psychiatric symptoms will be affected.

Part A is most useful to counselor for conceptualizing treatment; Part B is most useful to third-party payers who require a medical model assessment. When counselors write goals that address both A and B, they allow themselves maximum freedom and flexibility to work in their preferred way while translating their work so that third-party payers get their needs met as well.

Initial Phase Client Goals

During the initial phase of counseling (in most cases the first one to three sessions), client goals generally involve stabilizing crisis symptoms, such as suicidal and homicidal thinking; severe depressive or panic episodes; stabilizing eating and sleeping patterns; managing child, dependent adult, and elder abuse issues; addressing substance and alcohol abuse issues; and stopping self-harming behaviors, such as cutting. In addition to stabilizing crisis issues, some theories have specific clinical goals that should be addressed in the initial phases. For example, solution-based counselors begin working on clinical symptoms in the first session by setting small, measurable goals toward desired behaviors as well as increasing clients' level of hope (O'Hanlon & Weiner-Davis, 1989).

Working Phase Client Goals

Working phase client goals address the dynamics that create and/or sustain the symptoms and problems for which clients came to counseling. These are the goals that most interest third-party payers. The secret to writing great working phase client goals is framing the goal *in the theoretical language* used for conceptualization and then linking this language to the psychiatric symptoms. When counselors state the goal using theoretical language, it enables them to document a coherent treatment using their preferred language of conceptualization rather than language that is geared for those prescribing medication.

For example, when a client is diagnosed with depression, many counselors include a goal such as "reducing depressed mood." Let's not kid ourselves: a person does not need a master's degree and 2,000 to 4,000 hours of training to come up with such a goal. This medical model, symptom-based goal does not provide clues as to what the counselor will actually do. Furthermore, all documentation for the case will need to monitor the client's level of depression each week. In contrast, a clinical client goal should address the theoretical conceptualization that will guide the reduction of depression. Some examples include the following:

- *Psychodynamic:* Reduce rationalization to increase ability to directly experience emotions and reduce depressed mood.
- *Humanistic:* Increase ability to experience authentic emotions in the present moment to reduce depressed mood and increase sense of personal agency.
- *Cognitive-behavioral:* Reduce negative self-talk related to social acceptance to increase positive mood.
- *Narrative:* Reduce influence of family's and societal evaluations of self-worth to increase sense of autonomy and reduce depressed mood.

Each of these goals addresses a client's depressed mood as well as providing a clear clinical conceptualization and sense of direction, being much more useful to counselors than the medical goal of "reduced depressed mood."

Closing Phase Client Goals

Closing phase client goals address (a) larger, more global issues that clients bring to counseling and/or (b) moving the client towards greater "health" as defined by the counselor's theoretical perspective. The former type of goals often takes the form of clients presenting with one issue, perhaps marital discord, and then later wanting to also address their parenting issues in the later stages of counseling. Similarly, often a client may present with depression or anxiety and in the later phase want to address relationship issues or an unresolved issue with their family of origin. Also, a couple may present with several pressing issues, such as conflict and sexual concerns to be treated in the working phase, and in the later phase want to examine more global issues, such as redefining their identities and relational agreements.

The second type of client goal in the later phases is driven by the counselor's agenda. Some theories, such as humanistic and psychodynamic, have very clearly defined theories of health that counselors work toward. Other theories, such as systemic and solution-focused therapies, have less clearly defined long-term goals and theories of health for people. Thus, closing phase goals often include an agenda item that clients may not have verbalized. For example, in humanistic counseling, increased authenticity is a long-term goal that is embedded in the theory that should be included in long-term goals for clients. With such a general goal, it helps to add more detail, such as "increase sense of authenticity *in the marriage OR in career OR in social interactions.*" The more specific the goal, the more likely it is to be achieved.

Writing Useful Interventions

The final element of treatment plans is including interventions to support each counseling task or client goal. Once you have conceptualized treatment and identified counseling tasks and client goals, identifying useful interventions is generally quite easy (thankfully). The interventions should come from the counselor's chosen theory and be specific to the client.

Guidelines for Writing Interventions

- **Use Specific Interventions From Chosen Theory**: Interventions should be clearly derived from the theory used to conceptualize counseling tasks and client goals. If an intervention from another theory is integrated, the modifications should be clearly spelled out.
- **Make Specific to Client**: Use confidential notation (e.g., AF for adult female and AM for adult male) to make the goal as specific and clear as possible. For example, "Increase AF's ability to express emotions effectively with AM."
- **Include Exact Language When Possible**: Whenever possible, counselors should use the exact question or language a counselor would use to deliver the intervention (e.g., "On a scale from 1 to 10, how would you rate your current level of happiness?").

Do Plans Make a Difference?

Now that you know how to create a detailed treatment plan, I want to also let you in on a little secret: like most things in life, counseling rarely goes according to plan. Life happens, new problems arise, original ones lose their importance, and new stressors change the playing field. Does that make them useless? Absolutely not. Treatment plans help counselors in numerous ways, many of which are not obvious at first:

- Treatment plans help counselors think through which dynamics need to be changed and how.
- Treatment plans provide counselors with a clear understanding of the client situation so that they can more quickly and skillfully address new crisis issues or stressors that arise.
- Treatment plans give counselors a sense of confidence and increase clarity of thought that makes it easier to respond on the spot to new issues.
- Treatment plans ground counselors in their theory as well as understanding of how their theory relates to clinical symptoms.

All this is to say, do not be surprised when counseling does not go according to plan; instead, expect it. And know that the time you take to create a treatment plan makes you much better able to respond to the unplanned.

ONLINE RESOURCES

Symptom-Based Treatment Planners
www.jongsma.com

Theory-Based Treatment Planning
www.cengage.com/brookscole

References

Berman, P. S. (1997). *Case conceptualization and treatment planning*. Thousand Oaks, CA: Sage.

Dattilio, F. M., & Jongsma, A. E. (2000). *The family therapy treatment planner*. New York: Wiley.

Gehart, D. R., & McCollum, E. (2007). Engaging suffering: Towards a mindful re-visioning of marriage and family therapy practice. *Journal of Marital and Family Therapy, 33,* 214–226.

Gehart, D. R., & Tuttle, A. R. (2003). *Theory-based treatment planning for marriage and family therapists: Integrating theory and practice*. Pacific Grove, CA: Brooks/Cole.

Johnson, S. L. (2004). *Counselor's guide to clinical intervention: The 1-2-3's of treatment planning* (2nd ed.). San Diego: Academic Press.

Jongsma, A. E., Peterson, L. M., & Bruce, T. J. (2006). *The complete adult psychotherapy treatment planner* (4th ed.). New York: Wiley.

Jongsma, A. E., Peterson, L. M., & McInnis, W. P., & Bruce, T. J. (2006). *The child psychotherapy treatment planner* (4th ed.). New York: Wiley.

O'Hanlon, W. H., & Weiner-Davis, M. (1989). *In search of solutions: A new direction in psychotherapy*. New York: Norton.

O'Leary, K. D., Heyman, R. E., & Jongsma, A. E. (1998). *The couples psychotherapy treatment planner*. New York: Wiley.

Wiger, D. E. (2005). *The psychotherapy documentation primer* (2nd ed.). New York: Wiley.

Section II

Counseling and
Psychotherapy Theories

CHAPTER

4

Psychoanalytic and Psychodynamic Counseling and Psychotherapy

Analysis does not set out to make pathological reactions impossible, but to give the patient's ego freedom to decide one way or another.

—Sigmund Freud

Lay of the Land

Over a century in development, psychoanalytic and psychodynamic theories include a wide range of practices, including "blank-slate" analysts whose clients free-associate on a couch, empathetically engaged counselors who address early childhood relationships, relationally oriented therapists who coconstruct interpretations with clients, Jungian analysts who use mythic archetypes to conceptualize modern struggles, and brief psychodynamic practitioners who use manualized treatment with substance abuse. All these—along with Adler's individual psychology (Chapter 5)—are considered *depth psychologies* because they explore the *unconscious mind*, which is conceptualized as "deeper" than conscious mind. As they are not only "deep" but also have the longest history of all psychotherapies, let me warn you from the start that this chapter is correspondingly deep and long. So let's start at the beginning: with Freud himself.

The original psychotherapy, Freudian *psychoanalysis* is the root of all psychodynamic approaches, with ego psychology, object relations, self psychology, relational, and intersubjectivity theories being the most direct descendants. Although there is some debate over the terms, everyone agrees that *psychoanalysis* always refers to Freud's original approach, and most agree that it describes long-term counseling with multiple weekly sessions in which an analyst analyzes a person's personality using ego psychology, object relations, self psychology, or a relational approach. In psychoanalysis, the analyst is more likely to use a blank-slate approach, often uses a couch, and typically does not engage clients with warmth—an often mocked approach in Woody Allen movies and other Hollywood films. For better or worse, this form of treatment in contemporary contexts is increasingly rare.

In contrast, psychodynamic therapy or counseling refers to a more standard, shorter-term (but typically still long), one-session-per-week outpatient counseling approach that addresses a specific presenting problem, such as depression or anxiety, rather than the general project of personality analysis. To keep you thoroughly confused, ego psychology, object relationship, self psychology, and relational psychoanalysis can be used for either psychoanalytic or psychodynamic approaches. And if that wasn't complex enough, "analytic" and "psychodynamic" are sometimes also used to refer to the work of Carl Jung, who was a contemporary of Freud's.

In this chapter, I will introduce you to the more influential psychoanalytic and psychodynamic approaches and try to help you keep them straight. As the counseling processes for five of the major schools—Freudian drive theory, ego psychology, object relations, self psychology, and relational analysis—share many similarities and are often integrated by "psychodynamic" counselors, these will be discussed in the same section with differences highlighted throughout so that you can directly compare approaches. Emphasis will be placed on object relations, self psychology, and relational psychology, which are more common approaches in contemporary practice. Jungian theory and evidence-based brief psychodynamic therapies will be addressed in separate sections.

A quick glance of what's ahead:

- *Psychoanalysis:* Based on Freud's original theories, classic psychoanalysis is a relatively rare but still practiced approach that focuses on analysis of innate drives and transference issues.
- *Ego psychology:* Similar to Freudian theory in terms of the working relationship, ego psychology focuses on analysis of how the ego uses defense mechanisms to manage innate drives.
- *Object relations theories:* Using a more empathetic and warmer counseling relationship, object relations theorists focus on repairing the client's early "object" and relational patterns, often by promoting corrective emotional experiences in the counseling relationship. There are several schools of object relations theory, each using a unique system of analysis; however, they can generally be divided into schools that (a) integrate drive theory and (b) are purely relational.
- *Interpersonal analysis:* Related to object relations, Sullivan's (1953, 1954) interpersonal analysis is unique in that the analysis process relies heavily on observable data and focuses almost exclusively on interpersonal interactions rather than unconscious processes.
- *Self psychology:* Based on the work of Kohut, self psychology involves empathic immersion in the client's inner world, analysis of selfobjects, and a focus on building self-esteem.
- *Relational and intersubjectivity theories:* Recent approaches that emphasize the intersubjective nature of reality and employ a more collaborative counseling relationship, including the co-construction of interpretations with clients (Stolorow, Brandschaft, & Atwood, 1987).
- *Jungian analysis:* Jung's distinct approach posits a collective unconscious that shapes our personalities on the basis of universal, archetypical patterns and aims to help people self-actualize, living up to their full potential.
- *Brief psychodynamic theories:* Time-limited, evidence-based approaches that have been demonstrated effective with depression and substance abuse.

Basic Psychodynamic Assumptions

The vast majority of psychodynamic theorists share the following basic assumptions (Greenberg & Mitchell, 1983; Mitchell & Black, 1995; St. Clair, 2000):

- A person's history affects present behaviors and relationships.
- There is an unconscious mind that exerts significant influence over present behavior.
- The personality is structured into various substructures, such as ego, id, and superego.
- A person's personality is significantly impacted by early relationships in life, especially with one's mother or primary caretaker.
- Insight into one's personality and internal dynamics can help resolve various psychopathologies.
- Clients *project* onto the counselor interrelational patterns from earlier unresolved issues, most often with the clients' parents; the *transference* of these patterns can be analyzed and used to promote change in the counseling relationship.

Psychodynamic Theory

In a Nutshell: The Least You Need to Know

At its most basic level, psychodynamic theory is about analyzing an individual's personality—characteristic habits of mind—to better understand how these dynamics affect the presenting problem and general quality of life. Psychoanalytic and psychodynamic approaches share the basic practices of (a) analyzing or conceptualizing personality structures and functioning, (b) fostering client insight into their personality dynamics, and then (c) working through these insights toward action. The different schools vary in the quality of the counseling relationship (e.g., neutral vs. empathetic) and the preferred concepts for case conceptualization (e.g., defense mechanisms, ego/id/superego). For example, Freudian drive theorists and ego psychologists use a more dispassionate counseling relationship to encourage and use projection to promote change, whereas object relations, self psychologists, and intersubjectivity theorists use more empathy and warmth to create a relationship that can foster corrective experiences. The differences between major schools are summarized below.

	Drive Theory	Ego Psychology	Object Relations	Self Psychology	Interpersonal	Relational/ Intersubjectivity
Theorist	S. Freud	A. Freud, Erickson, Horney	Kernberg, Klein, Fairbairn, Mahler, Winnicott	Kohut	Sullivan	Mitchell, Greenberg, Stolorow
Focus of Analysis	Drive theory; id; instincts	Ego; defense mechanisms	Intrapsychic representations of caregivers	Relationship with self and selfobjects	Observable interactions; self system	Interpersonal world; relational matrix
Root Cause of Problems	Conflicts between id and superego	Defense mechanisms used to manage infantile drives	Pathological internal object relations	Distorted images of self	Keeping elements of interpersonal interactions out of awareness	Distorted expectations of interpersonal world
Mechanism of Change	Making unconscious conscious	Developing more mature defense mechanisms; increase ego strength	Integration of good and bad in objects; release bad objects from subconscious; realistic view of others	Developing a more realistic self-image and sense of self-worth	Developing the ability to maintain healthy interpersonal relations	Developing more realistic expectations and interpretations of relationships
Client–Counselor Relationship	Detached expert; blank slate for client	Detached expert; blank slate for client	Empathetic; uses relationship to reflect on object relation patterns	Empathetic; uses mirroring to help restore self-image	Uses relationship to explore interpersonal dynamics	Uses relationship to explore interpersonal relationship patterns
Commonly Used Techniques	Free association; dream analysis	Analysis of defense; free association; dream analysis	Analysis of early relationships, present relationship with counselor and others	Analysis of selfobject relations; mirroring; empathy	Analysis of behaviors in interpersonal relationships	Exploring client's experience of the relationship with counselor

The Juice: Significant Contributions to the Field
If you remember one thing from this chapter, it should be ...

Transference and Countertransference
Transference A classic psychoanalytic concept that has remained central to virtually all schools, *transference* refers to when a client projects on the counselor attributes that stem from unresolved issues with primary caregivers; therapists use the immediacy of these interactions to promote client insight and work through these conflicts (Kernberg, 1997; Luborsky, O'Reilly-Landry, & Arlow, 2008). The process of transference reveals unconscious templates that clients bring to relationships over and over again. For example, if a client had a critical parent, the client is likely to interpret silence, neutrality, and vague comments as critical. In extreme cases, without repeated, enthusiastic, over-the-top expressions of verbal confirmation (i.e., "you're amazing, fantastic—the *best* client I *ever* had"—and, no, such statements are not appropriate in counseling), these clients will always feel criticized and/or looked down on and will often desperately seek approval from the analyst.

Drive theorists and ego psychologists encourage transference by maintaining a strict neutral stance that encourages clients to project unresolved issues on to the counselor; the analyst can then interpret these for the client. For example, the analyst may analyze transference by stating, "When I sit here quietly listening, you seem to think that I am judging you to be inadequate, much the same way your father used to do when you were little." In object relations, self psychology, and relational approaches, the counselor uses transference slightly differently because they use a more empathetic relationship rather than neutrality to build their relationships with clients. When transference happens in these relationships, the counselor discusses the transference patterns with the client and explains how it emerged in the current relationship: "You seem to think that my quietly listening implies that I am somehow judging you. Would it surprise you to know that I am not? I am simply listening intently." Psychoanalysts also vary on their opinion about whether a "real" nontransference relationship is possible in treatment or whether all interactions are inherently a form of transference, with some arguing that even a positive therapeutic alliance "reflect(s) transference dispositions stemming from a normally achieved trusting relationship between the infant and the mother" (Kernberg, 1997, p. 10).

Recent scholars have added an important caveat to analyzing transference: the client might just be right! In most cases, there is usually a grain of truth in any perception (Gill, 1982). Thus, analysts should not consider all client perceptions and reactions as simply transference; in most cases, the client's perspective has trace to significant amounts of truth. In addition, relational theorists maintain that the analyst's personality unavoidably influences the client's transference: the analyst *cannot not* affect how the client behaves (Greenberg & Mitchell, 1983). Furthermore, analysts recognize that "the concept of 'resistance' as potentially fostering an adversarial relation between patient and analyst, and imposing the analyst's views on the patient" (Kernberg, 1997, p. 9). The process of sorting transference out from accurate description becomes particularly confusing when gender, age, culture, economic, educational, and other diversity issues are taken into consideration. What is accurately perceived as respectful in one culture (e.g., looking someone in the eye when you speak) is considered exceptionally rude in another; such minor differences quickly cascade into a series of misinterpretations on the part of both parties. Thus, it is imperative that counselors be cautious when examining transference, considering the contrasting of their gender, sexual orientation, culture, and economic status and that of the client's.

Countertransference As if matters were not complex enough, counselors also need to consider the issue of *countertransference*. Countertransference refers to when counselors project back onto clients, losing their therapeutic neutrality and having strong emotional reactions to the client. The understanding of countertransference has broadened over the years to include not only the analyst's problematic unconscious projections but also the total emotional reaction (Kernberg, 1997). Thus, countertransference can be used in two basic ways, with different schools of psychoanalysis emphasizing one over the other:

- *Countertransference as unconscious projection:* Especially early in training or around a personal issue for the counselor, the countertransference reaction represents an unconscious projection on the part of the analyst that needs to be explored in supervision, and it is often inappropriate to discuss with clients.
- *Countertransference as conscious experiencing of the other:* If the counselor has self-awareness and can accurately sort out the sources of countertransference, it can be used to help the counselor and client better understand how others experience the client and the reactions the client may trigger in others (Luborsky et al., 2008). In this case, countertransference is used with the client to promote insight.

More traditional approaches, such as ego psychology and drive theory–based object relations, focus primarily on the client's transference with less focused attention on the analyst's countertransference. In marked contrast, "interpersonal psychoanalysis gives almost symmetrical [equal] attention to transference and countertransference," giving it a more central role in the process of assessment and treatment (Kernberg, 1997, p. 7).

Corrective Emotional Experience   Once transference and countertransference patterns have been carefully considered and assessed, relationally focused analysts use this information to provide clients with a *corrective emotional experience* in which the analyst responds differently than the client experienced in childhood to facilitate resolution of an inner conflict. For example, if a client interprets the analyst's refusal to vociferously agree as an aggressive stance, the analyst can use the opportunity to help the client understand that her neutral stance is not an attack but simply another means of showing support and interest.

Self-Assessment Questions to Manage Transference and Countertransference

- What does the client perceive in me *specifically:* an attitude, emotion, behavior, or a thought?
- What behaviors, comments, nonverbals is the client responding to?
- Which elements of the client's experience are accurate descriptions of what is happening?
- Which elements of the client's experience seem to be related to one of the client's prior relationships or relationship with a caregiver?
- Are there differences between us that might explain the client's perception of me, such as age, gender, culture, sexual orientation, education, and so on?
- Do I have any inner emotional reaction to the client's transference? Do I feel angry, insulted, or self-righteous? Or am I able to maintain a calm, nonreactive empathy?
- Do I have any countertransference issues that I am aware of? May there be some that I am not aware of?
- Who does this client remind me of most? How do I react to that person? Is that repeating here?
- Is there anyone in the client's life who might also have a response similar to the response I am having? How does that person respond to the client? How can I use my response to provide a more effective response?

Rumor Has It: The People and Their Stories
Drive Theory
Sigmund Freud   Born into a Jewish wool merchant in 1856 in the Czech region of the Austrian Empire, Sigmund Freud developed the first psychoanalytic theory and was the first to use the "talking cure" that is common today. Most would claim that he is the grandfather of all the ideas in this book. Although some of his concepts have

fallen out of favor and many of his practices are inappropriate for current practice contexts, the majority of his ideas—such as the unconscious, transference, and defense mechanisms—are still at the heart of modern counseling practice and current understandings of the human psyche.

Freud grew up in Vienna in the late 19th century, which was an intellectual center of Europe and home to many of greatest thinkers of the 19th and 20th centuries (you will notice that it is home to many of the people in this book and the related text *Mastering Competencies in Family Therapy*). He was married to Martha Mernays for 53 years, and they had six children together, the youngest of whom was Anna, who became a well-known ego psychologist (see below). After graduating from high school in 1873, he began studying neurology at the University of Vienna under the mentorship of Ernest Wilhelm von Brüke, who had recently developed the concept of *psychodynamics*, proposing that psychological processes are a flow of energy that follows principles similar to other dynamic physical systems. After finishing a doctoral dissertation on the neurology of fish, Freud's career took a fateful turn when he received a fellowship to study with Jean Martin Charcot, a French hypnotherapist who studied hysteria (now known as somatization disorder), a disorder in which a person has a physical symptom with no identifiable physical cause; thus, a psychological cause is assumed to be the origin. This experience shifted Freud's research to psychopathology, and, as we know, the rest is history (but since this is a textbook, I will continue the story anyway).

Unlike Charcot, Freud found free association (see section "Free Association") and dream analysis to be more effective means for curing psychopathology. His pioneering work led him to theorize that there was an *unconscious mind* that played a significant role in the development and curing of psychological problems; this theory is still generally accepted by the vast majority of psychologically oriented professionals today. His other significant theories include the psychosexual theory of development, the structures of the personality (id, ego, and superego), and drive theory. He was a prolific author, with some of his major works including *The Neuropsychoses of Defense* (1974d), *Studies on Hysteria* (1974e), *The Interpretation of Dreams* (1974b), *Three Essays on Sexuality* (1974f), *On Narcissism* (1974c), and *The Ego and the Id* (1974a).

In 1902, Freud formed an informal discussion group, the *Mittwochsgesellschaft* (Wednesday Society), which met on Wednesdays in Freud's apartment to discuss emerging psychological theories and eventually became the Viennese Psychoanalytic Society. This group included Alfred Adler, whose ideas were more practical and family focused (see Chapter 5), and Carl Jung, whose ideas were more spiritual and cross-cultural (later in this chapter); both men parted ways with Freud to pursue their own counseling theories and methods. Historians debate whether they were more "students" or "colleagues" of Freud; however, it seems fair to say that if you did not agree with Freud, you were not invited to afternoon coffee or to join his circles, and there are numerous accounts of feuds with his colleagues and students. Many rumors about Freud abound; some of the better-documented ones include an affair with his client/sister-in-law Anna O., his own numerous phobias and psychosomatic disorders, and his experimentation with cocaine as an antidepressant and general panacea.

When the Nazis came to power in Germany in 1933, they burned Freud's writings. When they annexed Austria in 1938, Freud fled that June, reportedly with the help of a sympathetic Nazi officer who was a fellow physician and valued Freud's work. Freud and his family settled in Hampstead, London. After numerous failed operations on his oral cancer, Freud convinced his personal physician to assist him in suicide in September 1939.

Ego Psychology

Anna Freud   Freud's youngest daughter, Anna Freud, built on her father's work on the id and drive theory but added analysis of ego functioning and defense mechanisms; thus, her work is referred to as *ego psychology*. Working primarily with preschool children in London, Anna identified 10 defense mechanisms, extending the work begun by her father. In significant departure from her father, she also recognized that motivation can come from external sources, not just internal drives.

Erik Erickson   A student of Anna Freud and ego psychologist, Erik Erickson's most significant contribution was an eight-stage model of *psychosocial development* that is more widely used and accepted than Freud's psychosexual development model.

Karen Horney   Born in Hamburg, Germany, in 1885, Horney was a female pioneer in psychoanalysis, a founding member and first female instructor at the Berlin Psychoanalytic Institute. In the 1920s and 1930s, she critically examined Freud's theories and their applicability for women's psychosocial development. In 1932, she moved to the United States, where she became involved with the New York Psychoanalytic Institute, from which she was fired as an instructor because of her critique of Freud in her 1939 book *New Ways in Psychoanalysis*. She then founded the American Institute of Psychoanalysis, which is still active today.

Object Relations Theorists Who Incorporated Drive Theory

Otto Kernberg (American School of Object Relations)   Born in Vienna in 1928, educated in Chile, trained at the Menninger Clinic in Kansas, and based in New York, Kernberg integrated drive theory and object relations theory and focused his work on borderline personality disorder.

Melanie Klein (British School of Object Relations)   Born in Vienna in 1882 and resettled in London in 1926, Klein developed a unique form of object relations therapy that incorporates both Freud's drive theory and object relations theory and is considered to be the most influential person in the field since Freud (Mitchell & Black, 1995). Unlike Freud, she worked directly with troubled children, a pioneer in child and play therapy (Klein, 1975).

Margaret Mahler (American School of Object Relations)   Born in Vienna in 1897, Mahler was a Jewish physician and psychoanalyst who fled to New York in 1938 and became a consultant to the Children's Service of the New York State Psychiatric Institute. She developed a theory of separation and individuation that details the process of "psychological birth," by which an infant becomes psychologically separate from its caregivers in the first 3 years (Mahler, Pine, & Bergman, 1975).

Object Relations Theorists Who Did Not Use Drive Theory

William Ronald Dodds Fairbairn (British School of Object Relations)   Born in Edinburgh in 1889, Fairbairn developed a "pure" object relations model—purely psychological—without biological drive elements. He "understood ego in terms of the ego striving for a relationship with an object, not merely seeking satisfaction" (St. Clair, 2000, p. 50).

Donald Winnicott (British School of Object Relations)   An English pediatrician, Winnicott's "ideas have likely had more influence on the understanding of the common, significant issues met by psychoanalysts and psychotherapists in their everyday practice than anyone since Freud" (Bacal & Newman, 1990, p. 189). His concepts include the transitional object, good-enough mothering, true self, and false self.

Interpersonal

Henry Stack Sullivan   Born in 1892 in New York, Sullivan was one of the first American analysts, his work representing a more optimistic view of human nature as well as an approach that better reflects American ways of life. Although he employs a type of drive theory, his approach emphasized a drive for relatedness as the primary drive rather than sex or aggression and is referred to as *interpersonal theory*, a distinct form of object relations analysis (Mitchell & Black, 1995). His work was among the first to consider the impact of culture and relationships in understanding mental illness. Considered almost heretical by some because he did not emphasize "depth" and the unconscious, he advocated analyzing verifiable observable data rather than the unconscious mind (Greenberg & Mitchell, 1983). His approach was seminal in the development of other approaches, including relational psychoanalysis and systemic family therapy (see Chapter 10).

Self Psychology

Heinz Kohut Born in 1913 in Vienna, Kohut received his MD at the University of Vienna in neurology and fled like other influential Jews in Austria in 1939. He settled in Chicago and became a prominent member of the Chicago Institute for Psychoanalysis, developing the psychoanalytic approach of self psychology, which he developed primarily with narcissistic patients for whom traditional analysis did not work. He rejected Freud's structure of the self—id, ego, and superego—and instead focused on a person's sense of self and self-worth.

Relational Model

Jay Greenberg Coauthored with Stephen Mitchell, Greenberg's *Object Relations in Psychoanalysis* (Greenberg & Mitchell, 1983) laid the foundation for relational theory. In this classic text, they divided psychoanalysis into two broad and what they believe to be theoretically irreconcilable approaches: Freud's drive model and the relational model, which includes psychologically oriented object relations approaches, self psychology, and the newly emerging relational psychoanalysis. Greenberg is a training and supervising analyst at the William Alanson White Institute of Psychiatry, Psychoanalysis, and Psychology and is a clinical associate professor of psychology at New York University.

Stephen Mitchell After completing his work with Greenberg, Mitchell spent the remainder of his career detailing a *relational* model for psychoanalysis that focuses on the internal structures that are developed from the individual's interpersonal experiences (Mitchell, 1988; Mitchell & Black, 1995).

Robert Stolorow Stolorow was a leader in bringing the intersubjectivity perspective to psychodynamic work, a perspective that challenges the prevailing belief in a discrete, individual mind and instead posits that emotional experience occurs within interconnected psychological systems or fields that are created by two or more people in a relationship (Stolorow et al., 1987).

Big Picture: Overview of Counseling Process
Listening, Interpretation, and Working Through

In general, current psychodynamic counseling involves three generic phases:

1. Listening with empathy to reduce defensiveness and increase willingness to hear interpretations
2. Interpretation to promote insight
3. Working through insight to promote new action

- *Listening and empathy:* The primary tool of psychoanalytic therapists is listening objectively to the client's story without offering advice, reassurance, validation, or confrontation. Empathy may be used to help the client open to nondefensively hearing the therapist's interpretation of unconscious dynamics.
- *Interpretation and promoting insight:* In the next phase, the focus is to encourage insights into personal and interpersonal dynamics, which the counselor promotes by offering interpretations to the client using various case conceptualization approaches; the form of case conceptualization is the most distinguishing feature between the various schools.
- *Working through:* Finally, *working through* refers to the process of repeatedly getting in touch with repressed strivings and defense responses so that the unconscious can be made conscious (St. Clair, 2000). The counselor facilitates this process by providing a realistic ego to help the client tolerate delay and anxiety as the client revisits, explores, and struggles to accept and understand drives, urges, and patterns that have been unrecognized. However, this is just the first step of the working-through process. Working through ultimately involves translating these insights into action. Understanding that you are projecting onto your partner feelings and expectations that really belong in your relationship with your mother is not too difficult; changing how you respond to your partner when you feel rejected and uncared for is more challenging.

Basic Psychodynamic Process

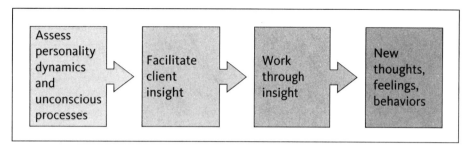

Psychoanalysis

Psychoanalysis refers to an intensive approach designed to create significant and sustainable personality change (Abend, 2001; St. Clair, 2000). Analysts typically meet with patients (preferred term) 3 to 5 days per week for several years. Thus, a person doesn't casually stumble into analysis, nor should an analyst slyly lure someone into long-term analysis. It should be a process that is entered on with full knowledge and consent (McWilliams, 1999). The counseling process in psychoanalysis follows the above process, with the basic process of analysis–insight–working through–action frequently repeating at deeper and more profound levels. As analysis progresses, the process should—if all is going well—accelerate, with the client relying less and less on the analyst for insight and becoming more adept at working through new insights and translating them to real-world change. Psychoanalysis is typically an expensive endeavor for patients, and therefore it tends to attract wealthier and psychologically minded people who highly value insight.

Psychodynamic Counseling and Psychotherapy

In contrast to analysis, psychodynamic counseling and psychotherapy target specific symptoms or problems, such as depression or recovering from a divorce, with sessions typically occurring once per week and lasting several months to a couple of years, depending on client needs (Altman, 2008). More recently, brief forms of psychodynamic counseling have been developed to last 12 to 16 sessions. Again, the same basic process is employed, but the goals are narrower, creating clearer criterion for termination (i.e., when the client is able to maintain prior level of work and social activity, counseling is done). As you can imagine, psychodynamic counseling is more common than psychoanalysis. Any of the schools in this chapter—drive theory, ego psychology, object relations, self psychology, and relational approaches—can be used in either psychoanalysis or psychodynamic counseling.

Making Connection: Counseling Relationship
Introduction to Psychoanalytic Relationships: One- and Two-Person Relationships

Each school of psychodynamic counseling has a differing approach to relationships, ranging from a highly distant blank-slate role of the drive theory analyst to a highly engaged, deeply human intersubjective approach. Mitchell (2000) differentiates these into two general types: *one-person* versus *two-person* psychology. In approaches that emphasize *one-person psychology*, the entire focus and process of analysis is on—you guessed it—one person, the client. Although historically the primary form of relationship in psychodynamic approaches, the one-person psychology relationship is increasingly rare and is typically used only in formal analysis that emphasizes drive theory and ego psychology (Marmor, 1997).

In *two-person psychology*, analysis includes—bet you can guess this—two people: counselor and client. In this approaches, counselors are keenly aware of their impact on clients. First articulated by object relations and self psychology practitioners and developed most fully by relationally oriented practitioners, two-person psychology is increasingly used by the majority of psychodynamic practitioners. That said, it is perhaps best to think of these existing on a continuum with newer forms of psychodynamic practice emphasizing the more relational two-person psychology and more traditionally oriented and analytically focused counselors emphasizing one-person psychology.

Transference and Countertransference (see "The Juice" above)

Neutrality and the Blank Slate (Drive Theory and Ego Psychology)

Freudian and ego psychology analysis typically maintain *neutrality* in relation to clients to provide a blank slate on which clients can project unconscious material that the analyst can then use to promote insight. This stance, sometimes referred to as the *rule of abstinence*, requires that the analyst not gratify the client's instinctual demands, such as wanting more connection with the counselor or for the counselor to agree with the client on various topics. Kernberg (1997) explains, "The psychoanalyst, I believe, should behave as naturally as possible, without any self-revelation and without gratifying the patient's curiosity and transference demands, and acting, outside his specific technical function, within ordinary norms of social interaction" (p. 12).

This neutral stance is *not* used simply to frustrate clients but is considered essential to helping clients. Especially in formal analysis, the analyst keeps responses short, offers little new information to the conversation, is slow to reveal personal information or opinions (either verbally or nonverbally), and avoids discussing topics unrelated to the process at hand. By being more of a recipient, the analyst can carefully observe clients to study their internal and unconscious processes and, most important, *allow for transference*. For example, if a client harbors fears of not being smart enough, the client is likely to project these fears onto the analyst's cool interactions and assume that the analyst thinks that she is dumb or that her fears are silly. The less-than-chatty approach is, when done well, done from a place of empathy (albeit unexpressed) and a desire to help clients more quickly gain insight into relational patterns and use these insights to make meaningful life change.

Holding Environment (Object Relations)

Winnicott (1965) originally discussed *holding environment* as it relates to good-enough mothering (see Good Enough Mothering and the True Self below) and refers to the nurturing environment provided by the mother that enables the child to move from an unintegrated state to having a structured, integrated self. A successful holding environment reduces overwhelming stimuli that the child cannot yet manage—thus requiring skillful empathy on the part of the mother/caregiver. By protecting the child against overwhelming events, the child avoids ego fragmentation and develops positive feelings about the self and sense of being real.

The concept of a holding environment is also used to refer to the counselor–client relationship in which the counselor provides a supportive, nurturing environment that enables the client to develop a structured, integrated self and a positive sense of self, which in the case of many clients did not happen as successfully as it could have in childhood (Brown, 1981). When applied to the counseling process, holding environment refers to providing structure, consistency, and routine to filter out overwhelming stimuli and enable the client to develop the ego strength to do the work of psychoanalysis. In this process, the structure of the counseling process takes care of ego maintenance functions so that the client has freed energy to work through and resolve conflicts and developmental crises.

Empathy (Object Relations, Self Psychology, and Relational Theory)

Empathy—the ability to grasp another's internal reality—is required of all good counselors. However, the counselor's use and demonstration of empathy varies dramatically, depending on the counselor's theory. For example, traditional Freudian analysis relies heavily on empathy, but empathy is expressed not as a warm, "I-feel-your-pain" manner but rather through highly logical interpretive insight that requires empathy to ascertain. Within the psychodynamic circles, Kohut was the first strong advocate for supportive expressions of empathy in psychoanalysis and used it primarily when there was tension between the client and the analyst to allow for corrective emotional experiences (Kohut, 1984). However, he was not the first to use it: "Although self psychology must not claim that it has provided psychoanalysis with a new kind of empathy, it can claim that I have supplied analysis with new theories which broaden and deepen the field of empathic perception" (Kohut, 1984, p. 175). Kohut described the practice of empathy as the analyst verbalizing to the client that he grasped what the client is feeling, demonstrating that the client has been understood. Thus, empathetic expression involves first grasping and then sharing aloud this understanding. The concept of empathy has been broadened to include empathizing with that which the client cannot tolerate in himself, projections, and other forms of dissociations from self (Kernberg, 1997).

Mirroring (Self Psychology)

A term from self psychology, *mirroring* refers to the counselor confirming the client's sense of self. Kohut believed that healthy adults "continue to need the mirroring of the self by selfobjects [persons experienced as part of self functioning and identity] throughout life" (St. Clair, 2000, p. 146). When met with indifference by someone with whom one is trying to connect, a person is left feeling helpless and empty and with a lowered sense of self-esteem. Thus, counselors provide mirroring for clients by confirming their worth, both verbally and nonverbally. In the case study at the end of this chapter, the counselor uses mirroring with Heidi, a 73-year-old retired banking executive whose family fled when the Nazis entered Austria while she was still an infant.

Relational Psychoanalysis and Intersubjectivity

Based on social constructionist theory (see Chapter 12), relational and intersubjective psychoanalysis approaches maintain that the analyst cannot be neutral but is an active agent in the dynamic interactions that occur in session (Stolorow et al., 1987). Greenberg (2001) identifies four assumptions that relational psychoanalysts use in understanding the counseling relationship; these are views that are not shared with any other psychodynamic school:

1. The analyst has a deep, personal influence on the client and has more influence than is typically acknowledged.
2. The impact of the analyst's behavior can never be understood while it is happening, if ever.
3. The analyst cannot adopt any posture, including neutrality or empathy, that guarantees a predictable atmosphere and relationship; instead, each relationship must be uniquely negotiated to suit both client and counselor.
4. The analyst is a subjective participant in the analysis process; objective neutrality is impossible.

In the relational psychoanalysis, the analyst's role is to provide useful ideas and explore their relational interactions to help clients reach their goals. Unlike other schools of psychoanalysis, they do not presume that they have a more accurate truth, understanding, or interpretation of the client's life than the client does. Relational psychoanalysts strive to create an intersubjective relationship with clients in which both the analyst and client mutually influence each other, cocreating interpretations and better understandings of self and other.

Personal Analysis

From its inception and perhaps more than any other approach, psychoanalysis has required that analysts go through analysis themselves in order to be helpful to clients. In fact, a person's credibility as an analyst is often established by whom one sought for analysis. If a counselor has not deeply explored unconscious patterns, he or she will inevitably project these onto clients, act out on the basis of these unconscious patterns, and/or misinterpret elements from clients' lives. Thus, in order to "train" to be a psychodynamic counselor, one must first go through what is typically several years of analysis oneself. In fact, many would consider it *unethical* (scope of competence issue) to practice analysis and psychodynamic counseling without having experienced the process oneself.

The Viewing: Case Conceptualization
Introduction to Psychodynamic Case Conceptualization

You will quickly note that "The Viewing" section is far, far longer and more complex than "The Doing" section in this chapter. Should you want to curse me halfway through, just remember that would be a form of "projection" (see "Defense Mechanisms"): I am just the messenger here. What is important to note is that most of the work in psychodynamic counseling is in the viewing, the case conceptualization. Admittedly, case conceptualization doesn't get more intricate than this; the upside is that it is one of the most comprehensive approaches available. Increasingly, when conceptualizing, psychodynamic practitioners borrow freely from one school or another—drive theory, ego psychology, object relations, self psychology, relational theory, and even brief approaches (Jung is generally left out of this)—rather than stay rigidly wedded to one theory or another (McWilliams, 1999). This enables counselors to custom tailor case conceptualizations for a single client; it also means that they must master many more concepts, which generally are not all used with every client. Hang tough for what is a case conceptualization half marathon (13 areas for potential assessment).

Levels of Consciousness: Conscious, Preconscious, and Unconscious (Drive Theory)

Freud described three levels of consciousness: the conscious, the preconscious, and the unconscious, considered one of his earliest and most enduring contributions. The *conscious* mind includes sensations and experiences that the person is aware of, such as awareness that you are tired, hungry, and/or currently reading a long (hopefully not too boring) chapter on psychoanalysis. Freud believed the conscious mind comprised a small part of mental life. The *preconscious* holds memories and experiences that a person can easily retrieve at will, such as what you ate for dinner last night, lines from your favorite song, or elements of this chapter for your final exam. The *unconscious* holds memories, thoughts, and desires that the conscious mind cannot tolerate and is the source of innate drives; Freud believed this to be the largest level of consciousness and focused his work on making conscious material conscious. Thus, most Freudian techniques are methods for making the unconscious conscious, such as dream analysis and free association. More recent practitioners distinguish the "present" unconscious from a person's childhood or "past" unconscious and often begin treatment by analyzing here-and-now unconscious meanings that are more experience near and easier for clients to relate to (Kernberg, 1997). Let's just hope that the contents of this chapter do not remain deeply hidden in your unconscious when it comes time to take the final exam.

Structures of the Self: Id, Ego, and Superego (Drive Theory)

The psychodynamic term *self* refers to the organization and integration of all psychic structures that make up the individual (St. Clair, 2000). An object relationship always takes place between the entire self and an object, not between elements of the self—such as ego or id—and an object. Freud conceptualized the self as having three structures that are used to conceptually understand and discuss psychodynamics and are not thought of as actual "things":

- *Das Es* ("The It"): Latinized for English speakers as *id* (the Latin term makes it sound more technical and mysterious than simply saying "the it"): Unorganized part of the personality that is motivated by instinctual drives; it inspires us to act according to the "pleasure principle." This part of the personality is almost if not exclusively unconscious. Infants are born with only id impulses and develop other personality structures in the first few years of life.
- *Das Ich* ("The I"): Latinized for English speakers as *ego*: The ego operates according to the "reality principle," striving to meet the needs of the id in socially appropriate ways. More a part of a person's conscious mind, the ego is the part of the personality that involves intellect, cognition, defense mechanisms, and other executive functions and serves as a mediator between the id and the superego.
- *Das Über-Ich* (The Over/Above-I): Latinized for English speakers as *superego*: Always striving for perfection, the superego represents ego and social ideals and generally prohibits the id's drives and fantasies that are not socially acceptable.

Freudian analysts conceptualize client problems by examining how the ego manages the ongoing conflicts between the id's drives and the superego's prohibitions. In many cases, the ego "manages" these tensions using a defense mechanism.

Drive Theory (Drive Theory and Ego Psychology)

Freud conceptualized the human psyche as a type of machine: "he built his theory on a vision of man emphasizing the internal workings of a psychic apparatus fueled by the energy of instinctual drive" (Greenberg & Mitchell, 1983, p. viii). When energy within this system arises that cannot be "discharged," it must be managed and/or channeled in some fashion, such as denying or redirecting it. Freud identified the energy of the system as *libido*, a sexual energy, and after World War I added the *death drive*, the source of aggressive energy, as another form of energy that must be similarly managed. These energies are *instinctual drives* that are an inherent part of being human, experiences shared by all; however, when these drives are not properly acknowledged and managed, symptoms can develop. Freud's *psychosexual developmental model* (see below) described the development and maturation of libido energy. Although Freud did not develop a parallel model for the death drive, Melanie Klein, an object relations theorist, developed her ideas around the concept of the aggressive death drive (Altman, 2008). Other object relations theorists developed alternative drive theories that posited the drive for relationship; however, these relational drive theories are used primarily to describe the human need to seek relationship and generally do not include the mechanistic elements of Freud's drive theory.

Psychosexual Stages of Development and the Oedipal Complex (Drive Theory)

Based on drive theory and some of his most controversial ideas, Freud's *psychosexual stages of development* describe how the personality—id, ego, and superego—developed during the first 5 years of life. Freud believed that children experience general sexual/sensual gratification through various parts of the body until they reached adolescence, when sexuality pleasure becomes localized in the genitals. He acknowledged that this theory "may indeed sound strange enough … [but] we shall indeed be … richer by a motive for directing our attention to these most significant after-effects of infantile impressions which have hitherto been so grossly neglected" (Freud, 1963b, p. 13).

Contemporary practitioners are frequently divided into two general "camps": those who use drive theory and the psychosexual stages (Freudian drive theory analysis, ego psychologists, and some object relations practitioners) and those who believe drive theory and the psychosexual stages to be incompatible with object relations theory (self psychologists, interpersonal theorists, and the remaining object relations practitioners; Greenberg & Mitchell, 1983; Kernberg, 1997). There is also debate as to how literally versus metaphorically to interpret the psychosexual stages, with Americans tending to be more literal than their continental counterparts. Feminists have long critiqued Freud's psychosexual stages on numerous fronts, including the unabashed male bias that assigns a higher value to masculinity and uses masculinity as the standard by which females are understood (Friedan, 1963). Nonetheless, Freud's psychosexual stages provide a template for understanding how sexuality and aggressive drives may shape the personality and, more important, shape the development of the superego and morality.

Oral Stage: Dependency and Security (Birth to 18 Months)   During this period, infants are dependent on their mothers to gratify their needs, which they do orally: sucking, biting, and spitting. If infants rely too heavily on the mother during this stage, they become *dependent* in adulthood. On the other hand, infants who too infrequently have their needs met may become *insecure* as an adult. In case formulation, psychodynamic counselors may refer to "orally dependent" personalities that have an exaggerated need to be nurtured.

Anal Stage: Control (18 months to 3 Years)   During the anal stage, toddlers learn to control their sphincters, thus learning to manage the polarities of relaxation and rigidity. Children who become fixated in this stage may be *anally retentive*, developing an overly strong need to control urges and maintain control, or *anally expulsive*, unable to maintain control over instinctual urges.

Phallic Stage: Morality and Superego (3 to 6 Years)   The most controversial of Freud's theories and a surefire way to add zest to any conversation that lacks enthusiasm, the phallic stage is marked by the Oedipus/Electra complexes, castration anxiety, and penis envy. Named after Sophocles' famous Greek tragedy, the *Oedipal complex* refers to what Freud believed to be a universal pattern in which boys directed their sensual impulses toward their mothers and had aggressive impulses toward their fathers; similarly, the *Electra complex* refers to girls who desire their fathers and want to eliminate their mothers. Children successfully resolve these libidinal instincts by developing a *superego* that enables them to identify with the same-sex parent and change from erotic to nonsexual love for the opposite-sex parent. *Castration anxiety* refers to a boy's fear that he may be castrated as punishment for masturbating, Oedipal urges, or other expressions of libidinal energy, all of which were strictly prohibited in Freud's era when boys were frequently warned that their penises would fall off if they played with them. On the other hand, girls may develop *penis envy*, wondering if they had done something wrong and already lost theirs. These theories developed from his early female patients reporting sexual advances by older men. Initially, Freud believed the reports to be what we now call sexual abuse, but later he believed that they must have been fantasies. As you might imagine, modern feminists as well as gay/lesbian advocates vociferously object to these theories, as they imply that homosexuality is a failure in development, that young children sexually desire their parents, and that sexual abuse can be blamed on children who "seduce" their parents.

Perhaps best understood in a more metaphoric sense, the important outcome of the phallic stage is the development of the superego and a sense of morality: "The superego embodies a successful identification with the parents' superego and gives permanent expression to their influence" (St. Clair, 2000, p. 26). Freud similarly emphasized the importance of the ultimate outcome as developing a conscious or superego so that one can successfully participate in society: "Whether one has killed one's father or has abstained from doing so is not really the decisive thing. One is bound to feel guilty in either case" (Freud, 1961, p. 89).

Latency Stage: Sexuality Latent (6 to 12 Years)   In the latency period, libidinal energy is channeled to normal childhood activities, such as school, friendship, and hobbies; this is a period in which libidinal sexual conflicts are not typically present.

Genital Stage: Adult Sexuality (12 or More Years)   In this stage, sexual energy is focused on members of the opposite sex. If issues were not appropriately resolved in earlier stages, they are likely to create difficulties and symptoms in adulthood.

Symptoms as Intrapsychic Conflict: Primary and Secondary Gains

Presenting symptoms, such as a phobia, depression, or psychosomatic complaint, are viewed as expressions of inner or *intrapsychic conflict*, often a metaphor for emotions that cannot otherwise be consciously acknowledged and/or expressed (Luborsky et al., 2008). The analyst views these symptoms as clues to the client's underlying inner conflicts. The goal of therapy in such cases is to gain awareness and enable safe expression of these emotions. For example, a client who complains of chronic back pain may be feeling burdened in a relationship or at work, or a client who has a fear of heights may be afraid of realizing his full potential.

Primary gains and *secondary gains* of a particular symptom are also considered in assessment (McWilliams, 1999). Primary gains refer to the primary benefit of the symptom. For example, the primary gain of a teen's depression may be that the loss of energy and interest enables him to avoid an activity that causes distress in some way (e.g., he may feel that he is not good at sports, and being too depressed to go to practice allows him to get out of this). In addition, there are often *secondary gains*, which are benefits that are not immediately related but a natural consequence nonetheless. For example, the depression may get him attention from girls at school, released from normal chores, out of visits to extended family, or—whoops!—whatever he wants because a counselor takes his side against his parents. Thus, professionals need to be careful that they don't inadvertently create secondary gains in the name of being helpful, which requires careful thought because what might be therapeutic for one client is a secondary gain for another.

Defense Mechanisms (Drive Theory, Ego Psychology, Object Relations, and Self Psychology)

Defense mechanisms are automatic responses to perceived psychological threats and are often activated on an unconscious level (Luborsky et al., 2008). When the ego is unable to reconcile tensions between the id and the superego and/or manage unacceptable drives, it may use one or more defense mechanisms to manage the seemingly irreconcilable conflict. When used periodically, defense mechanisms can be adaptive ways of coping with stress; when used regularly, they become quite problematic. Freud began identifying these early in his work, and later theorists have continued adding to the list. Following are some of the more common forms of defense mechanisms (see also Chapter 15 for additional discussion of defense mechanisms). In the case study at the end of this chapter, the client's long-term reliance on several defense mechanisms to suppress emotions resulted in chronic worry that has only gotten worse over the years; the counselor helps her bring these emotions into her consciousness so that she can more effectively deal with them.

Denial   One of the first defenses identified by Freud, denial is the refusal to accept an external reality or fact because it is too threatening and may involve the reversal of facts (Luborsky et al., 2008). Denial is commonly seen in families with substance and alcohol abuse as well as people in dead-end jobs and relationships.

Introjection   The earliest form of identification used by infants, introjection describes when one "takes in whole" behaviors, beliefs, and attitudes of another. In the case of infants, their earliest object relations are formed by introjections of their caregivers. Introjections can have positive or negative emotional valence. Initially, infants "split" these into two sets of memories, and in healthy development these become integrated (Kernberg, 1976). Adults who use the defense of introjection "swallow whole" the opinions, style, and characteristics of others in order to identify with them or gain their approval.

Splitting (Object Relations and Self Psychology)   A defense that is of particular interest to object relations and self psychologists, splitting refers to the inability to see an individual as an integrated whole that has both positive and negative qualities (St. Clair, 2000). Splitting is normal for infants, but as they mature, infants are better able to understand that the mother who feeds them when they are hungry ("good" mother) is the same as the one who straps them into an uncomfortable car seat ("bad" mother). When an adult uses splitting as a defense mechanism, the person switches from seeing people as all-good or all-bad: idealizing and then villainizing. In some cases, they can rapidly alternate between an all-good or all-bad view of the same person, creating significant chaos in relationships. As you can imagine, this results in very difficult interpersonal relationships; my teen clients refer to them as the "drama queens and kings." Splitting is a defense that is commonly seen in borderline personality disorder.

Projection   Projection refers to falsely attributing one's own unacceptable feelings, impulses, or wishes onto another, typically without being aware of what one is doing (e.g., seeing others as greedy but not recognizing this characteristic in oneself; Mitchell & Black, 1995). In clinical practice, this is often seen in the case where one partner thinks of cheating and then projects these intentions onto the faithful partner.

Projective Identification   Similar to simple projection, projective identification involves falsely attributing to another one's own unacceptable feelings. However, in this case, "what is projected is not simply discrete impulses, but a part of the self—not just aggressive impulses, for example, but a bad self, now located in another" (Mitchell & Black, 1995, p. 101). Since what is projected is part of the self, there is a continued unconscious identification that maintains a typically strong and animated connection and control. Furthermore, in many cases the person's controlling behaviors often result in the other person acting in such a way as to confirm the projection, making it difficult to clarify who did what to whom first. The classic example of this is jealousy: a person is jealous of his partner's relationship with other men but claims that is because of her behavior. His jealousy causes her to be more secretive to avoid conflict, which further confirms his hypothesis about her, quickly creating a negative, downward spiral. Projective identification can also take the form of a radical activist against violence (pick one: animal, child, embryo, women, etc.) who projects aggressive impulses on others and then puts obsessive effort into promoting nonviolence, often using violent metaphors and sometimes violent means. Even when advocating noble causes, such a person tends to recklessly pursue the perceived evil in others to the point where their personal relationships, career, and well-being are harmed.

Repression A central concept in Freud's approach and considered one of the two basic defenses by Kernberg (along with splitting; 1976), repression describes the *unconscious process* that occurs when the superego seeks to *repress* the id's innate impulses and drives (St. Clair, 2000). In drive theory, repression is the cause of a wide range of neurotic symptoms, such as obsessions, compulsions, hallucinations, psychosomatic complaints, anxiety, and depression. Because it happens outside of awareness, repression is considered more pathological than *suppression*, in which the person consciously pushes the impulse out of mind.

Suppression Unlike repression, suppression is the *intentional* avoidance of difficult inner thoughts, feelings, and desires. When thoughtfully chosen, this defense can be very useful when facing difficult emotions over extended periods of time, such as grief, complicated loss, and so on.

Erickson's Psychosocial Stages of Development (Ego Psychology)

One of the most widely used developmental models, Erickson's (1994; Erickson & Erickson, 1998) eight-stage psychosocial model of development describes developmental crises that must be negotiated at eight significant points in life (see also Chapter 15). If these crises are not mastered, difficulties are encountered in subsequent stages. His stages closely parallel Freud's psychosexual stages initially but then extend across the life span.

Trust Versus Mistrust: Infant Stage Applicable to the first year or two of life, infants in this stage develop a healthy balance of trust and mistrust based on their experiences with early caregivers. A healthy balance of trust translates to a general sense of hope and safety in the world while simultaneously knowing when caution is warranted. Persons who have had traumatic childhoods or whose parents overly protected them often have confusion over when, where, and who to trust, resulting in a sense of being either unrealistically entitled or needlessly afraid.

Autonomy Versus Shame and Doubt: Toddler Stage During toddlerhood, children develop a sense of autonomy and influence in their lives while also learning the limits of their abilities. If caretakers are either neglectful or overly protective, children become overburdened with a sense of shame and may grow up to have lingering issues that manifest as extreme self-doubt or debilitating shame and/or shyness. Alternatively, if parents do not allow their children to experience shame and self-doubt, these children tend to become impulsive and inconsiderate of others.

Initiative Versus Guilt: Preschool and Kindergarten Age During preschool and kindergarten, children transition through a developmental stage in which they develop a sense of initiative and purpose tempered by guilt when their actions hurt others. Children who have either overly protective or neglectful parents may develop a strong sense of guilt and insecurity about making their own choices, leading to risk avoidance and inhibition. Alternatively, children who have an underdeveloped awareness of guilt and how their actions affect others become overly aggressive and even ruthless.

Industry Versus Inferiority: School Age In the early years in school, children learn new skills, developing a sense of competence from which they build their sense of self-worth; thus, the task at this stage is to engage in industrious activities to build confidence in their abilities. Children who are frequently criticized or compared to others and found to be lacking develop a pervasive sense of inferiority. Recent research also shows that overly praised children who are protected from experiencing failure and obstacles also develop a sense of inferiority because they are thwarted from developing a genuine sense of mastery (Seligman, 2002). Thus, contrary to their parents' intentions, children who are constantly sheltered from the feelings of losing a game, getting bad grades, being left out, and similar feelings of inferiority are actually likely to develop a lingering sense of inadequacy as they get older that can manifest as "underachieving" down the road. Alternatively, overly identifying with one's industriousness can result in obsessiveness in their activities.

Identity Versus Identity Confusion: Adolescence Few developmental stages are more fabled—or as well researched—as adolescence. Erickson saw this as a time of identity development when a person first begins to answer questions, such as who am I and how do I fit in? Developmentally, this is a time of exploring possible identities and social roles, which often takes the form of wild outfits, colorful hair, rebellious music, rotating social groups, and other ways to magnificently annoy one's parents. Teens who are not allowed to explore their identity or are made to feel guilty for not pursuing certain life paths may experience role confusion, failing to identify a clear or viable sense of identity. Alternatively, role confusion can also take the form of failing to adopt viable social role and instead developing a reactive identity that is based on a rebellious need to "not be" what someone wants, often taking the form of drug use, a radical social group, gang membership, or high school dropout. In such cases, teens are not able to conceive of themselves as productive members of their family or society.

Intimacy Versus Isolation: Young Adulthood In recent generations, young adulthood has become much longer than in years prior because of more people seeking higher education and changing views of marriage and "settling down." During this time, a person establishes intimate relationships in their personal, social, and work lives, developing their own families and social network. People who struggle at this stage can become either overly focused on their relationships, possibly becoming sexually promiscuous, or overly identified with being in a relationship or becoming increasingly socially isolated.

Generativity Versus Stagnation: Adulthood The developmental tasks of adulthood focus on feeling as though one meaningfully contributes to society and the succeeding generations and is often measured by whether one is satisfied with life accomplishments. A midlife crisis refers to feeling as though one's life is stagnant, off course, and/or in need of fixing, which some pursue by trying to make radical life changes—sometimes these help and at other times get a person even more off course. Often, the consequences of developmental deficiencies from prior stages come to a head during this time and can now be worked through and more readily addressed. Additionally, developmental issues at this stage can take the form of being overly involved and extended in one's social or work world or, alternatively, becoming cynical and disconnected.

Integrity Versus Despair: Late Adulthood The final developmental stage is an increasingly important one for counselors to understand as more elderly are receiving professional services. During this stage, a person balances a sense of integrity with a sense of despair as one looks back over one's life and faces the inevitability of death. Those who are able to face the end of life with a greater sense of integrity and wisdom are able to integrate the experiences of their lives to make meaning and accept what and who they have been. In contrast, others struggle to make peace with their lives and with life more generally and experience inconsolable sadness and loss or, alternatively, develop a false sense of self-importance that is conveyed as arrogance and self-righteousness.

Object Relations Theory

A term first coined by Freud and objectionable (no pun intended) to modern ears, *object* in psychodynamic theory is used to refer to the "object" of a person's desire, attention, or "drive" (think "object of my affection"; St. Clair, 2000). So, yes, it often refers to a person, most often one's mother. It derives from subject/object distinction in classic grammar: the subject (of the sentence) does something (verb) to an object. Objects can be *internal* (operating in one's internal world) or *external* (existing in the "real" world). Freudian drive theory analyzes how a person relates to the "objects" of his or her psychosexual and life/death drives. In contrast, object relations theory explores how a person relates to external and internal objects to understand personality dynamics. Object relations theorists believe that the personality results from the *internalization* and *introjection* of external interaction patterns with objects, namely, primary caregivers (Fairbairn, 1954; Kernberg, 1976; St. Clair, 2000). *The relationships with caregivers become the templates for all future relationships* and hence are carefully assessed and analyzed to understand problems later in life.

Object relation theorists are most concerned with how the infant internalizes relationships in the first 3 years of life and analyze how this affects adult personality development. Initially, "introjections [of caregivers] with positive valence and those with negative valence are thus kept complete apart ... simply because they happen separately and because of the ego's incapacity to integrate introjections not activated by similar valences" (Kernberg, 1976, p. 35). The most critical task in the first 3 years then becomes to integrate "good" and "bad" objects into a coherent, realistic understanding of another and avoid the defense mechanism of *splitting* and *repression* (see preceding text). When a young child is abused or frustrated and lacks any control over the situation, a common coping strategy is to "split" the object into "good" and "bad" aspects and then internalize the "bad" aspect, making the external and uncontrollable object "good" and the self "bad." Thus, to emotionally survive, abused children may hate themselves and love their abusive caregivers, resulting in a pattern of continued victimization in adulthood. The focus of treatment in such cases is to identify, make conscious, and integrate these good and bad parts to create a more coherent identity, realistic expectations of others, and new relationship patterns.

Good-Enough Mothering and the True Self (Object Relations)

Good news for perfectionists, Winnicott's (1965) observations revealed that mothers who were generally (but not perfectly) able to respond to their infants' communication and needs while allowing them to move toward independence provided "good-enough" mothering, allowing the child to develop a *true self*. When relating from the true self, a person can spontaneously express needs and desires while maintaining a clear distinction between self and other. In contrast, if the mother is too cold and distant and/or too chaotic, good-enough mothering does not occur, and the child may develop a *false self* that is overly anxious to comply with others, feels "unreal," and struggles in relationships. Winnicott's goal in therapy was to help clients repair parenting damage and restore a sense of true self. Modern research on brain development provides support for Winnicott's theory by linking healthy brain development with the quality of parental interaction with infants (Siegel, 1999).

Stages of Separation and Individuation (Mahler's Object Relations)

Margaret Mahler described a *separation–individuation* process during the first 3 years of life during which time the infant develops an intrapsychic sense of self that gives the child a sense of being an independent entity. Thus, her theory describes how a person is "psychologically born." She described a three-phase developmental process (St. Clair, 2000):

Stage 1: Normal infant autism: During the first month, newborns are unable to differentiate their actions and that of their caretakers; the primary task is to maintain a homeostatic equilibrium outside the womb.

Stage 2: Normal symbiosis: During the second month of life, a psychological shell begins to form for the infant that encloses the symbiotic relationship of mother and child as a dual entity. From this point on, infants begin to be aware of the need-satisfying object (i.e., mother). Mahler believed that severely disturbed children regressed to this mental state of fusion. Good mothering encourages the child toward sensory awareness of the environment.

Stage 3: Separation and individuation: In the final phase, which begins at 5 months and continues until 3 years of age, the child both (a) individuates, developing intrapsychic autonomy, and (b) separates, creating psychological differentiation from the mother. This third stage has four subphases:

> *Subphase 1: Differentiation and body image:* The child begins to physically distance slightly from the mother when practicing motor skills, often "checking back" to make sure the mother is still there.
>
> *Subphase 2: Practicing:* Once infants begin to walk, they increasingly venture away with periodic returns for emotional connection. This is a period in which the child feels omnipotence and a peak in an idealized state of self.
>
> *Subphase 3: Rapprochement:* During the second half of the second year, toddlers become more aware of physical separateness, their sense of omnipotence declines, and they reexperience separation anxiety. This phase is marked by inner conflicts, resulting in demands for closeness alternating with demands for autonomy.
>
> *Subphase 4: Emotional object constancy and individuality:* Beginning in the third year of life, children begin to develop emotional object constancy, using an integrated inner image of the good and bad aspects of mother that provides comfort in her physical absence. This whole-object representation allows children to develop a unified self image.

Narcissism and Selfobjects (Self Psychology)

Kohut's self psychology is a unique form of object relations that he developed from his work with persons diagnosed with narcissistic personality disorder (St. Clair, 2000). Freud implied that narcissistic people could not be treated because they could not form relationships with others. In contrast, Kohut (1977) conceptualized such persons as having narcissistic object relations, viewing objects (i.e., others) as if they were parts of the self and/or performing a crucial function for the self. Kohut reversed Freud's assumptions that drives preceded a sense of self: "In Kohut's theorizing it is the self that develops and is the motivational centre of the person. Evidence of the 'drives,' 'drivenness,' rage, or perversions are the manifestations of structural vulnerabilities, experiences of selfobject failures, a breakdown of the self. That was the direction in which Kohut led psychoanalytic exploration" (Lachmann, 1993, p. 227).

As conceptualized by Kohut, the selfobjects are those persons or objects that are experienced as part of the self or are used in service of the self to provide identity (Kohut, 1984; St. Clair, 2000). They are not whole objects but rather a series of unconscious patterns and themes. Young children develop selfobjects on the basis of two things: (a) the *idealized image of the parents* ("my parents are perfect") and (b) the *grandiose part of the self* ("I deserve to get what I want"). These two create a tension between what the child should do (what the parent would do: the idealized selfobject) and what the child wants to do (the grandiose self). The empathetic relationship between the parents and child helps the child develop a *cohesive self*. Nontraumatic failures of parental responsiveness—minor delays in responding to needs, such as a delay in getting a hot meal to a hungry child—actually serve to develop the nuclear self. In contrast, childhood traumas and deprivation prevent the healthy development of self; thus, "the grandiose self and idealized objects continue in an unaltered form and strive for the fulfillment of their archaic needs" (St. Clair, 2000, p. 144). In these circumstances, the "selfobject experiences of all the preceding stages of his life reverberate unconsciously" (Kohut, 1984, p. 50), and these become the focus of self psychology treatment.

Relational Matrix

Abandoning drive theory, relational psychoanalysts use the *relational matrix* to organize, frame, and interpret clinical information (Mitchell, 1988). This matrix includes the self, the object, and transactional patterns and redefines the how "mind" is defined: "*Mind has been redefined from a set of predetermined structures emerging from inside an individual organism to transactional patterns and internal structures derived from an interactive, interpersonal field*" (p. 17; emphasis in the original). According to relational theory, the "self" cannot be understood or even meaningfully experienced outside of interpersonal relationships. In fact, for relation theorists, "*all* meaning is generated in relation, and therefore nothing is innate in quite the same way as it is in the drive model" (p. 61).

The relational approach conceptualizes the individual embedded within a web of relationships called the *relational matrix* or *interactional field,* in which an individual connects with and differentiates from others. Rather than the individual, the basic unit of analysis is the interactional field, considering the *person-in-context* at all times, making it more applicable for diverse clients. Both intrapsychic and interpersonal dynamics are part of the field, and each affects the other. In the interactional field model, the self is experienced differently in each relationship, in each selfobject relation. Thus, the self is discontinuous, with different selves experienced in different relationships. For example, you may be confident with your best friend, insecure with a partner, and difficult to please with your parents.

Unconscious Organizing Principles and Culture

A particular form of relational theory, intersubjectivity theory draws on constructivist theory, self psychology, and relational analysis (Stolorow et al., 1987). Based on postmodern constructivist philosophy, intersubjectivity theory posits that "people experience the world through the lens of their particular organizing frameworks—unique unconscious principles or templates—that formed based on early relational experiences" (Leone, 2008, p. 83). These unconscious principles are not a distortion or projection but rather an inescapable lens that each person develops in order to interpret his or her experiences. One *cannot not* have these principles or templates; without them, a person cannot organize his or her experiences.

These unconscious organizing principles are shaped not only by early childhood relationships but also by culture. Culture by definition is a set of shared unconscious organizing principles (Rubalcava & Waldman, 2004; Waldman & Rubalcava, 2005). Each person within a given culture develops his or her own set of unconscious organizing principles based on early relationships as well as other diversity variables, such as gender, age, education, and so on. During every moment of one's life, these unconscious organizing principles are used to inform one's sense of self, emotions, and behaviors. For example, whether a person interprets a friend's pat on the back as kind, rude, or inappropriate depends on these unconscious templates. Thus, intersubjectivity theorists radically redefine transference as a normal process that involves the client using unconscious organizing principles to interpret the counselor's behavior; the client cannot avoid doing this, nor can the counselor avoid countertransference. Intersubjectivity theorists use the immediacy of the counseling relationship to explore these principles and revise them as necessary to address current problems and relationships. In the case study at the end of this chapter, the counselor explores Heidi's unconscious organizing principles about the importance of achievement in defining self that were shaped by her early traumas and family losses.

Targeting Change: Goal Setting
General Goals of Psychoanalysis

Having specific theories of health, psychodynamic approaches share similar long-term goals. These are general goals that define "mental health." They include the following:

- Decreased irrational impulses (early and middle phase)
- Increased ability to manage stress; decreased use of defense mechanisms (early and middle phase)
- Increased ego strength, self-esteem, and self-cohesion (middle and late phase)
- Increased insight followed by agency (middle and late phase)
- Increased emotional maturity and intelligence (middle and late phase)
- Decreased perfectionism (middle and late phase)
- Decreased internal conflict and personality integration (late phase)
- Increased ability to experience mature dependency and intimacy (late phase)

Irrational Impulses   Often, the earliest goals in treatment involve decreasing irrational impulses that result in compulsive or obsessive behaviors, self-destructive behaviors, substance abuse, depressive thinking, inappropriate, sexual impulses, and so on (Messer & Warren, 1995). These impulsive behaviors and obsessive thoughts are typically what cause many clients to seek treatment; thus, they are often highly motivated or at least somewhat eager to see a quick reduction in frequency. Goals can be written to target a simple decrease, especially initially (e.g., reduce binge eating to no more than once per week), or total elimination of the behavior (e.g., no episodes of binge eating to be sustained for 2 months).

Stress Management and Defenses   Early goals also target decreasing a client's use of defense mechanisms and increasing the client's ability to manage stress without them. When writing goals, the specific defense mechanisms being targeted should be specific because most of us have a wide variety of favorites for use in different circumstances and relationships, each potentially requiring different interventions (e.g., denial, projection, introjection, passive aggression).

Ego Strength, Self-Esteem, and Self-Cohesion   As the mediator between the id's pleasure-seeking impulses, the superego's moral injunctions, and reality, the ego needs to be strong to keep a healthy balance. "Having ego strength" means that a person does not deny difficult realities but rather finds ways to cope that integrate the conflicting needs of the id, superego, and external world (McWilliams, 1999). By definition, the person does not blindly follow the id's pleasure-seeking drives, the superego's strict rules and dictates, or reality's most recent limits. Instead, the ego proactively engages the tension created by these opposing forces and seeks to find reasonable ways to mediate the differences and meet the various demands and needs without denying any. For example, when struggling with reading a difficult chapter, a person with ego strength may honor the needs of the id to find something better to do, the superego's demands to work harder, and reality's demands to prepare for a quiz by taking small breaks, asking for help, and/or setting aside extra time to study (so, go ahead, and enjoy your break; we'll be right here waiting for you).

Insight Followed by Agency   "After the insight: agency." If agency, action, and change follow insight, then it is meaningful counseling. Therapeutic insight should strike like lightning, making it hard to return to one's old ways afterward. If a client has only insight after insight after insight and nothing changes, then you need to work on the defense of intellectualization that is preventing the message from hitting home. Although Freud and many who came after him considered insight "curative," practitioners in more recent decades agree that if insight is not followed by change, then it is not enough (McWilliams, 1999). Furthermore, relational and more modern practitioners believe that insight is best arrived at collaboratively—counselor and client working together—rather than the traditional analyst *providing* the insight for the client.

Emotional Maturity and Intelligence   Psychoanalytic practices help develop emotional maturity, which closely correlates to what Daniel Goleman (1995) recently called *emotional intelligence* (McWilliams, 1999). Emotional maturity or intelligence involves being aware of what one is feeling, understanding why one feels that way, and managing the emotions in a mature and intelligent way—rather than blindly reacting based on id-like impulses or rigid superego codes of morality. Recent neurological research supports the practice of finding words to express emotion because emotional memories stored in more primitive, nonlinguistic parts of the brain can be brought to the prefrontal cortex, where it can be explored, understood, and transformed with language and greater understanding.

Perfectionism   Another desired outcome of psychoanalytic counseling is to reduce the punitive nature of the superego, which typically takes the form of perfectionism (Messer & Warren, 1995). When a person's superego dominates the personality, the person becomes obsessed with following socially imposed rules and definitions of success without balancing the person's personal needs and drives. Although initially perfectionism often has many benefits in the form of worldly success, over time this strategy ultimately results in numerous potential neuroses, such as eating disorders, depression, and anxiety.

Personality Change   Psychodynamic counseling approaches are designed to change personality and character structures; that is always the long-term goal and arguably the most essential. Personality change is achieved by resolving internal and often unconscious conflicts, and this involves a process of better understanding the self. Although initially Freud believed that insight was curative, most analysts today believe that insight is not enough: insight must be demonstrated by meaningful change in behaviors, thoughts, and feelings (Abend, 2001). Additionally, one of the most notable changes is in interpersonal relationships: clients should be able to have more meaningful and less conflictual relationships with significant people in their lives.

Mature Dependency and Intimacy   By working through infant and childhood dependency issues, psychoanalysis enables adults to develop a mature and health dependency on others and the capacity for intimacy (McWilliams, 1999; Messer & Warren, 1995). Mature dependency involves acknowledging the human need for community, selecting supportive partners and friends, being emotionally vulnerable, and experiencing emotional and physical intimacy while still maintaining a clear identity. The other person is not expected to be all-nurturing or the panacea to life's problems but instead is accepted as an integrated whole: both the good and the bad parts. Furthermore, through psychoanalysis, clients develop the capacity for adult intimacy, which involves psychological and sexual vulnerability.

The Doing: Interventions
Interpretation and Working Through Resistance
The most basic technique, all psychoanalytic approaches use interpretation of unconscious material to facilitate client insight. Numerous possibilities exist for interpretation:

- Dreams, fantasies, and daydreams
- Symptoms
- Transference and countertransference
- Favorite metaphors and word choice
- "Freudian" *slips of the tongue* (accidentally misspoken words that reveal unconscious motivations)
- Jokes and asides

Depending on the analyst's style of case conceptualization and analysis, the analyst may interpret sexually repressed material (drive theory), defense mechanisms (ego psychology), early childhood events (object relations), or selfobject conflicts (self psychology).

Like most things in life, the key to successful interpretation is timing! If the client is not ready, be prepared for *resistance*. In this case, the client is not ready to bring unconscious material to conscious awareness. In most cases, the closer the material is to preconsciousness, the more ready the client is for interpretation. For example, if the analyst has not felt that the client was ready to hear an interpretation that she is angry at her partner but then she reports that she was "shaken" by a dream in which she was yelling at a character who represents her husband, the analyst may use this moment to present the interpretation.

Although initially interpretation was used to promote cognitive insight, increasingly analysts from all schools of psychoanalysis also attend to clients' affective experience in making and assessing the effectiveness of interpretation: "in the clinical situation the dominance of affective investment has come to be accepted almost universally as the most appropriate point for analytic intervention" (Kernberg, 1997, p. 8). The "affective investment" does not simply refer to the most readily visible emotions; rather, it refers to a holistic analysis of where emotional energy is invested across the entire range of conscious and unconscious processes, including transference, infantile material, counter-transference, and so on.

Steps to Providing Effective Interpretation

1. *Begin with case conceptualization*: Interpretation should not be made willy-nilly, off-the-cuff, or as the spirit moves. Instead, as a first step, the counselor needs to develop a well-crafted case conceptualization that thoughtfully reveals where the client invests most emotional energy (see "The Viewing" section for numerous options).

2. *Wait for the "moment"*: Once you have a clear sense of the client's dynamics and issues, don't rush into the next session ready to proclaim your insightful truth. In fact, it is hard to prepare a well-crafted interpretation because, to be effective, most need to be done when the client is ready to hear it, which is often after relating a new, often painful, difficult, or challenging event. In the struggle to understand what has just happened, most clients will then be more open to hearing an alternative perspective. The key is that when clients are still in the thralls of emotional upheaval, they are more likely to resist interpretation. So there is a sweet spot—somewhere between emotional turmoil and getting over it (by getting the defenses back on line), where clients pause to wonder, reflect, and ask why—that's the moment they are ready. Trust me, with time, you get better at finding this moment—it's generally obvious when you miss it.

3. *Work from the present to past*: In most cases—and certainly no single set of steps will work for all forms of interpretation—begin by describing dynamics in the present issue (e.g., what just happened in session, what happened at work, between counselor and client, or whatever is most upsetting)—and then make links to the past (e.g., relationship with mother, father, past abuse; Kernberg, 1997).

4. *Assess client response*: Finally, you need to assess how clients respond to the interpretation. Do they resist: "I don't think that is what is happening at all"? Or do they agree: "Wow. I never thought of it before, but I think you are right"? Or do they fall somewhere in between: "I don't know. Some of that might be true"? Different schools and individual practitioners have different approaches to responding to each type of response. New counselors are probably safest using a more collaborative, relational approach to work with the client's reality to reinterpret the interpretation in such a way that it not only "makes sense" in the client's subjective world but also translates to changes in action, feelings, and thoughts in their everyday life.

Empathy: Understanding–Explaining Sequence

Kohut (1984) describes an *understanding–explaining sequence* to both solidify the counseling relationship and provide meaningful interpretation. Most often, these two are presented together in a single utterance by the counselor. However, he emphasizes that in some cases, especially with people who have been severely traumatized, this phase may remain the only phase for a very long time.

Empathetic Understanding–Explaining Sequence

This process involved two phases: understanding and explaining.

1. *Understanding*: The understanding phase was an expression of empathy: "I can understand how my being late must have been upsetting for you."

2. *Explanation*: The second phase, explaining, provides some form of interpretation that helps the client understand the source of the emotion: "We all care about how those around us see us and treat us, especially those who are important to us, much

(*continued*)

like our parents were to us years ago. Given your mother's unpredictability and your father's disinterest in you, my actions must have been especially upsetting."

Kohut used these two together to express a therapeutic expression of empathy that provides a corrective emotional experience and helps clients develop more cohesive sense of self.

Kohut (1977) cautioned practitioners to look for evidence that a particular empathetic interpretation was correct. He states, "We also know that there is one attitude that, after it has become an integral part of our clinical stance, provides us with an important safeguard against errors arising in consequence of our instinctive commitment to established patterns of thought: our resolve not to be swept away by the comfortable certainty of the 'Aha-experience' of intuited knowledge but to keep our mind open and to continue our *trial empathy* in order to collect as many alternatives as possible" (Kohut, 1977, p. 168). Kohut believed that only a gradual change in symptoms and behavior patterns provide evidence that one's empathetic interpretations are correct. In the case study at the end of this chapter, the counselor uses the understanding–explaining sequence to help Heidi understand why she chose to pursue a career rather than a family and why she has had difficulty maintaining intimate relationships.

Free Association

Developed by Freud, free association involves asking a client to "just say what comes to mind" on a given topic, such as "your mother," allowing unconscious material to arise. The client may describe recent events, memories, feelings, fantasies, bodily sensations, or any other material. Analysts may have clients lay on a couch rather than sit in a chair to encourage a more relaxed and free-flowing thought process to encourage unconscious thoughts to emerge. The analyst listens carefully for unusual connections, idiosyncratic logic, slips of the tongue, and efforts to edit or hold back. After this process, the analyst may provide interpretations to help promote insight into the client's process.

Dream Interpretation

"Dreams in general can be interpreted, and that after the work of interpretation has been completed they can be replaced by perfectly correctly constructed thoughts which find a recognizable position in the texture of the mind" (Freud, 1963a, p. 29).

Freud's approach to dream interpretation was revolutionary in his time, a period when scientists viewed dreams as a "somatic expression." In contradiction to the medical establishment, he proclaimed, "I must insist that the dream actually has significance, and that a scientific procedure in dream interpretation is possible" (Freud, 1974b, p. 83). Dubbed by Freud "the royal road to the unconscious," dream interpretation has been a key intervention since the beginning of psychoanalysis (Luborsky et al., 2008). In the tradition of Freud, the dreamer—not the analyst—is the key to symbolic meaning of the dreams; there are no predetermined meanings: "some times a cigar is just a cigar!" The dreamer's associations with symbols in the dream provide clues to underlying unconscious meaning of the dream. In dream analysis, dreams have two layers of meaning: the *manifest content* is the literal content of the dream, and the *latent content* is the underlying, unconscious material that must be interpreted to be accessed.

Intersubjective Responding

Relational psychodynamic counselors rely on the counseling relationship itself to create opportunities for clients to gain insight and make change, referred to as *intersubjective responding*. Using a postmodern approach, they do not necessarily relate every experience in the counseling relationship to childhood experiences but instead stay focused on the present relationship and the client's interpretations of it, which may be related to culture, gender, economic status, or education as well as childhood experiences. For example, if a client comments that she is frustrated because she does not feel like the counselor is telling her what he really thinks, the counselor will approach this comment from a nondefensive and nonassuming position, curiously exploring her perception, the expectations behind it, and their antecedents, which may be related to numerous factors, including childhood relationships.

Putting It All Together: Psychodynamic Treatment Plan Template

Use this treatment plan template for developing a plan for clients with depressive, anxious, or compulsive types of presenting problems. Depending on the specific client, presenting problem, and clinical context, the goals and interventions in this template may need to be modified only slightly or significantly; you are encouraged to significantly revise the plan as needed. For the plan to be useful, goals and techniques should be written to target specific beliefs, behaviors, and emotions that the client is experiencing. The more specific, the more useful it will be to you.

Treatment Plan

Initial Phase of Treatment (First One to Three Sessions)
Initial Phase Counseling Tasks

1. *Develop working counseling relationship. Diversity note:* Adapt style for ethnicity, gender, age, and so on.
   Relationship-building approach:
   a. Use **empathy** and **mirroring** to provide a supportive, holding environment for client.

2. *Assess individual, systemic, and broader cultural dynamics. Diversity note:* Adapt for family structure, ethnic/religious norms, gender, age, ability, sexual/gender orientation, and so on.
   Assessment strategies:
   a. Analyze **unconscious conflict** underlying symptoms and role of **defense mechanisms** in managing them.
   b. Analyze **object relations** and **selfobjects** patterns, including expressions in current relationships and historical development during infancy.
   c. Assess **relational matrix** and culturally defined unconscious organizing principles that shape the client's worldview.

Initial Phase Client Goal (One to Two Goals): *Manage crisis issues and/or reduce most distressing symptoms*

1. *Decrease* emotional reactivity to perceived **threats to self** to reduce [specific crisis symptoms].
   Interventions:
   a. Provide **empathy** using **understanding–explaining sequence** to reduce client's inaccurate perceptions of external threat to self.
   b. **Interpretation** to reduce need to use reactive **defense mechanisms** in response to incorrectly perceived threats.

Working Phase of Treatment (Three or More Sessions)
Working Phase Counseling Task

1. *Monitor quality of the working alliance. Diversity note:* Remain sensitive to relationship and conflict management patterns that may be related to gender, cultural, socioeconomic status, family dynamics, and so on.
   Assessment Intervention:
   a. Monitor and work through transference and countertransference.

(continued)

Working Phase Client Goals (Two to Three Goals). Target individual and relational dynamics using theoretical language (e.g., decrease avoidance of intimacy, increase awareness of emotion, increase agency)

1. *Decrease* use of [specify **defense mechanism**] to protect self from [specify perceived threat] to reduce [specific symptom: depression, anxiety, etc.].
   Interventions:
   a. **Interpretation** of role of **defense mechanism** and how it developed in early childhood experiences and is being inappropriately used currently.
   b. Analysis of **transference** in session when defenses are used in relationship to counselor.

2. *Increase* **ego strength** and **self-cohesion** to reduce [specific symptom: depression, anxiety, etc.].
   Interventions:
   a. **Mirroring** to confirm client's sense of worth and value.
   b. **Empathy** using the **understanding–explaining sequence** to increase client's sense of cohesion.
   c. **Dream interpretation** and **free association** to bring sources of inner conflict to conscious awareness.

3. *Increase* sense of personal agency informed by emotional intelligence to reduce [specific symptom: depression, anxiety, etc.].
   Interventions:
   a. **Intersubjective responding** to increase client's awareness of self in sessions versus various emotional-relational contexts.
   b. **Working through resistance** to translating insight into action.

Closing Phase of Treatment (Last Four or More Sessions)
Closing Phase Counseling Task

1. *Develop aftercare plan and maintain gains. Diversity note:* Manage end of counseling by adjusting for sociocultural and gender expectations for handling loss.
   Intervention:
   a. Analyzing **transference** and abandonment issues as impending termination approaches.

Closing Client Goals (One to Two Goals): Determined by theory's definition of health and normalcy

1. *Decrease* internal conflict while increasing **personality integration** to reduce potential for relapse in [specific symptom: depression, anxiety, etc.].
   Interventions:
   a. **Dream analysis, free association,** and **analysis of transference** to identify internal conflicts generally and those related to ending treatment specifically.
   b. Enable client to identify, consciously contain, and successfully manage internal conflicts to allow for fuller personality integration.

2. *Increase* ability to experience **mature dependency** and intimacy to reduce potential for relapse in [specific symptom: depression, anxiety, etc.].
   Interventions:
   a. Analyze **transference** and **work through resistance** to intimacy in in-session and out-of-session relationships.
   b. **Intersubjective responding** to critically examine the **unconscious organizing principles** the client uses to relate to others.

Evidence-Based Treatment: Brief Psychodynamic Counseling

In a Nutshell: The Least You Need to Know

Several "brief, psychodynamic" approaches have been developed and validated through research (Book, 1998; Messer & Warren, 1995). These approaches use many of the same case conceptualization skills as traditional psychodynamic approaches; however, they differ in the quality of the counseling relationship, the specificity of the goals, and the directiveness of the interventions. These "brief" approaches may require from 12 to 50 sessions but typically end after 20. Similar to other psychodynamic approaches, they believe that early childhood relationships significantly affect problems later in life and that defense mechanisms should be targeted in treatment. Thus, most brief psychodynamic approaches aim to strengthen the ego so that it can better manage problem impulses and resolve inner conflicts. The counselor is more active in these approaches, quickly identifying core dynamics that are targeted for intervention; the counselor–client relationship is used as a learning forum for *corrective emotional experiences*, in which the counselor's response helps correct old traumas.

Big Picture: Overview of Counseling Process

Sifneos (1979) identifies five phases of brief psychodynamic counseling and psychotherapies:

1. *Client-counseling encounter:* The client and counselor develop a working rapport and mutually agree on a focus of treatment. During this time, the counselor develops a case conceptualization of the client's dynamics, focusing on those that are related to the identified problem.
2. *Early treatment:* The counselor confronts idealistic, positive transference and helps the client distinguish wishful thinking from realistic expectations of the counselor and the counseling process.
3. *Height of treatment:* During this working phase, the past is explored to better understand current problems and transference issues that arise in session; clients are encouraged to use new ways of relating both in and out of session.
4. *Evidence of change:* Clients begin to apply what they learn in session to everyday life.
5. *Termination:* Once goals have been reached, counselors help them move toward termination rather than look for new goals. Careful attention is paid to issues of loss and separation as treatment ends.

Making Connection: Counseling Relationship

Corrective Emotional Experience

Rather than using transference and countertransference to promote insight into early childhood relationships, brief psychodynamic counselors use these immediate in-session interactions to promote *corrective emotional experiences*. Corrective emotional experiences involve using the counseling relationship to work through old childhood traumas and relational patterns (Mallinckrodt, 2010). For example, if a client perceives the counselor's professional mannerism as also implying disapproval, the counselor can use this opportunity to clarify that the professional boundaries are just that—professional boundaries—and do not imply any judgment or valuing of the client as a person, as may have been the case with the client's father or mother. When this is done with sincerity and without reactivity on the part of the counselor, this can be a profound healing experience for the client.

Specific Brief Psychodynamic Approaches

Interpersonal Psychotherapy

Originally developed for treating depression, *interpersonal psychotherapy* has been used with couples, older adults, bipolar disorder, eating disorders, anxiety disorders, and borderline personality disorder (Weissman, Markowitz, & Klerman, 2000, 2007). In one of the largest mental health studies conducted in the United States, interpersonal psychotherapy was compared with cognitive therapy and antidepressant medication and found to be as effective (Krupnick, Elkin, Collins, Simmens, Sotsky, et al., 1994); thus, it has a well-respected evidence base. The approach is based on the assumption that stressful interpersonal experiences in adulthood trigger childhood attachment issues, resulting in depression or similar disorder. The approach focuses on building strong interpersonal relationships to reduce the likelihood of relapse.

Treatment is time limited and focuses on the following four areas:

1. Interpersonal deficits (i.e., lack of skills or knowledge)
2. Role expectations and conflicts (i.e., creating realistic expectations)
3. Role transitions (i.e., redefining relationships based on developmental and contextual needs)
4. Grief issues (i.e., dealing with past and current relational loss)

Interpersonal psychotherapy has three phases:

Phase 1: Initial sessions: Focuses on identifying one or two concerns from the four areas listed above. The counseling process and diagnosis are explained so that the client fully understands the process and how it will help.

Phase 2: Intermediate phase: During this working phase, the counselor actively helps the client address the targeted problems using a wide range of interventions that include psychoeducation, interpretation of patterns, advice giving, insight-stimulating questions, and behavior change techniques.

Phase 3: Termination: Termination requires two to four sessions to help the client develop confidence that he or she can handle future problems using the skills that he or she has learned.

Core Conflictual Relationship Theme Method

Luborsky and colleagues (Luborsky & Crits-Christoph, 1998; Luborsky & Luborsky, 2006; Luborsky et al., 2008) have developed the Core Conflictual Relationship Theme method to operationalize transference in their brief, psychodynamic method. The method involves analyzing all accounts clients share about their interactions with others to identify core relationship themes that create conflict and problems. Counselors do this by analyzing three elements in each encounter reported by the client:

- W: The client's wish (W), either stated or implied (e.g., wanting to be loved, appreciated, acknowledged)
- RO: The response of others (RO), either real or imagined (e.g., rejection, disapproval, criticism, ignoring)
- RS: The response of self (RS) (e.g., anger, sadness, withdrawal, attacking other, blaming self, feeling trapped).

The counselor tracks these three elements in each problem encounter described by the client and help the client to gain insight into these patterns and change their responses. Research shows that clients' wishes generally remain the same, but their responses and those of others change.

Time-Limited, Dynamic Psychotherapy

Designed for persons diagnosed with personality disorders, time-limited dynamic psychotherapy uses the counseling relationship to encourage corrective emotional experiences (Levenson, 2003). Clients interact with counselors the same way they do with others in their lives. Counselors using a time-limited, dynamic approach use their responses within the counseling relationship to provide new experiences for clients that enable them to change how they interact with others outside of session. The counselor has a positive, supportive approach that provides clients safety in exploring these long-standing relational patterns. Initially, counselors begin by identifying present relationship patterns but then move toward exploring the early origins of these patterns. Counselors can help clients see how these patterns may have been adaptive earlier in life but no longer serve their purpose.

Jungian Analytic Psychology

In a Nutshell: The Least You Need to Know

A distinctive approach that emphasizes cultural and spiritual elements, Jungian analysis is premised on the *collective unconscious*, a store of universal archetypes, myths, fairy tales, and experiences that are part of each individual's psyche and that can be used for psychological healing (Douglas, 2008). The goal of counseling is to build a relationship between the conscious and unconscious and the *ego* (how one sees and experiences the self) and the *Self* (a higher-order self that is whole and complete) to create a unique sense of individuality and connection with life, the cosmos, and the divine. Jungian counselors analyze dreams, synchronicity experiences, and life patterns by analyzing the archetypical, mythic, and legendary themes to help clients become more aware of material in the personal unconscious and collective unconscious.

The Juice: Significant Contributions to the Field

If there is one thing you remember from this part of the chapter, it should be ...

Archetypes

Archetypes are unconscious universal patterns that can be traced across cultures and influence how people think, feel, and behave. Jung (1959a) defined them as typical modes of apprehension. They are powerful forces that can be either destructive or healing, depending on how a person relates to it. Certain archetypes exist in everyone, such as the Self, anima/animus, and shadow. Others express themselves only in certain people at certain times, such as the divine child, hero, trickster, mother, father, and so on. Some of the key archetypes are discussed next.

Ego   Using the term differently than Freud, Jung's ego refers to a complex set of representations of oneself that has both conscious and unconscious elements that are both personal and collective (Hopcke, 1989). "Simply put, too simply perhaps, the ego is how one sees oneself, along with the conscious and unconscious feelings that accompany that view ... [which] represents the very hard won self-awareness that makes us human" (p. 77). He believed that the modern idealization of the ego could lead to an imbalance with other elements of one's being, most notably the Self.

Self   The Self (with capital S) is an archetype of wholeness that stems from a deeper connection with life and all humanity (Harris, 1996; Hopcke, 1989). The Self is a supraordinate, organizing principle of the psyche, in many ways incorporating all the others. The Jungian counseling process is designed to help people become more aware of the Self.

Shadow   "The shadow is a moral problem that challenges the whole ego-personality, for no one can become conscious of the shadow without considerable moral effort. To become conscious of it involves recognizing the dark aspects of the personality as present and real" (Jung, 1983, p. 91). The shadow archetype represents the typically unpleasant, socially unacceptable, and immoral aspects of a person that are suppressed and/or unconscious; these can become the source of neurosis, psychosis, or compulsive behavior (Douglas, 2008; Hopcke, 1989). The process of counseling typically involves the process of addressing the shadow and its contents—which may or may not be negative—and learning to own them as part of the self even if not acted on.

Persona   One of Jung's more practical and down-to-earth concepts, the *persona* is "the part of the personality developed and used in our interactions, our conscious outer face, our social mask" (Hopcke, 1989, p. 86). Serving as one's "public face," the persona plays an important role of mediating between the outer world and the inner world (Douglas, 2008). The persona is not inherently good or bad, but frequently it is the source of trouble when a person identifies with it rather than the Self.

Anima/Animus   One of Jung's more controversial ideas, anima/animus developed from his observation that below the conscious masculine personality was a feminine side (anima); he later added but did not as fully develop the idea that women also have a masculine side (animus; Harris, 1996). The exploration of this archetype has had profound effects on our contemporary understandings of gender, and increasingly it is acceptable for both men and women to get in touch with and express qualities typically associated with the other gender. Jung believed that these remained primarily unconscious yet were important mediators between the ego and one's inner life.

Hero   One of the most clear and undeniable universal archetypes, the hero plays an important role at a personal level as well as societal level and often serves as a persona (Harris, 1996). Jung identified several universal elements of the hero's story: a divine birth, descent into the underworld, overcoming near-impossible obstacles, and helpful companions as well as themes of defeat, death, and rebirth. Although, like all archetypes, neither inherently good nor bad, Jung believed that overidentification with the hero often leads to problems commonly associated with hubris and overconfidence, namely, ultimate defeat and disgrace (Hopcke, 1989).

Wise Old Man or Woman   Another readily identifiable archetype, the *wise old man* is found in most world cultures and represents humanity's collective wisdom as well as certain qualities of masculinity, namely, strength, quietness, and fortitude (Harris, 1996; Hopcke, 1989). The wise old woman, often appearing in the form of the Virgin Mary or Kwan-Yin, typically demonstrates feminine qualities, such as nurturance and forgiveness. The wise old man or woman archetype often makes an appearance toward the end of the counseling process as a client moves toward greater inner awareness.

Trickster   Ah, the trickster! The trickster often pulls one over on the counselor too! The trickster is found in most world cultures: the court jester in Europe, the mythic Milarepa in Tibet, the Native American Kokopelli, and the Greek Hermes (Harris, 1996; Hopcke, 1989). The trickster is a master of speaking truth through paradox, is the first to proclaim that "the emperor has no clothes," and is the one laughing at a funeral. The quintessential shape-shifter, the trickster represents unexpected reversals and thus is a harbinger of transformation and change. In counseling, the trickster makes many appearances, often the unfortunate cause for seeking a counselor, the source of unexpected positive and negative turns during the process, and sometimes even the reason for a speedy end.

Rumor Has It: The People and Their Stories
Carl Gustav Jung

Born in 1875 in a northeastern province of Switzerland, Carl Gustav Jung was born to a minister in the Swiss Reformed Church. Jung was a quiet and introverted child who was interested in anthropology, mysticism, and philosophy, interests that are clearly evident in the counseling approach he later developed. His mother was an eccentric woman who claimed to see and communicate with spirits and was often unavailable for her son.

Although Jung began studying medicine, he later switched his study to the less respected subject of psychiatry. In 1903, he published his dissertation, *On the Psychology and Pathology of So-Called Occult Phenomena*. In 1906, he sent a copy of a paper, "Studies in Word

Association," to Freud, initiating a significant, productive, and historic—yet short—6-year friendship between the two men. Their friendship ended in 1912 when Jung published *Psychology of the Unconscious,* in which he diverged from Freud's thinking.

After serving as an army doctor in World War I, Jung returned home to marry Emma Rauschenbach, and they had five children. He continued to develop his theory, which was deeply spiritual, influenced by Christianity, Buddhism, Hinduism, Daoism, and other world religions that were just being explored in the West. He wrote the introduction to many of the first English translations of works, such as *The Tibetan Book of the Dead* and *I Ching.* He was a mystic, believing that each individual could have direct contact with the divine, and his approach is an expression of this belief.

Big Picture: Overview of Counseling Process

Although many elements of the theory may seem too abstract and a far cry from typical presenting problems, in practice Jungian analysis is down-to-earth and practical, focusing on relieving suffering (Hopcke, 1989). Like Freud, Jung believed that resolution of client problems involved resolving unconscious conflicts by bringing to awareness repressed and suppressed thoughts and feelings. More so than Freud and other psychodynamic theorists, Jung was quick to abandon preconceived theory if doing so benefited an individual's treatment because he believed that each person's journey toward individuation or wholeness was truly unique. Thus, rather than adhere to a strict set of interventions, Jung was creative and adaptive, using whatever seemed to be most useful to a particular client. He saw his role as more of a healer or guide, helping a client move toward greater integration of their inner polarities, of their unconscious and conscious minds, and of their ultimate connection to the cosmos.

Jung (1956a) identified four stages of counseling:

1. *Confession:* In this first stage, clients recount or "confess" their life stories, which often creates a sense of *catharsis,* or emotional release. The counselor listens empathetically and nonjudgmentally, helping the client feel reconnected to another.
2. *Elucidation:* In the second stage, the counselor helps the client gain insight about the transference relationship as well as childhood memories that are related to the problem.
3. *Education:* Jung explains that the stage of education involves "pointing out that no amount of confession and no amount of explaining can make the crooked plant grow straight, but that it must be trained upon the trellis of the norm by the gardener's art. Only then will normal adaptation be reached" (p. 68). In this phase, insight is translated into meaningful new action.
4. *Transformation:* The final phase of transformation applies only to those clients who desire to seek individuation rather than simply symptom relief, which is generally achieved in the third stage. Jung focused the later half of his career on this phase and compared it to the medieval art of *alchemy,* in which alchemists tried to turn base metals into gold. Similar to alchemists who changed themselves as part of the process of transforming metals, Jung believed that the counselor must simultaneously make personal life changes before clients can achieve personal transformation. In this phase, clients become more consciously connected with their Selves and the collective unconscious.

Making Connection: Counseling Relationship
Collaborative Educators

The Jungian style in the counseling room is one of fellowship, the counselor *collaboratively* working with clients in pursuing their unique journeys of individuation. At times, the Jungian counselor also plays the role of *educator,* offering information and insight regarding the role of archetypes and meaning. In comparison to Freud, Jung maintained a more pragmatic "whatever-works" attitude that required a flexible role on the part of the counselor (Hopcke, 1989).

Healer, Heal Thyself

Jung viewed counselors as archetypal healers, and as such they must engage in the archetypal journey of healers to heal themselves. Jung emphasized that analysts must also go on this journey to help guide clients in this process. One's personal work with archetypes, the unconscious, and collective unconscious is the only way to help others do the same. Without intimate and personal knowledge of these vast, mysterious realms, counselors will quickly get lost. Since many elements of the journey of individuation are archetypal, once the counselor has made significant progress on his or her own journey, it becomes much easier to help clients on theirs. Thus, similar to other depth psychologists, Jungian counselors engage in their own analysis as part of their training.

The Viewing: Case Conceptualization
Collective Unconscious

A significant departure from other forms of depth psychology, Carl Jung posited the *collective unconscious*, which exists beyond the individual and represents the evolutionary mind of humanity, including archetypes, myths, images, and symbols that can be traced in cultures throughout the world. Jung believed that the universal unconscious was *in addition to* the conscious and unconscious mind described by Freud. Jung states, "I have chosen the term 'collective' because this part of the unconscious is not individual but universal; in contrast to the personal psyche, it has contents and modes of behaviour that are more or less the same everywhere and in all individuals. It is, in other words, identical in all men and thus constitutes a common psychic substrate of a suprapersonal nature which is present in every one of us" (Jung, 1959a, pp. 3–4).

The structure of the personality as described by Jung included the following:

- *Conscious mind:* The part of the mind that one is aware of; contains the ego
- *Personal unconscious:* Includes forgotten elements, repressed memories, and elements that never were conscious (Harris, 1996)
- *Collective unconscious:* A universal consciousness made up of archetypes that all individuals have access to

Complexes and Catharsis

Early in his career when working with spontaneous word association, Jung noticed that certain emotionally charged patterns emerged that were clearly related to a person's pathology (e.g., themes of sadness and loss in response to words like "hopscotch" or "jungle gym"; Harris, 1996; Hopcke, 1989). He referred to these emotionally charged sets of responses as *complexes*. Potentially conscious but more typically unconscious, Jung believed that all complexes have archetypal elements that need to be explored. The analysis process brings these complexes to conscious awareness so that the person can reinterpret, make new associations, and experience *catharsis*, or emotional release.

Polarities and Enantiodromia

Jung believed that many forms of psychopathology developed around *polarities*: personality traits that get magnified or minimized (Hopcke, 1989). For example, working too hard without creating space for play and relaxation quickly leads to an unbalanced life and eventually pathology, such as depression, anxiety, or social withdrawal. Thus, even a virtuous quality—such as a "good work ethic"—can be the source of problems if it becomes polarized. In his conceptualization of psychological types, Jung conceptualized personality elements as polarities and believed that maturity involved a healthy balance of any two polarities. A related concept, *enantiodromia,* refers to Heraclitus' law that "everything sooner or later turns into its opposite" (Douglas, 2008, p. 117). This process is commonly seen in those who try to pursue ultrapure forms of spirituality and abstinence; they often are caught indulging in extreme forms of sexual misconduct, substance abuse, or frivolous extravagance (I won't name names, but you can probably call to mind a few examples from yesterday's paper). Similarly, many who pursue extreme forms of fame often find themselves in a similar situation.

Psychological Types

One of Jung's most enduring works, his theory of psychological types involves three elements, each consisting of two polarities:

- *Extravert/Introvert: Describes general attitude and orientation*
  Terms now used by nonprofessionals, Jung originally used the terms *extravert* and *introvert* to refer to a person's basic approach to libidinal energy. Extraverted refers to the individual's energy more typically being directed from inside the self to the outer world: "Extraversion is characterized by interest in the external object, responsiveness, and a ready acceptance of external happenings, a desire to influence and be influenced by events, a need to join in" (Jung, 1983, p. 140). In contrast, the introvert's libidinal energy more often moves from the outer world toward the self: "Introversion ... being directed not to the object but to the subject ... holds aloof from external happenings, does not join in. ... For him self-communing is a pleasure. His own world is a safe harbour, a carefully tended and walled-in garden" (pp. 141–142). Neither being better than the other and each having an important role in psychological health, the focus in counseling is to find a healthy balance between the two.
- *Thinking/Feeling*
  Jung described how people organize information and make decisions on the basis of two styles: thinking or feeling. Thinking types prefer analysis and logic, whereas feeling types focus on values and morality (not necessarily emotion). Understanding a person's type helps to better understand his or her motivations and reasons for making a decision.
- *Intuitive/Sensing*
  Finally, Jung characterized a person's typical style of "experiencing" the world as either intuitive—relying heavily on unconscious and collective unconscious information—or sensing—relying more on information through the senses. Counselors can use the knowledge of a person's preference for experiencing to develop interventions that "make sense" to the client.

Myers-Briggs   Developed by a mother–daughter team, the well-known Myers-Briggs typology used in business, college counseling, and numerous other arenas are based on Jung's personality characteristics. They have developed instruments that are commonly used to determine a person's type (Myers, 1998). Myers and Briggs added one more dimension to Jung's three: judging/perceiving:

- *Judging/Perceiving*
  Judging and perceiving refer how one orients to outer life. Judging types prefer to have things planned, ordered, and organized; they feel most at ease after a decision has been made. In comparison, perceiving types enjoy the process of exploring possibilities and have a spontaneous approach to life; they like to take in new information and experiences.

Targeting Change: Goal Setting
Individuation

The goal of Jungian analysis is to build a relationship between the conscious and unconscious and the ego and Self to create a unique sense of individuality while still connected to the larger human experience (Hopcke, 1989); this process is called *individuation.* Like humanists (Chapter 9), Jung believed that the human spirit naturally moves toward and seeks wholeness, which is represented in the archetype of the Self and is fundamental to his approach. The journey toward wholeness involves reconciling polarities and opposites within the psyche, increasingly bringing to consciousness the multifaceted elements of one's humanity. Jung saw the individuation process as the primary focus during the second half of life, after the achievements of young adulthood are well established (Jung, 1956b).

Example of Goals
- Facilitate catharsis related to childhood experiences (early phase)
- Increase awareness of persona and how it is maintained (early and middle phase)
- Increase awareness and acceptance of shadow elements of the self (middle and late phase)
- Integrate shadow elements into conscious understanding of self (middle and late phase)
- Increase sense of wholeness and well-being (late phase goal)
- Increase sense of connection to others, humanity, and/or the divine (late phase)

The Doing: Interventions
Symbols
Jungian counselors attend to *symbols* in clients' dreams (see below), choice of metaphors, synchronistic events (see section "Synchronicity"), symptoms, fantasies, and other material. Jungians view symbols as pointing to meanings that are not yet fully understood, which they distinguish from signs that are simply representational of a known thing: "Symbols provide the way out of a dilemma, a transcendent coming together of the opposites" (Harris, 1996, p. 56). Clinicians help clients (a) identify personally relevant symbols, (b) decode their personal meaning for clients, and (c) use them to promote healing. For example, a swan may become an important symbol for a woman who is struggling to accept her body image; the symbol may appear in her dreams, be part of synchronistic chance happenings, and become a personal symbol of healing for her. The fairy tale *The Ugly Duckling* may be an inspirational story for the woman as she embraces her physical beauty in new ways. The counselor can help guide her in how to use the symbol to help her interpret her life and inform new attitudes and behaviors.

Dream Analysis
As in Freudian psychoanalysis dream analysis is a hallmark technique of Jungian analysis. Both Freud and Jung agreed that dreams revealed unconscious material, but because they had quite different definitions of the unconscious mind, they approached dreams quite differently. Freud believed that dreams served the purpose of dealing with suppressed libidinal and aggressive impulses that the dreamer could not consciously recognize; Freud analyzed virtually all dreams through this lens. In contrast, Jung had a more intuitive and varied approach to dreams. He believed that the dreams were the unconscious expressing itself—sometimes expressing repressed material, sometimes foreshadowing the future, and sometimes providing direction to the individuation process—using its native language: symbols. The dream needed to be interpreted for the conscious mind to understand it and use it in the individuation process. "The point of dream work for Jung was to arrive at an interpretation or a set of interpretations that united conscious understanding and unconscious processes in a way that was intellectually, emotionally, and intuitively satisfying" (Hopcke, 1989, p. 26).

Jung's dream analysis employs a combination of using universal archetypal symbols and myth combined with the dreamer's unique associations and meanings. Ultimately, as in Freud's approach, the dream must be interpreted using the dreamer's unique meanings. Generally, Jungian dream interpretation involves three phases:

Jungian Dream Interpretation

Step 1: Identify dreamer's associations: As or after the dreamer shares the dream, the counselor asks about the dreamer's associations to significant people, places, events, and items in the dream.

(continued)

- What were the details that stood out in the dream and/or continue to linger (size, shapes, colors, objects, places, general feeling)?
- Were the elements of the dream familiar or unfamiliar?
- Were the elements new, old, current, future, or of a distant time?
- What was the dreamer's emotional state(s) in the dream?
- After waking (and in session), what emotional response did the dreamer have?
- Even if the dream does not have specific references, does the dream remind the dreamer of anyone, a place, or time in any way?

Step 2: Identify universal symbols/symbol amplification: In a process called *symbol amplification,* the analyst identifies potential archetypal elements in the dream (Hopcke, 1989).

- Are elements of the dream reminiscent of myths, legends, or folktales?
- Do any of the characters or elements represent an archetype? If so, how are these elements represented—positively, negatively, traditionally, untraditionally?
- Are there specific symbols that stand out, especially elements that had a strong emotional charge?

Step 3: Consolidation of interpretations: Finally, the counselor and dreamer work together to consolidate the two possible sets of interpretations into one or more interpretations that resonate and have significant personal meaning for the dreamer.

Active Imagination: Dreaming the Dream Onward

A technique related to dream work, *active imagination* helps develop a person's relationship to their unconscious mind and archetypes (Hall, 1986; Harris, 1996; Hopcke, 1989). In most dreams, the dreamer is a passive recipient of the unconscious, which writes the story, casts the parts, and directs the show. In active imagination, the client uses content that has been received from the unconscious through dreams or other means and combines it with conscious intent to promote healing and transformation. The goal is to have the conscious and unconscious minds work in tandem to balance and correct problematic polarities. Thus, it is not allowing the ego to have wild fantasies or simply replaying dreams. Instead, it is typically a visualization technique in which the person bridges these two worlds. For example, new endings can be created for nightmares that enable the dreamer to experience a new response to a frightening situation. The person begins by imagining herself back in the dream, calling to mind the various elements, and then allowing the mind to spontaneously play with the scene and explore what unfolds when the conscious mind is allowed to spend time in this environment.

Jungian Analysis of Transference

Like other depth psychologists, Jungians believe that transference plays an important role in the counseling process, but they have a unique three-stage approach (Douglas, 2008; Jung, 1959b). In the first stage, the clients' projections relate to their personal histories, typically from childhood. During this phase, the counselor helps the client recognize that these projections belong to the client and has the client withdraw them from the counselor and integrate them into their own personalities. For example, if a client projects harshness onto the counselor, the counselor helps the client recognize the projection and to accept the harsh aspects of the self, whether directed at the self or others. In the second phase, the client learns to discern which elements of projection are personal and which are archetypal, a unique element in Jungian analysis of transference. This phase involves identifying cultural, gender, and archetypal elements of projections. In the final phase, the personal reality of the counselor is differentiated from the projected image, and a human-to-human connection is made.

Jung further clarifies that counselors have a profound and deeply personal responsibility related to transference. At one level, the counselor must be aware of typical countertransference issues, as is common in all psychodynamic approaches. But Jung goes further: "The doctor knows—or at least he should know—that he did not choose this career by chance; and the psychotherapist in particular should clearly understand that psychic infections, however superfluous they seem to him, are in fact the predestined concomitants of his work, and thus fully in accord with the instinctive disposition of his own life. The realization also gives him the right attitude to his patient. The patient then means something to him personally, and this provides the most favourable basis for treatment" (1959b, p. 177).

Synchronicity

Synchronicity refers to uncanny and meaningful coincidences that cannot reasonably be explained by chance: "When coincidences pile up in this way one cannot help being impressed by them—for the greater the number of terms in such a series, or the more unusual its character, the more improbable it becomes" (Jung, 1960, p. 105). For example, you think of a friend you have not spoken to in years, and the next day he calls; you have a dream about a diamond, and the next day you find yourself stuck in traffic behind a Diamond Plumbing truck while passing a Diamond Cleaners, and later that day your coworker shows you her new diamond ring; or your Jungian analyst explores your hero archetype, and you find yourself coming across superheroes in various media for the rest of the week. Jung believed that these experiences could not be explained without the hypothesis of the collective unconscious. Counselors interpret synchronistic events as information from the collective unconscious about what themes or archetypes the person should be attending to in order to facilitate the process of individuation.

Interventions for Special Populations

Sand Play

A distinct form of intervention, sand play is a highly developed Jungian approach to using a sand tray with miniature figures; it is distinct from the more generic use of sand tray that can be used from any counseling approach. Sand play was originally developed by Dora Kalff, a Jungian analyst with an interest in Buddhism "who recognized that Sandplay provided a natural therapeutic modality for the child, allowing the expression of both the archetypal and intra-personal worlds, as well as connecting the child to outer everyday reality" (Mitchell & Friedman, 1994, p. 50). Kalff believed that sand play could activate the psyche toward wholeness and healing by reestablishing a connection between the ego and Self (Boik & Goodwin, 2000). Although originally developed for children, sand play is commonly used with adults, especially those working through trauma and loss, as well as couples and families. In contrast to more generic forms of sand tray work, in sand play the counselor quietly observes as the client develops a scene in the sand with the figurines without offering interpretations until after several trays have been completed.

The Sand Trays Sand play counselors use specific dimensions for the sand tray, dimensions that allow the mind to easily "take in" the scenes created in the sand. Sand trays should be 28.5 inches by 19.5 inches with a depth of 3 inches and set on a table with a height of approximately 30 inches. The trays are typically painted blue on the inside to represent water or sky, and a very fine grade of sand fills the tray. A formal sand play room has both a "dry" and a "wet" sand tray (and a frequently used vacuum for between sessions).

Figurines The figurines in sand play are typically kept on open shelves so that each is easily visible. In the Jungian approach, they are organized in "evolutionary" order with inanimate, natural objects at the bottom (e.g., rocks); then plants and foliage; and then dinosaurs, sea creatures, reptiles, birds, mammals, humans, and finally divine beings on the top shelf. (note: Sand play requires more tidiness than most other forms of intervention.)

Introducing the Tray   Once the counselor has established rapport and believes that sand play would be an appropriate intervention, the counselor introduces the activity using nondirective prompts, such as "Would you like to do a Sandplay? ... Put in what speaks to you" (after pointing to the collection of figurines) (Mitchell & Friedman, 1994, p. 54).

Counselor Role   The counselor's primary task is to create a free and protected psychological space in which the client feels comfortable exploring and yet protected and within safe limits (Mitchell & Friedman, 1994). Typically, the counselor sits off to the side and silently observes while the client works in the sand creating a scene with the figurines. Interpretations are *not* offered at the time the scenes are completed; instead, the counselor waits until after several trays have been completed to discuss them with clients. The counselor's quiet, supportive, and trusting presence enables the client to more easily access and express their unconscious to facilitate a healing process.

Recording   In most cases, the counselor will take a photograph of each tray after the client leaves for use later in the counseling process when the client is ready to explore the symbols and meaning in the tray. If a camera is not available and/or in addition to the photograph, the counselor can also make a sketch of the tray while the session is in progress (Mitchell & Friedman, 1994).

Putting It All Together: Jungian Treatment Plan Template

Use this treatment plan template for developing a plan for clients with depressive, anxious, or compulsive types of presenting problems. Depending on the specific client, presenting problem, and clinical context, the goals and interventions in this template may need to be modified only slightly or significantly; you are encouraged to significantly revise the plan as needed. For the plan to be useful, goals and techniques should be written to target specific beliefs, behaviors, and emotions that the client is experiencing. The more specific, the more useful it will be to you.

Treatment Plan

Initial Phase of Treatment (First One to Three Sessions)
Initial Phase Counseling Tasks

1. *Develop working counseling relationship. Diversity note:* Adapt for ethnicity, gender, age, and so on.
   Relationship-building approach:
   a. Create a "**collaborative educator**" relationship in which client views counselor as a resource on personal journey of healing and individuation.

2. *Assess individual, systemic, and broader cultural dynamics. Diversity note:* Adapt to client's sociocultural norms and other diversity factors.
   Interventions:
   a. Assessment strategy: "**Confession**" or telling of unedited life story.
   b. Assessment strategy: Identify prominent conflicts related to **archetypes, polarities, complexes,** and **shadow** elements of self.
   c. Assessment strategy: Identify **Myers-Briggs psychological type.**

Initial Phase Client Goals *(One to Two Goals): Manage crisis issues and/or reduce most distressing symptoms*

1. *Decrease* **unconscious conflicts** that escalate to crisis to reduce [specific crisis symptoms].

(continued)

Interventions:
a. Analysis of **complexes, polarities,** and **archetypal** patterns that fuel crisis.
b. **Active imagination** to increase coping skills and develop alternative responses to crisis.

Working Phase of Treatment (Three or More Sessions)
Working Phase Counseling Task

1. *Monitor quality of the working alliance. Diversity note:* Account for diversity issues and personality types in maintaining working alliance.
   Assessment Intervention:
   a. Monitor and analyze **transference**; adapt relationship to accommodate **personality type**.

Working Client Goals (Two to Three Goals). *Target individual and relational dynamics using theoretical language (e.g., decrease avoidance of intimacy, increase awareness of emotion, increase agency)*

1. *Decrease* **unconscious conflict** and **complexes** related to [specify problem or context] to reduce [specific symptom: depression, anxiety, etc.].
   Interventions:
   a. Analysis of **childhood experiences, symbols, dreams,** and **archetypes** to bring unconscious conflicts to conscious awareness and allow for catharsis.
   b. Analysis of **synchronicity** of conflict to understand conflicts and identify their role in individuation process.

2. *Increase* awareness of role of **persona, shadow,** and **Self** as well as role of [specify **archetype**] to reduce [specific symptom: depression, anxiety, etc.].
   Interventions:
   a. Analysis of **childhood experiences, symbols, dreams,** and **archetypes** to bring unconscious **archetypal conflicts** and **shadow** elements of self to conscious awareness.
   b. Sand play to explore dynamics of persona, shadow, Self, and other archetypes.

3. *Increase* **integration of polarities** in personality and consciousness to reduce [specific symptom: depression, anxiety, etc.].
   Interventions:
   a. Analyze **transference** to identify and integrate polarities.
   b. Analyze **synchronistic** events to facilitate integration of polarities.

Closing Phase of Treatment (Last Two or More Sessions)
Closing Phase Counseling Task

1. *Develop aftercare plan and maintain gains. Diversity note*: Integrate religious and community resources.
   Intervention:
   a. Educating client on how to use analysis of **synchronicity, dreams,** and **symbols** to independently continue lifelong process of **individuation**.

Closing Phase Client Goals (One to Two Goals): *Determined by theory's definition of health and normalcy*

1. *Increase* ability to consistently connect with and act from **Self** to reduce potential for relapse in [specific symptom: depression, anxiety, etc.].
   Interventions:
   a. Educating client on how to analyze **dreams, symbols,** and **synchronistic** events with increasingly less assistance from counselor.

(continued)

      b. **Active imagination** to consciously transform conflicts and complexes.

      c. Use of personally meaningful **symbols** to solidify connection with **Self**.

2. *Increase* sense of connection to others, humanity, and the divine to reduce potential for relapse in [specific symptom: depression, anxiety, etc.].
   Interventions:

   a. Educating client on how to increase tolerance of other **personality types** and alternative ways of being in the world.

   b. Use of personally meaningful **symbols** and **synchronicity** to solidify connection with divine.

Snapshot: Research and the Evidence Base

Quick Summary: Evidence-based brief psychodynamic approaches have the best empirical support; psychodynamic counseling has generally been found to be as effective as other approaches, such as cognitive-behavioral therapy; traditional psychoanalysis has the most scant evidence base for its efficacy.

Although often having a reputation for little research support, psychodynamic counseling has a respectable and growing evidence base (Leichsenring, 2009; Shedler, 2010). The best and most rigorously researched psychodynamic approaches are the brief psychodynamic methods, many of which are recognized as evidence-based approaches by the U.S. National Institutes of Health (Luborsky et al., 2008; Weissman et al., 2000, 2007). The strongest support for the effectiveness of general psychodynamic counseling comes from large-scale studies comparing psychodynamic to other approaches, such as cognitive-behavioral and humanistic, as was recently done in the United Kingdom, indicating no significant difference in outcome between theories (Stiles, Barkham, Mellor-Clark, & Connell, 2008). More recent studies show a trend for sustained gains and even *increasing* gains after counseling has ended (Abbass, Hancock, Henderson, & Kisely, 2006; Leichsenring, 2009). In addition, there is support for specific psychodynamic concepts. For example, using the Core Conflictual Relationship Theme model, Luborsky and associates (Luborsky & Crits-Christoph, 1998; Luborksy & Luborksy, 2006; Luborsky et al., 2008) have researched and found evidence that supports the psychoanalytic concept of transference. Additional research is needed to compare the different models or schools of psychodynamic theory to determine if they vary in effectiveness generally or for specific issues (Leichsenring, 2009). Finally, newer areas of research in psychodynamic counseling focus on the neurological and physiological correlates of psychodynamic processes and inform new ways of conceptualizing unconscious process and attachment (Marci & Riess, 2009; Roffman & Gerber, 2009).

Snapshot: Working With Diverse Populations

Quick Summary: These insight-oriented approaches should be carefully adapted when working with diverse populations, attending to the client's attitude toward introspection, rationality, and psychological analysis; the more recently developed relational and intersubjective approaches are more easily adapted than traditional approaches.

As traditionally practiced, psychoanalysis is considered not easily adaptable to other cultures (Luborsky et al., 2008) or sexual minorities (Glassgold & Iasenza, 2004) and has long been critiqued even from within the field as biased against women (Horney, 1939). In particular, there is continued concern about the appropriateness of adapting psychodynamic approaches to gay and lesbian clients, especially given the inherent heterosexual assumptions of drive theory as well as the limited number of diverse psychodynamically oriented practitioners (Glassgold & Iasenza, 2004; Greene, 2004). Some practitioners, such as Fred Pine (1990), have adapted psychoanalytic work to be more "supportive" when working with poor clients and clients with limited educational backgrounds. Pine uses "ego-building" interventions, such as naming feelings and alerting clients before offering a potentially difficult-to-hear interpretation. In addition, the more recently developed relational approaches enable psychodynamic practitioners to use a contextually sensitive approach that carefully incorporates the client's unique interpersonal context into the counseling process (Altman, 2008; Waldman & Rubalcava, 2005). Relational and intersubjectivity approaches recognize that both counselor and client "make sense of the other's affect, behavior, and expression in terms of their own unconscious cultural organizing principles" that is considered when assessing the intersubjective field (Rubalcava & Waldman, 2004, p. 138). Jungian analysis is an excellent option for clients desiring a more spiritual approach to counseling. In general, counselors should proceed mindfully, paying careful attention to countertransference when implementing these approaches with diverse clients and consider adapting case conceptualization and interventions to client needs and realities.

Psychodynamic Case Study

Heidi, a 72-year-old woman, reports that her habit of worrying has gotten worse in recent years. She was a banking executive for years and retired at 68. Her parents fled Austria during World War II, settling in the United States after living for some years in South America. She describes her parents as proud people who worked hard to make a good life for her. Although they were ethnically Jewish, she says they were not very religious. She was born right before they fled, and thus her early years were turbulent, as her parents were focused on rebuilding their lives and mourning the loss of their parents in the camps; she does not have any siblings. She says that she was closest to her father, who was a quiet but warm person who encouraged her professionally. Her mother was stern and strict, focusing on her schoolwork and chores. Heidi still feels that her mother was disappointed that she did not do enough with her life. Heidi never got married or had a family but has several close friends whom she now considers family.

Case Conceptualization

This case conceptualization was developed by selecting key concepts from "The Viewing: Case Conceptualization" section of the psychodynamic part of this chapter. You can use any of the concepts in that section to develop a case conceptualization for this or other cases.

Levels of Consciousness

Because Heidi's anxiety and worry have a long history (she says that she has worried a lot most of her life), it is likely that there is a fair amount of unconscious material related to her current situation. In addition, given the intergenerational history of trauma and trauma at a young age, much of this may also be more unconscious than conscious.

Structures of the Self

As evidenced by Heidi's symptoms, history, and career choice as is common in her cultural background, Heidi has an overactive superego that in many ways helped her succeed professionally. However, at this point, it is creating increasing suffering. She describes her mother's criticalness as the primary source of her overpowering superego.

Drive Theory (Drive Theory and Ego Psychology)

In many ways, Heidi has redirected her libidinal energy into her work to avoid relationships and to find a consistent means of self-validation. After retirement, she has now lost this, and it is now causing her to doubt herself and self-worth more.

Secondary Gains

A secondary gain of her worrying is that she always has something to talk about with friends and a means to stay connected with them. She calls or asks to visit to share her latest concerns about finances, health, and so on. She generally gets sympathy or, if not, at least some social connection.

Defense Mechanisms

Heidi has a history of *splitting* in her adult life as well as her childhood, where she saw her father as all-good and mother as all-bad. In her adult life, she periodically ends friendships when she feels that someone has not shown enough loyalty or caring. She also *represses* many of her more vulnerable feelings to avoid appearing weak and needy; although she worries, she does so with more anger and frustration than fear. She also *projects* a sense of being criticized onto others, often feeling insulted when no insult was intended.

Erickson's Psychosocial Stages of Development

In terms of her psychosocial development, two key issues stand out. First, she never developed a strong capacity for intimacy and instead focused on being a productive professional. Now that she is entering later life, she is struggling with feelings of despair and struggling to make sense of her life; she has repressed many of her earlier dreams and longings in favor of security but now is dealing with the repercussions of repressing these for so many years.

Object Relations Theory/True Self

Because of the upheaval and trauma in Heidi's family during her early years as well as her mother's emotional distance, Heidi has not resolved many of these early issues. She has internalized her mother's criticism and is quick to hear it from others. Although her father was more supportive, his approval never seemed enough to outweigh her mother's disapproval. In many ways, she still lives from the false self that she developed to please her mother.

Relational Matrix

Heidi's relational matrix has shrunk dramatically in recent years; thus, she has fewer people (or activities) to reflect back her worth. As she and her friends are older, she worries about her network of friends shrinking even more. Most of her friends are bright, former professionals who are active in local arts and music, as is she. This network creates a common bond that gives her something to look forward to.

Unconscious Organizing Principles and Culture

Heidi's father was a medical doctor in Austria before he fled with his young family early during World War II. The loss of their way of life and other family members has created a family expectation that ruin and doom are right around the corner. Having emigrated from Austria to South America and then to the United States, there was never a sense of being rooted or deeply connected. Their greatest joy—and a deep sense of safety—was derived from having a prestigious and lucrative career that creates stability and financial security.

Treatment Plan

Initial Phase of Treatment (First One to Three Sessions)
Initial Phase Counseling Tasks

1. *Develop working counseling relationship. Diversity note:* Adapt relationship style to honor immigration, ethnic/religious background, trauma history, and age.
    Relationship-building approach/intervention:
    a. Use **empathy** and **mirroring** to provide a supportive, holding environment for the adult female (AF), maintaining awareness of her cultural/family background that devalued demonstrative emotional expression.

2. *Assess individual, systemic, and broader cultural dynamics. Diversity note:* Attend to issues of immigration, Holocaust, and Austrian, South American, and American social norms, especially in childhood.
    Assessment strategies:
    a. Analyze **unconscious conflicts** underlying anxiety and role of **defense mechanisms** in managing them.
    b. Assessment strategy: Analyze **object relations** patterns, including expressions in current relationships and historical development during childhood years when family fled from Nazis.
    c. Assessment strategy: Assess **relational matrix** and **culturally defined unconscious organizing principles** that shape the client's worldview, with careful attention to Austrian/Jewish values, legacy of the Holocaust, and her family's traumatic immigration story.

Initial Phase Client Goal

1. *Decrease* emotional reactivity to perceived criticism to reduce anxiety and worry.
    Interventions:
    a. Provide **empathy** using **understanding–explaining sequence** to reduce client's inaccurate perceptions of criticism from others.
    b. **Interpretation** of relational patterns with parents to reduce need to use splitting and repression in response to incorrectly perceived threats.

Working Phase of Treatment (Two or More Sessions)
Working Phase Counseling Task

1. *Monitor quality of the working alliance. Diversity note:* Carefully adapt expectations for her age, cultural, and professional norms for relating.
    Assessment Intervention:
    a. Monitor and work through **transference** and **countertransference**.

Working Phase Client Goals

1. *Decrease* use of splitting, repression, and projection to protect self from feeling criticized by self and others to reduce worry/anxiety.
    Interventions:
    a. **Interpretation** of role of **defense mechanisms** and how it developed in early childhood immigration and trauma experiences and is being inappropriately used currently.
    b. Analysis of **transference** in session when AF perceives counselor as critical and/or sees counselor as all-good or all-bad.

2. *Increase* **ego strength** and **self cohesion** to reduce worry/anxiety.
    Interventions:
    a. **Mirroring** to confirm AF's sense of worth and value, with an emphasis on acknowledging vulnerable emotions.

(continued)

    b. **Empathy** using the **understanding–explaining sequence** to increase client's sense of cohesion.

    c. **Dream interpretation** and **free association** to bring sources of inner conflict to conscious awareness, especially as they relate to early childhood/family traumas related to fleeing from the Nazis and immigrating.

3. *Increase* sense of personal agency informed by emotional intelligence to reduce social conflicts and engagement.
   Interventions:

    a. **Intersubjective responding** to increase client's awareness of self in sessions versus various emotional-relational contexts.

    b. **Working through resistance** to translating insight into action.

Closing Phase of Treatment
Closing Phase Counseling Tasks

1. *Develop aftercare plan and maintain gains. Diversity note:* Manage end of counseling by adjusting for sociocultural and gender expectations for handling loss.
   Intervention:

    a. Analyzing **transference** and abandonment issues as impending termination approaches.

Closing Phase Client Goals

1. *Increase* sense of **integrity** related to past and current life decisions to reduce sense of **despair** as she faces end of life.
   Interventions:

    a. **Dream analysis, free association,** and **analysis of transference** to identify regrets and unresolved past traumas and losses.

    b. Enable client to **work through** past losses and traumas related to childhood as well as choosing to focus all her energies in her career and ignore her desire for relationship/family.

2. *Increase* ability to experience **mature dependency** and intimacy to reduce potential for using her anxiety to stay connected to friends.
   Interventions:

    a. Analyze **transference** and **secondary gains** and **work through resistance** to intimacy in in-session and out-of-session relationships.

    b. **Intersubjective responding** to critically examine the **unconscious organizing principles** the client uses to relate to others and how she builds relationships.

ONLINE RESOURCES

Associations

Diversity note: In addition to those listed, most major cities have an association or institute for psychoanalytic studies, and many also have an institute dedicated to the work of C. G. Jung.

American Institute of Psychoanalysis
www.aipnyc.org

American Psychological Association, Division 39, Psychoanalysis
www.apa.org

American Psychoanalytic Association
www.apsa.org

C. G. Jung Institute of Chicago
www.jungchicago.org

C. G. Jung Institute of Los Angeles
www.junginla.org

C. G. Jung Institute of New York and CG Jung Foundation
www.cgjungny.org

Center for Applications of Psychological Types (Myers-Briggs)
www.capt.org

Chicago Institute for Psychoanalysis
www.chicagoanalysis.org

International Psychoanalytic Association
www.ipa.org.uk

International Association for Relational Psychoanalysis and Psychotherapy
www.iarpp.org

Jungian Society for Scholarly Studies
www.thejungiansociety.org

Los Angeles Institute and Society for Psychoanalytic Studies
www.laisps.org

Myers-Briggs
www.myersbriggs.org

Psychoanalytic Institute of New York
www.psychoanalysis.org

Society of Analytical Psychology
www.jungian-analysis.org

Journals

Contemporary Psychoanalysis

Journal of Analytical Psychology
www.wawhite.org

Journal of the American Psychoanalytic Association
www.jungian-analysis.org/journal-of-analytical-psychology

Psychoanalytic Dialogues
www.apsa.org
www.theanalyticpress.com

References

*Asterisk indicates recommended introductory readings.

Abbass, A. A., Hancock, J. T., Henderson, J., & Kisely, S. (2006). Short-term psychodynamic psychotherapies for common mental disorders. *Cochrane Database of Systematic Reviews*, Issue 4, Article No. CD004687. doi:10.1002/14651858. CD004687.pub3

Abend, S. M. (2001). Expanding psychological possibilities. *The Psychoanalytic Quarterly, 70*, 3–14.

Altman, N. (2008). Origins and evolution of psychoanalytic theory. In J. Frew & M. D. Spiegler (Eds.), *Contemporary psychotherapies for a diverse world* (pp. 41–92). Boston: Houghton Mifflin.

Bacal, H. A., & Newman, K. M. (1990). *Theories of object relations: Bridges to self psychology.* New York: Columbia University Press.

Boik, B. L., & Goodwin, E. A. (2000). *Sandplay therapy: A step-by-step manual for psychotherapists of diverse orientations.* New York: Norton.

Book, H. E. (1998). *How to practice brief psychodynamic psychotherapy: The core conflictual relationship theme method.* Washington, DC: American Psychological Association.

Brown, L. J. (1981). The therapeutic milieu in the treatment of patients with borderline personality disorder. *Bulletin of the Menninger Clinic, 45*, 377–394.

Douglas, C. (2008). Analytical psychotherapy. In R. J. Corsini & D. Wedding (Eds.), *Current psychotherapies* (8th ed.). Pacific Grove, CA: Brooks/Cole.

Erickson, E. (1994). *Identity and the life cycle.* New York: Norton.

Erickson, E., & Erickson, J. (1998). *The life cycle completed: Extended version.* New York: Norton.

Fairbairn, W. R. D. (1954). *An object relations theory of the personality.* New York: Basic Books.

Friedan, B. (1963). *The feminine mystique.* New York: Norton.

Freud, S. (1961). *Civilization and its discontents (standard edition)* (J. Strachey, Trans.). New York: Norton. (Original work published 1931)

Freud, S. (1963a). *Dora: An analysis of a case of hysteria* (P. Rieff, Ed.). New York: Collier.

Freud, S. (1963b). *Sexuality and the psychology of love* (P. Rieff, Ed.). New York: Collier.

Freud, S. (1974a). *The ego and the id*. In J. Strachey (Ed.), *Standard edition of the complete psychological works of Sigmund Freud, Vol. 19*. London: Hogarth Press. (Original work published 1923)

Freud, S. (1974b). *The interpretation of dreams*. In J. Strachey (Ed.), *Standard edition of the complete psychological works of Sigmund Freud, Vol. 4*. London: Hogarth Press. (Original work published 1900)

Freud, S. (1974c). *On narcissism*. In J. Strachey (Ed.), *Standard edition of the complete psychological works of Sigmund Freud, Vol. 14*. London: Hogarth Press. (Original work published 1914)

Freud, S. (1974d). *The neuropsychoses of defense*. In J. Strachey (Ed.), *Standard edition of the complete psychological works of Sigmund Freud, Vol. 3*. London: Hogarth Press. (Original work published 1894)

Freud, S. (1974e). *Studies on hysteria*. In J. Strachey (Ed.), *Standard edition of the complete psychological works of Sigmund Freud, Vol. 2*. London: Hogarth Press. (Original work published 1895)

Freud, S. (1974f). *Three essays on sexuality*. In J. Strachey (Ed.), *Standard edition of the complete psychological works of Sigmund Freud, Vol. 7*. London: Hogarth Press. (Original work published 1905)

Gill, M. (1982). *The analysis of transference (Vol. 1)*. New York: International Universities Press.

Glassgold, J. M., & Iasenza, S. (Eds.). (2004). *Lesbians, feminism, and psychoanalysis: The second wave*. Binghamton, NY: Harrington Park Press.

Goleman, D. (1995). *Emotional intelligence*. New York: Bantam.

Greene, B. (2004). African American lesbians and other culturally diverse people in psychodynamic psychotherapies: Useful paradigms or oxymoron? In J. M. Glassgold & S. Iasenza (Eds.), *Lesbians, feminism, and psychoanalysis: The second wave* (pp. 57–77). Binghamton, NY: Harrington Park Press.

Greenberg, J. R. (2001). The analyst's participation: A new look. *Journal of the American Psychoanalytic Association, 49*, 417–426.

*Greenberg, J. R., & Mitchell, S. A. (1983). *Object relations in psychoanalytic theory*. Cambridge, MA: Harvard University Press.

Hall, J. A. (1986). *The Jungian experience: Analysis and individuation*. Toronto: Inner City Books.

*Harris, A. S. (1996). *Living with paradox: An introduction to Jungian psychology*. Pacific Grove, CA: Brooks/Cole.

Hopcke, R. H. (1989). *A guided tour of the collected works of C. G. Jung*. Boston: Shambhala.

Horney, K. (1939). *New ways in psychoanalysis*. New York: Norton.

Jung, C. G. (1983). Psychological types and the self-regulating psyche. In A. Storr (Ed.), *The essential Jung* (pp. 129–146). Princeton, NJ: Princeton University Press. (Original work published 1921)

Jung, C. G. (1956a). Problems of modern psychotherapy. In R. F. C. Hull (Trans.), *The practice of psychotherapy: Essays on the psychology of the transference and other subjects* (2nd ed., *The collected works of C. G. Jung, Vol. 16*, Bollingen Series XX, pp. 53–75). Princeton, NJ: Princeton University Press. (Original work published 1933)

Jung, C. G. (1956b). The stages of life. In R. F. C. Hull (Trans.), *The structure and dynamics of the psyches* (2nd ed., *The collected works of C. G. Jung, Vol. 8*, Bollingen Series XX, pp. 53–75). Princeton, NJ: Princeton University Press. (Original work published 1930)

Jung, C. G. (1959a). Archetypes of the collective unconscious. In R. F. C. Hull (Trans.), *The archetypes and the collective unconscious* (2nd ed., *The collected works of C. G. Jung, Vol. 9*, Bollingen Series XX, pp. 3–41). Princeton, NJ: Princeton University Press. (Original work published 1934)

Jung, C. G. (1959b). The psychology of transference. In R. F. C. Hull (Trans.), *The practice of psychotherapy: Essays on the psychology of the transference and other subjects* (2nd ed., *The collected works of C. G. Jung, Vol. 16*, Bollingen Series XX, pp. 163–201). Princeton, NJ: Princeton University Press. (Original work published 1946).

Jung, C. G. (1960). *Synchronicity: An acausal connecting principle*. R. F. C. Hull (Trans.). Princeton, NJ: Princeton University Press.

Kernberg, O. (1976). *Object relations theory and clinical psychoanalysis*. New York: Jason Aronson.

*Kernberg, O. (1997). Convergences and divergences in contemporary psychoanalytic technique and psychoanalytic psychotherapy. In J. K. Zeig (Ed.), *The evolution of psychotherapy: Third conference* (pp. 3–18). New York: Brunner/Mazel.

Klein, M. (1975). *The psychoanalysis of children* (A. Strachey, Trans.; H. A. Thorner, Rev.). New York: Delacorte Press. (Original work published 1932)

Kohut, H. (1977). *The restoration of the self*. New York: International Universities Press.

Kohut, H. (1984). *How does analysis cure?* Chicago: University of Chicago Press.

Krupnick, J., Elkin, I., Collins, J., Simmens, S., Sotsky, S., Pilkonis, P., et al. (1994). Therapeutic alliance and clinical outcome in the NIMH Treatment of Depression Collaborative Research Program: Preliminary findings. *Psychotherapy: Theory, Research, Practice, Training, 31*(1), 28–35. doi:10.1037/0033-3204.31.1.28

Lachmann, F. (1993). Self psychology: Origins and overview. *British Journal of Psychotherapy, 10*(2), 226–231. doi: 10.1111/j.1752-0118.1993.tb00651.x

Leichsenring, F. (2009). Psychodynamic psychotherapy: A review of efficacy and effectiveness studies. In R. A. Levy & J. S. Ablon (Eds.), *Handbook of evidence-based psychodynamic psychotherapy: Bridging the gap between science and practice* (pp. 3–28). New York: Humana Press.

Leone, C. (2008). Couple therapy from the perspective of self psychology and intersubjectivity theory. *Psychoanalytic Psychology, 25*, 79–98. doi:10.1037/0736-9735.25.1.79

Levenson, H. (2003). Time-limited dynamic psychotherapy: An integrationist perspective. *Journal of Psychotherapy Integration, 13*(3–4), 300–333. doi: 10.1037/1053-0479.13.3-4.300

Luborsky, E. B., O'Reilly-Landry, M., & Arlow, J. A. (2008). Psychoanalysis. In R. J. Corsini & D. Wedding (Eds.), *Current psychotherapies* (8th ed.; pp. 15–62). Pacific Grove, CA: Thompson.

Luborsky, L., & Crits-Christoph, P. (1998). *Understanding transference: The Core Conflictual Relationship Theme method* (2nd ed.). Washington DC: American Psychological Association.

Luborsky, L., & Luborsky, E. (2006). *Research and psychotherapy: The vital link.* Lanham, MD: Jason Aronson.

Mahler, M., Pine, F., & Bergman, A. (1975). *The psychological birth of the human infant.* New York: Basic Books.

Mallinckrodt, B. (2010). The psychotherapy relationship as attachment: Evidence and implications. *Journal of Social and Personal Relationships, 27*(2), 262–270. doi: 10.1177/0265407509360905

Marci, C. D., & Riess, H. (2009). Physiologic monitoring in psychodynamic psychotherapy research. In R. A. Levy & J. S. Ablon (Eds.), *Handbook of evidence-based psychodynamic psychotherapy* (pp. 339–358). New York: Humana Press.

Marmor, J. (1997). The evolution of an analytic psychotherapist: A sixty-year search for conceptual clarity in the Tower of Babel. In J. K. Zeig (Ed.), *The evolution of psychotherapy: Third conference* (pp. 23–33). New York: Brunner/Mazel.

*McWilliams, N. (1999). *Psychoanalytic case formulation.* New York: Guilford.

Messer, S. B., & Warren, C. S. (1995). *Models of brief psychodynamic therapy: A comparative approach.* New York: Guilford.

*Mitchell, R. R., & Friedman, H. S. (1994). *Sandplay: Past, present, and future.* New York: Routledge.

*Mitchell, S. A. (1988). *Relational concepts in psychoanalysis: An integration.* Cambridge, MA: Harvard University Press.

*Mitchell, S. A., & Black, M. J. (1995). *Freud and beyond: A history of modern psychoanalytic thought.* New York: Basic.

Myers, I. B. (1998). *Introduction to type: A guide to understanding your results on the Myers-Briggs Type Indicator* (6th ed.). Gainesville, FL: Center for Applications of Psychological Types.

Pine, F. (1990). *Drive, ego, object, and self.* New York: Basic Books.

Roffman, J. L., & Gerber, A. J. (2009). Neural models of psychodynamic concepts and treatments: Implications for psychodynamic psychotherapy. In R. A. Levy & J. S. Ablon (Eds.), *Handbook of evidence-based psychodynamic psychotherapy* (pp. 305–338). New York: Humana Press.

Rubalcava, L. A., & Waldman, K. M. (2004). Working with intercultural couples: An intersubjective-constructivist perspective. In W. J. Corbin (Ed.), *Transformations in self psychology: Progress in self psychology* (Vol. 20, pp. 127–149). Hillsdale, NJ: Analytic Press.

Seligman, M. E. P. (2002). *Authentic happiness: Using the new positive psychology to realize your potential for lasting fulfillment.* New York: Free Press.

Siegel, D. (1999). *The developing mind: How relationships and the brain interact to shape who we are.* New York: Guilford.

*Shedler, J. (2010). The efficacy of psychodynamic psychotherapy. *American Psychologist, 65*(2), 98–109. doi:10.1037/a0018378

Sifneos, P. E. (1979). *Short-term dynamic psychotherapy: Evaluation and technique.* New York: Plenum.

*St. Clair, M. (2000). *Object relations and self psychology: An introduction.* Belmont, CA: Brooks/Cole.

*Stiles, W., Barkham, M., Mellor-Clark, J., & Connell, J. (2008). Effectiveness of cognitive-behavioural, person-centred, and psychodynamic therapies in UK primary-care routine practice: Replication in a larger sample. *Psychological Medicine: A Journal of Research in Psychiatry and the Allied Sciences, 38*(5), 677–688. doi:10.1017/S0033291707001511

Stolorow, R. D., Brandschaft, B. & Atwood, G. E. (Eds.). (1987). *Psychoanalytic treatment: An intersubjective approach.* Hillsdale, NJ: Analytic Press.

Sullivan, H. S. (1953). *The interpersonal theory of psychiatry.* New York: Norton.

Sullivan, H. S. (1954). *The psychiatric interview.* New York: Norton.

Waldman, K., & Rubalcava, L. A. (2005). Psychotherapy with intercultural couples: A contemporary psychodynamic approach. *American Journal of Psychotherapy, 59,* 227–245.

Weissman, M., Markowitz, J., & Klerman, G. (2000). *Comprehensive guide to interpersonal psychotherapy.* New York: Basic Books.

Weissman, M., Markowitz, J., & Klerman, G. (2007). *Clinician's quick guide to interpersonal psychotherapy.* New York: Oxford University Press.

Winnicott, D. W. (1965). *The maturational processes and the facilitating environment: Studies in the theory of emotional development.* New York: International Universities Press.

CHAPTER
5

Adlerian Individual Counseling

The chief danger in life is that you may take too many precautions.

—Alfred Adler

And my personal favorite:
The only normal people are the one's you don't know very well.

—Alfred Adler

I first studied Alfred Adler while studying abroad at the University of Salzburg in Austria. In my "Tiefenpsychologie" (depth psychology) course, we covered Freud, Jung, and Adler. I was well acquainted with the first two from my 2 years of psychology undergraduate course work at the College of William and Mary, but who was Adler? The "Eagle"? Apparently, some guy the Austrians thought played in the same league of Freud and Jung. I was suspicious that Adler was more of a local hero—or one who no longer had much influence. As with most thoughts I had as an undergraduate, I was wrong. *Very* wrong. It turns out that Adler's ideas lay the groundwork for the majority of theories practiced in the 21st century, and, as many Adlerians lament, his work is rarely cited by later generations—and, apparently, my cognitive-behavioral faculty at William and Mary (Sweeney, 2009). To be fair, the later generations may not have immediately read his work when they developed their theories—and so academics have a lot to bicker about in this regard—but in the big scheme of ideas, Adler was first to put pen to paper and describe many of the counseling principles we find common today. So, I hope you take careful note of his work and look for its quiet influence in the chapters that follow.

Lay of the Land

The unsung hero of counseling and psychotherapy, Alfred Adler's work laid the foundation for most forms of modern counseling. Even when not directly cited, elements of his ideas are identifiable in object relations, self psychology, humanistic, cognitive, behavioral, family systems, feminist, multicultural, and postmodern approaches. His approach has been characterized as an analytic-behavioral-cognitive approach that also incorporates systemic elements (Mosak & Maniacci, 1999). A contemporary of Freud and Jung who also worked at the University of Vienna, Adler developed a unique approach to counseling that is quite distinct from the psychoanalysis of Freud. Although modern practitioners have adapted his work for current times (Carlson, Watts, & Maniacci, 2006; Sweeney, 2009), for the most part Adler's individual psychology is practiced using the same key principles and practices identified by Adler in the 1910s. Adler's work has also been applied to group counseling and education (Adler, 1978; Carlson et al., 2006; Sweeney, 2009).

In a Nutshell: The Least You Need to Know

Adler's Individual Psychology departed from his colleagues Freud and Jung on numerous issues, including the following:

- *Holistic view:* Adler posited that a person must be seen *holistically*, as a unified personality or "individual."
- *Social factors:* Also departing from Freud's deterministic view, Adler emphasized that a person's *social environment* was a determining factor influencing personality development.
- *Choice:* He believed people have *choices* in how they approach their lives and that their past does not determine their future.
- *Social motivation:* He believed that people were motivated primarily by social connections, which he called *social interest*, rather than innate instinctual drives; he believed that high levels of social interest and prosocial behavior were signs of psychological health.
- *Teleological and goal oriented:* Adler believed that behavior was *purposeful* and *goal oriented* and that people strive toward meaningful activity, success, and achievement.
- *Subjective and phenomenological:* In addition, unlike Freud, Adler was interested in understanding and valuing a person's *subjective reality*, a principle emphasized in phenomenological approaches (see Chapter 6).

Adlerians believe that in striving for *superiority* and betterment of self, each person develops a *style of life* or *lifestyle*, a characteristic set of attitudes and assumptions that help a person make sense of life. This style of life clearly emerges in the first 6 years of life, but later development and events also shape a person's lifestyle. A person's style of life is the template through which all life events are interpreted; faulty interpretations and mistaken notions cause problems and difficulties. The process of counseling aims to help people correct these *basic mistakes* or faulty notions, enabling them to *consciously choose* a new style of life (you can now understand why Adler and Freud had bitter disagreements over espresso and strudel at Café Landtmann).

The counseling process itself is brief (generally fewer than 20 sessions; Bitter & Nicoll, 2000), present- and future-oriented (with some assessment of the past), and directive (Carlson et al., 2006). The counselor's primary role is *educational*, the counselor helping clients to understand the mistaken beliefs that inform their lifestyle and to help them improve their social relatedness, strive for goals that have meaning, and master the self. Counselors use *encouragement* to help clients move in the direction of their goals. Through a process of understanding *early recollections*, the *family constellation*, *sibling position*, and *style of life*, clients gain insight and self-understanding. Once insight is achieved, counselors help clients to develop the courage to take new action and make new decisions in their life and relationships.

The Juice: Significant Contributions to the Field

If there is one thing you remember from this chapter, it should be ...

Social Interest and Community Feeling

Adlerians believe that humans are innately social creatures (modern translation "genetically wired") (Adler, 1924, 1959; Dreikurs, 1989). As a species, humans need each other to survive. *Social interest* or *community feeling* (literal translation of the German *Gemeinschaftsgefühl*) refers to a person subjectively experiencing a sense that he or she has something in common with other people, is a part of a community, and benefits from cooperating with others in the community (Mosak & Maniacci, 1999). Moreover, Dreikurs (1958) emphasized that it is more than just the feeling of belonging: "The ideal expression of social interest is the ability to play the game [of life] with existing demands for cooperation and to help the group to which one belongs in its evolution closer toward a perfect form of social living. This implies progress without creating unnecessary antagonism" (p. 8).

In part, social interest is demonstrated by a willingness to *give more to the community than one receives in return* (i.e., have a generous spirit; Dreikurs, 1989). More important, the draw toward connection is a central organizing value in a well-adjusted person's life. In contrast, those who "measure their happiness and satisfaction only by what they get ... pay [for their error] in unhappiness and suffering" (p. 6). Laying the foundation for social justice and multicultural awareness, Dreikurs (in translating Adler's words) acknowledges that "sometimes the interests of various groups conflict. ... In such perplexing situations the social interest causes us to see that the interests of the super-ordinate group, which are justified on the ground of objective needs, have the first claim on us. We certainly want to do what we can to help men to found a society embracing the whole human race" (p. 8).

Adler identified three primary areas of social life in which social interest plays a central role: (a) communal life, (b) work, and (c) love relationships (Ansbacher & Ansbacher, 1956) and maintained that a person must be successful in all three areas to be well adjusted. Modern Adlerians have added three other areas: (d) self-acceptance, (e) spirituality, and (f) parenting (Carlson et al., 2006; Dreikurs & Mosak, 1967; Mosak & Dreikurs, 1967; Sweeney, 2009). Healthy adaptation within each of these realms involves striving for the goal of *perfection* (in a positive sense), becoming one's best self in each of these realms. In contrast, those who are more poorly adjusted strive for the goal of *personal superiority*, trying to be better than others, a critical distinction in Adlerian theory.

Adler explains that a sense of *individual inferiority* impairs a person's social interest. *Individual inferiority* is one of three forms of inferiority posited by Adler (Dreikurs, 1989):

1. *Biological inferiority:* Based on the need to form groups for physical survival; this form of inferiority promotes social interest.
2. *Cosmic inferiority:* Recognizing the inevitable death and the limitations of human existence; this form of inferiority also promotes social interest.
3. *Personal inferiority:* Feeling less powerful, able, or valued than others; this form of inferiority *inhibits* social interest because one does not feel as if he or she belongs to the community.

This sense of personal inferiority is the source of clients presenting problem: "any person who labors under a sense of inferiority always tries to obtain power of some kind in order to cancel the supposed superiority of other people. His feeling of inferiority impels him to strive for significance" (Dreikurs, 1989, p. 22); when this becomes a pattern, it is called an *inferiority complex*, a term that has trickled into popular vernacular (Mosak & Maniacci, 1999).

People respond to inferiority in primarily two ways: (a) to gain significance by achievement or (b) to avoid obligation, risky decisions, and connection with others. The pursuit of outstanding achievement can contribute to society even if fueled by fear; however, people who are ruthless and unethical in these pursuits waste their lives on what Adler terms "the useless side of life" (Dreikurs, 1989, p. 24). The counselor's role is to encourage people to transform their sense of inferiority to more effectively promote their social interest and eventually to reduce their overall sense of inferiority.

Assessing for Social Interest

When assessing for social interest, Adlerian counselors listen carefully to how clients describe their lives and problems. The three general types of social interest are as follows (Sweeney, 2009):

	Organizing Question	Content of Conversation
High Social Interest	What am I doing?	Sharing, enjoying, creating
Low Social Interest: "Successful person"	How am I doing?	Power, position, possessions
Low Social Interest: "Failure"	How am I doing?	Complaining, blaming, fears, excuses

---

Rumor Has It: The People and Their Stories

Founding Figures

Alfred Adler Born in Vienna, Austria, in 1870 to a Jewish merchant family, Alfred Adler's early years were difficult: he had rickets, nearly died of pneumonia, and was run over by two vehicles. He was an average student who was competitive with his older brother (Alfred was the second oldest of six children; this is an important side note, as his theory emphasizes the importance of birth order; Carlson et al., 2006; Sweeney, 2009). After receiving his medical degree, he practiced as a general physician and ophthalmologist in Vienna near the Prater, the central amusement park. His patients included many of the Prater's circus workers, and this most likely enabled him to learn to appreciate unusual strengths in people. During this time, he met Raissa, who was a Russian socialist and activist who was studying in Vienna; they then married and had four children.

In 1902, Freud invited Adler to join Freud's informal discussion group with other leading psychiatrists. This group, the Wednesday Society (German *Mittwochsgesellschaft*), became the beginning of the psychoanalytic movement. Most biographers agree that Adler's ideas differed from Freud's from the beginning. After serving as president of the Vienna Psychoanalytic Society, Adler and a group of his supporters left in 1911, the first to leave from Freud's group. Most scholars agree that Adler was never Freud's pupil; rather, they were early colleagues (Sweeney, 2009) initially sharing similarities as they developed a new form of treatment: "talk therapy." Their mutual dislike was well documented and is not surprising given the radically different approaches to psychotherapy; nonetheless, Adler respected Freud for his contributions, most notably his work on dream interpretation. The fundamental difference (which is a major) between their two theories is that Adler believed that the *social realm* was as important as the *inner world*, while Freud concerned himself only with the latter.

In 1912, Adler founded the Society for Individual Psychology and lectured internationally for 25 years promoting his socially oriented approach. In the 1920s, he established numerous child guidance clinics, which were later closed because of his Jewish heritage. In the 1930s, as World War II approached, he accepted an appointment at the Long Island College of Medicine in New York. He died in 1937 of a heart attack during a lecture tour.

Rudolf Dreikurs Born in Vienna in 1897 and a student of Alfred Adler, Dreikurs (1958, 1989; Dreikurs & Loren, 1968; Manaster & Corsini, 1982) continued promoting individual psychology after Adler's death and is credited as the principal person who promoted Adler's work in the United States. In particular, Dreikurs communicated Adler's ideas in pragmatic terms, making them useful to the average practitioner. Dreikurs specialized in working with preadolescent children, promoting cooperative behavior without punishment or reward (i.e., behavioral interventions). He was a significant force in the development of child guidance centers. In addition, he also used individual psychology principles to improved children's learning in the classroom (Dreikurs, 1968).

Modern Practitioners

Heinz and Rowena Ansbacher Heinz and Rowena Ansbacher have collected and edited many of Adler's original writings for English audiences (Ansbacher & Ansbacher, 1956, 1964). Their work preserves and explicates Adler's original writings and helps translate and clarify them for everyday practice.

James Bitter James Bitter is an influential Adlerian counselor who has developed Adlerian counseling as a brief approach and family approach (Bitter, Christensen, Hawes, & Nicoll, 1998; Bitter & Nicoll, 2000).

Jon Carlson Jon Carlson has developed Adlerian counseling for couples, families, and diverse populations (Carlson et al., 2006). He is also the host for several video training series, including the *APA Psychotherapy Video Tape Series III, Brief Therapy Inside and Out, Family Therapy With the Experts,* and *Psychotherapy With the Experts* (Carlson, n.d.).

Don Dinkmeyer, Gary McKay, and Joyce McKay Don Dinkmeyer, Gary McKay, and Joyce McKay (Dinkmeyer, McKay, & McKay, 2007) developed the *Systematic Parenting for Effective Parenting (STEP) Program*, an evidence-based parenting program based on Adlerian principles.

Harold Mosak Harold Mosak has written numerous primers and texts that offer practical descriptions of how to use Adler's approach in modern contexts (Mosak & Di Pietro, 2006; Mosak & Dreikurs, 1967; Mosak & Maniacci, 1999; Mosak & Sculman, 1988).

Thomas Sweeney Sweeney (2009) has developed a modern Adlerian approach that integrates elements of positive psychology and includes applications for career, couple, family, and group counseling.

Big Picture: Overview of Counseling Process

Adlerian counseling involves four stages (Sweeney, 2009):

- *Phase 1:* Establish an egalitarian relationship
- *Phase 2:* Assess lifestyle and private logic
- *Phase 3:* Encourage insight and self-understanding
- *Phase 4:* Educate and reorientate

Phase 1: Establish an Egalitarian Relationship

The first phase, described in detail in the "Making Connection" section, involves making a positive, warm connection with clients in which the counselor focuses on strengths and abilities. Adlerian counselors have the utmost hope that every person can find better ways of coping, improve their sense of belonging, and become meaningful contributors to the community.

Phase 2: Assess Style of Life and Private Logic

In the second phase, counselors assess clients' style of life and private logic, which is described in detail in the "Viewing: Case Conceptualization" section. Typically, the assessment period involves reviewing the following:

- Level of social interest
- Style of life and private logic

- The family constellation and sibling position
- Early recollections
- *Diagnostic and Statistical Manual of Mental Disorders (DSM)* diagnosis

Phase 3: Encourage Insight and Self-Understanding

In the third phase, counselors help clients gain better self-understanding, promoting *insight*, albeit a different form of insight that is typical in psychoanalytic approaches. In Adlerian work, counselors use insight as an *impetus* and source of positive motivation to take action and make changes rather than being an end in itself. In this phase, the counselor offers possible *interpretations* of behavior by identifying underlying motivations for problems, such as feelings of inferiority motivating a person's avoidance of commitment in a love relationship. Unlike Freudian interpretation, Adlerians *collaboratively* work with clients to find useful, meaningful interpretations of client motivations rather than relying on the counselor's objective perspective to determine the correct interpretation.

Phase 4: Educate and Reorientate

The final phase involves taking action! Counselors challenge clients to develop the *courage* it takes to make life changes based on their insights. These changes in behavior are referred to as a *reorientation*, referring to the fact that a person must "reorient" to life by correcting *basic mistakes* in his or her *style of life*. This phase involves primarily motivating the client to take action based on education regarding more accurate and effective approaches to life.

Making Connection: Counseling Relationship
Egalitarian

> The psychotherapist must lose all thought of himself and all sensitiveness about his ascendancy, and must never demand anything of the patient. ... The patient's social interest, which is always present in some degree, finds its best possible expression in the relation with the psychologist. The consultee must under all circumstances get the conviction that in relation to the treatment he is absolutely free. He can do, or not do, as he pleases. (Ansbacher & Ansbacher, 1964, p. 341; translation of Adler's 1933 article "Sinn des Lebens, What Life Should Mean to You")

A radical position during a time when psychoanalysis dominated the field, Adler promoted *egalitarian* relationships with clients that allowed them to maintain a sense of agency and choice (Sweeney, 2009). Counselors should not see themselves as superior even though they are in a helping position. Instead, Adlerian counselors—who do offer interpretations and education—approach clients from a more humble position of having something of potential usefulness for clients understanding that what is offered may or may not be actually useful in the client's subjective world.

Encouragement

One of its most distinguishing elements, "the Adlerian approach is characterized by its deliberate efforts to encourage the patient" (Dreikurs, 1989, p. 88). However, Adlerian encouragement should not be confused with a Pollyanna, cheerleaderish, "just-do-it" form of encouragement. Instead, Adlerian encouragement comes from a philosophical presupposition that life problems are not the result of personal failure or innate character flaws, as it may seem to a person experiencing a sense of *personal inferiority*; rather, they are the result of mistaken beliefs about life (a position also adopted in cognitive counseling). Thus, Adlerians are optimistic and hopeful about helping clients resolve their problems and thus believe beyond a shadow of a doubt that clients can improve their lives and therefore encourage them to do so.

Described as "a friendly, jovial, concerned person, filled with common sense, an ideal 'uncle'" (Manaster & Corsini, 1982, p. 168), Adler's style of encouraging fuses warmth, honesty, and practicality. To effectively convey encouragement, counselors must do it both verbally and nonverbally, which includes smiling, listening attentively, being patient, and taking action when needed (Sweeney, 2009). In the case study at the end of this chapter, the counselor uses encouragement extensively to help Budi, an Indonesian immigrant who became disabled because of a rare neural disorder.

Strategies for Conveying Encouragement

- Curiously asking about unique hobbies, abilities, or interests: "Tell me more about how you learned to do X."
- Verbally saying, "This is something I believe you can do."
- Complimenting and commenting on existing coping abilities: "You have done a remarkable job thus far raising two children without a partner."
- Hopeful comments when discussing new behaviors: "Doing X [new action—such as going to social events] is going to be far easier than what you have been doing to simply limp along all these years fearing failure."
- Correcting mistaken impressions in a hopeful way: "You may *feel* inferior, but it doesn't seem like your fears are based on a realistic assessment of your abilities."

Empathy and Social Interest

Counselors should be role models for social interest. As defined by Adler, social interest inherent requires empathy. Adler refers to an "English author" (this was before the *APA Manual of Style* requirements for direct quotation; he would have lost points on his paper for this glaring omission) who provides the best definition of social interest and social feeling that he could find at that time: "To see with the eyes of another, to hear with the ears of another, to feel with the heart of another" (Ansbacher & Ansbacher, 1956, p. 135). Carlson et al. (2006) liken this quality of social interest on the part of the counselor to Carl Rogers's empathy (see Chapter 6). Similarly, Carlson et al. (2006) link Adler's concept of encouragement to Rogers's core condition of unconditional positive regard because both approaches share a fundamental assumption: valuing of clients for their humanity.

Directive

The final aspect of the counseling relationship initially seems at odds with the preceding three. Adlerian counselors are directive (Carlson et al., 2006). How can a counselor be egalitarian and at the same time be directive? The catch is that their directiveness comes in the form of *education*: providing practical and helpful information. The key is a teaching style that is "encouraging" and nonhierarchical. The underlying message is that "I am offering you some information I believe to be useful; you can take it or leave it." Thus, they are not pushy salespeople. They educate with enthusiasm and hope, and thus their clients are generally willing pupils.

The Viewing: Case Conceptualization
Lifestyle Assessment

Lifestyle assessment is the heart of Adlerian assessment. *Style of life* or *style of living* is perhaps the closest modern translation of Adler's original German term *Lebensstil*. Lifestyle has been defined as *how* a person characteristically responds to others and the environment (Manaster & Corsini, 1982). Mosak and Maniacci (1999) define lifestyle as "the individual's characteristic way of thinking, seeing, and feeling towards life and is synonymous with what other theorists call 'personality'" (p. 31).

Adler thought of lifestyle as *the individuality of person expressing itself in its social environment* (Ansbacher & Ansbacher, 1956). Adler uses a pine tree as a simile for understanding the development of lifestyles: a pine that lives in the protection of a valley expresses itself quite differently from one growing on a mountaintop even though they have the same genetics. So too, humans express their individuality differently, depending on their social environment. Unlike the pine tree, humans have more choice in how they choose to express themselves: our mobility gives us a "leg up" on those trees (how could I resist such a pun?).

Adler used style of life liberally and variously to refer to the self, personality, unity of the personality, individuality, method of facing problems, opinion of self, view of life problems, and general attitude toward life (Ansbacher & Ansbacher, 1956). So, if it seems like the term is a bit general and all-encompassing, you're catching on. Most commonly in modern Adlerian counseling, a person's style of living refers to his or her fundamental beliefs about what is valuable in life, what is ideal, and what is to be avoided. Adler cautions that a person's style of living is not immediately apparent: "As long as a person is in a favorable situation, we cannot see his style of life clearly. In new situations, however, where he is confronted with difficulties, his style of life appears clearly and distinctly" (Ansbacher & Ansbacher, 1956, p. 173). Adler believed that a person's style of life becomes fixed by age 5, and general research on personality development supports this claim (Manaster & Corsini, 1982).

Both Sweeney (2009) and Carlson et al. (2006) have developed contemporary approaches to lifestyle assessment. Typically, the following areas are assessed:

- Parenting style
- Family constellation and birth order
- Early recollections
- Basic mistakes
- Organ inferiority or physical weak points
- "The question": function of the symptom
- Dreams

Parenting Style

Adler was particularly concerned about two parenting styles: pampering and neglect, with the former having more detrimental effects than the latter (Mosak & Maniacci, 1999). His concern with pampered children was that they are accustomed to "getting" and demand whatever they want and thus develop low levels of social interest and do not thrive as adults. In contrast, a neglected child may suffer but is more likely to develop social interests and to pursue self-improvement. However, he noted that children were not passive recipients; rather, children and parents mutually shaped each others' behavior. Adler believed that it was the child's *subjective* perception of the parenting style that ultimately most affected a person's style of life.

Questions for Assessing Parenting Style

- Describe your relationship to your parents as a child? Were they indulgent? Strict? Inconsistent? Supportive?
- How did you get what you needed? How did you get what you wanted?
- Did you have favorite strategies for getting your way?
- Which child was able to influence your parents the most? The least?

Family Constellation and Birth Order

As alluded to in "Rumor Has It" above, Adler put considerable emphasis on the socio-psychological configuration or *constellation* of a person's family, with an emphasis on birth order (Sweeney, 2009). Adlerians believe that the sibling closest in age and *most different* is the sibling that most affects how one defines the self. Above all, it is a person's *subjective* interpretation of the family constellation that has lasting impact on the style of life.

Debated for over 134 years, little consensus has emerged on the effect of birth order on personality (Hartshorne, Salem-Hartshorne, & Hartshorne, 2009). Adler considered birth order an important—but not determining (remember, it was Freud who believed in determinism)—variable in understanding human behavior (Sweeney, 2009). However, research over the years has yielded no definitive answer as to whether and how birth order affects development in part because many past studies did not control for socioeconomic status and ethnicity, both of which are frequently correlated with larger family size (Hartshorne et al., 2009; Sweeney, 2009). However, better-controlled research continues on birth order. For example, a recent study supports the idea that people are more likely to form close friends and romantic relationships with persons of the same birth order (Hartshorne et al., 2009).

- *Oldest child:* The oldest child generally begins life as the center of attention and typically learns to take the "newcomers" in stride if the parents provide encouragement for them to recognize their place in the family structure (Sweeney, 2009). Oldest children tend to relate well with adults, assume social responsibility, and develop socially appropriate forms of coping. Their lifestyle often includes striving for superiority, which may be a problem if not moderated over time.
- *Second child:* Second children will typically pursue an opposite position than the first because that is the role most readily available to them. On average, they may be less responsible, more independent, or more demanding than their older sibling. In some cases, the second child strives to be number one, creating *sibling rivalry*, especially if parents do not discourage the competition and comparisons. Some give up in discouragement, while others are socially productive even though they are motivated by the mistaken belief that their value comes from their achievements.
- *Middle child:* Families of three or more have middle children, who may feel "squeezed" between the others. Being neither the first nor the youngest child, many feel like they do not have a clear or unique role to play in the family. Similar to second children, middle children generally tend to define themselves in the opposite direction of their older sibling(s). They may be more independent, sensitive, or even rebellious, and some may directly ask parents for reassurance of their love. A benefit of their position, many learn to be skilled mediators, cope well with social stress, and learn from the mistakes of others (namely, their older siblings)—often with minimal gloating or name-calling.
- *Youngest child:* Perhaps the most frequently referred to family role, the "baby of the family" tends to enjoy being the center of attention and indulgence given that there are so many people in the family to take care of their needs. Youngest children often grow up to be charming or even manipulative and often avidly seek life's pleasures. If the parents emphasize achievement, they may become the hardest working of all to prove their place and ultimate worth.
- *Only child:* Only children are much like older children except that they are never dethroned and generally do not have the pressure of a close competitor. Only children tend to be inducted into the adult world early, becoming responsible, cooperative, and mature for their age. However, many have difficult relating to their peers, especially in the area of sharing.

To assess for birth order, counselors shouldn't simply ask, Were you the oldest or youngest in your family? Meaningful assessment requires more follow-up than that.

Questions for Assessing Birth Order and Family Constellation

- Do you have any siblings? If so, who was oldest, second oldest, and so on?
- Can you describe the role of each child in the family? How did your parents encourage or discourage these roles?
- Describe your parents' relationship as a couple and as a coparenting team?
- Who was most like your mother/father? Which siblings were most similar/dissimilar? Were there "favorites" or "teams"? Did the roles change over the years?
- Do you remember your attitude toward your siblings at various points in your childhood: preschool, school age, high school, and adulthood?
- What are the favorite family stories, sayings, or nicknames around sibling rivalry and differences?
- What do you think you learned from your role in the family?

Early Recollections

Adler used early childhood recollections as a means for understanding a person's style of life (Ansbacher & Ansbacher, 1956). *Early recollections* refer to a person's earliest clear memories of an event or situation. Often these reveal the source of fundamental beliefs about one's value, others, or life more generally. They tend to be definitive moments that often play a mythic role in a person's life: feeling left out at the playground, picking apples with your mother, or going for a car ride with dad. Generally, a minimum of three memories is required to identify a pattern. However, depending on the complexity of themes, more may be necessary to get to obtain a clearer understanding of how various elements of the lifestyle were developed.

Questions for Assessing Earliest Recollections

- "When you think back over your childhood, what are your earliest memories (generally before the age of 7)?" *or* "Describe what you believe to be your earliest memory from when you were a child, perhaps before you entered school or in preschool."

- "What were you feeling at that time? What were others feeling?"

- "What did you understand or not understand about what was going on? What were others thinking?"

- "What is the most vivid part of the memory? Why do you think that stands out?"

- "What do you think you learned from this experience?"

Basic Mistakes

Basic mistakes are faulty assumptions that develop in childhood as children make sense of their experiences, such as loneliness, parental anger, disappointment, traumas, and loss. To some extent, everyone enters adulthood with mistaken notions. However, when basic mistakes lead to a sense of *inferiority* and *low social interest*, a person is more likely to develop symptoms and end up in a counselor's office. Adler noted that in these situations, "the apperception-schema of the patient evaluates all impressions as if they were fundamental matters and dichotomizes them in a purposeful manner into above-below, victor-vanquished, masculine-feminine, nothing-everything, etc." (Ansbacher & Ansbacher, 1956, p. 333). In simpler terms, basic mistakes involve seeing life in either-or, black-and-white terms in which one side is valued as "better" than the other. As you can imagine, this quickly leads to feelings of inferiority on multiple fronts.

Mosak and Maniacci (1999) elaborate on this by identifying five types of basic mistakes:

1. *Overgeneralizations*: People who overgeneralize tend to exaggerate contextual truths into global all-or-nothing truths (e.g., "my boyfriend cheated on me" gets translated into "men can't be trusted").

2. *False or impossible goals of security*: Some people try to find ways to remove all risk from life, often making unreasonable demands on others (e.g., "If you love me, you will never hurt me"—even unintentionally—a great romantic ideal but difficult to achieve if flesh-and-blood humans are involved. Virtual realities may eventually hold different possibilities).

3. *Misperceptions of life and life's demands*: Some basic mistakes boil down to not really understanding the inescapable rules of life: people die, survival takes effort, survival requires cooperation, kindness matters, laws of nature apply evenly, hurting another ultimately hurts you, life doesn't come with guarantees, and so on (e.g., "I want to fall in love with someone who I know won't hurt me": again, a Labrador retriever may be your best option).

4. *Minimization or denial of one's basic worth*: In other cases, a person has gladly owned their sense of personal inferiority and deny their own intrinsic worth (e.g., "Why would anyone want to love me? I am inherently flawed").

5. *Faulty values*: Alternatively, some people cope with life by identifying with faulty values, values that are not in line with social interest but instead self-promotion (e.g., "If I am successful enough and achieve enough, people will *have to* love me").

Assessing a person's basic mistakes is tricky in that there isn't a simple set of questions to ask. The counselor must tease it out by asking about the family constellation, early recollections, and current problems. However, a careful and thoughtful initial assessment process with an eye toward identifying basic mistakes generally makes this process far easier.

Organ Inferiority or Physical Weak Points

Odd to the modern English ear, *organ inferiority* is term used by Adler to refer to physical weak points in the body. They are the physical parallel to the basic mistake: "what organ inferiorities are to the body, basic mistakes are to the mind" (Carlson et al., 2006, p. 90). Either actual physical problems or the belief that one is physically inferior can have significant impacts on one's style of life. When Adler used the term, he typically referred to children who were blind, had physical deformities, or had chronic illnesses that characterized the turn of the 20th century. In modern contexts, these physical issues often include a person's perception of weight, looks, or athletic ability in comparison to peers—or, in the case of most young American women, airbrushed supermodels.

Dream Analysis

Like Freud, Adler believed that dream analysis provided insight into a client's inner processes; however, unlike Freud, he didn't believe that they were related to infantile sexual wishes (Ansbacher & Ansbacher, 1956). Instead, he used the themes of dreams as clues to help analyze a client's style of life and to help identify potential solutions to problems. Furthermore, Adler believed that *the meaning of a dream was specific to the dreamer* and that the counselor was not in the position to have the final determination of their interpretation. For example, people who have dreams with themes of being hampered by obstacles, being unable to reach destinations, or being unable to meet up with an important person will likely have similar themes of feeling that the *world* (not their choices or actions) is keeping them from achieving their goals.

"The Question": Purpose of Symptom

Saving the best for last, *"the question"* is used to assess the underlying purpose and need for the symptom (Ansbacher & Ansbacher, 1964; Carlson et al., 2006). The question is as follows:

> "What would be different in your life if you didn't have this problem?" (Carlson et al., 2006, p. 110)

The client's response often provides clues as to what is being avoided by having the symptoms. For example, one depressed person may say that he would be more successful at work, while another may state that she would "be the old self" again who used to spend time with friends. The first response belies insecurities in his ability to succeed at work, and in the second she may fear that enjoying herself apart from her family reflects on her poorly as a mother and wife. More recently, solution-based counselors use the *miracle question,* which is a variation of Adler's original question (see Chapter 11). In the case study at the end of this chapter, the counselor uses "the question" to assess the purpose of Budi's depression, which he has experienced in various forms over the years.

Psychodynamic Formulation

When assessing a person's style of life, Adlerians also consider basic psychodynamic formulation in the function of symptom (Carlson et al., 2006). They use three general categories for clients in their psychodynamic formulation: neurotic (emotional disturbance expressed through physical or mental disturbance; behavior is generally within social norms), psychosis (loss of contact with reality), or personality disorder (chronic behavioral pattern that significantly impedes relationships). Adlerians use the basic guidelines for understanding the client's style of life.

Type of Person	Response to Challenge:
Encouraged person	"Can-do" attitude. Able to take needed action without worrying about what others think.
Persons with neurotic symptoms	"Yes-but" attitude: "I would take action if I didn't have this problem." They use their symptoms to get away with doing what they want (avoiding social interest) while still receiving social approval ("my symptom is the problem").
Persons with psychotic symptoms	Escapist attitude. They live in fantasy rather than reality to escape life's demands. They say "no" to society's demands.
Persons with personality disorders	"My-way-or-the-highway" attitude. They try to convince others that their way is the right way regardless of what others want or evidence to the contrary: "I'll cooperate if we use my rules."

Life Tasks and Social Interest

Adlerian assessment also involves identifying a person's level of social interest in the six life tasks (Ansbacher & Ansbacher, 1956; Carlson et al., 2006; Dreikurs & Mosak, 1967; Mosak & Dreikurs, 1967; Sweeney, 2009):

- *Work:* Not limited to gainful employment, "work" refers to a person's primary means of being a contributing member of society and can include education, household chores, child care, homemaking, and volunteer activities.
- *Communal life and friendship:* Connecting socially with others and enjoying connections with others is an important life task and measure of a person's social interest.
- *Love relationships:* Perhaps the most challenging of all, love relationships require courage and the greatest level of social interest to sustain.
- *Self-acceptance:* A modern addition that is implied in Adler's original work; developing an accepting relationship of the self as well as self-awareness is foundational to successful relating to others.
- *Spirituality:* More recently, Adlerians have added developing a relationship to something greater than the self as a critical life task.
- *Parenting:* Although not applicable to everyone, parenting requires a particular set of social skills and functioning that should be assessed separately from others.

A balanced life involves active and successful involvement in all these areas of life. Thus, in assessment, counselors should identify the areas in which a person functions best and areas where there are the most problems. In treatment planning, specific goals should be written for each area. Manaster and Corsini (1982) have their clients rate the percentage of happiness in each area before and after counseling to measure progress.

DSM Diagnosis

Adler did not use diagnostic classification for the treatment of individuals (Ansbacher & Ansbacher, 1956). However, true to their principle of social interest, contemporary Adlerians have chosen a proactive approach to *DSM* diagnosis because it enables them to better communicate with other professionals who use this language (Sweeney, 2009). Numerous differences exist between the *DSM* approach and Adlerian theory (Carlson et al., 2006; Sweeney, 2009):

	DSM	Adlerian
Approach to pathology	Descriptive: Identifies symptoms	Explanatory: Explains causation
Language	Pathology and deficit-based	Encouraging; positive
Focus	External, measurable behaviors	Subjective experiences

Maniacci (2002, p. 360) proposes a unique approach to integrating Adlerian practice with the *DSM:*

Axis I: The arrangement (how the client has "arranged" symptoms to cope; corresponds to clinical syndromes and areas of clinical focus)

Axis II: The lifestyle (corresponds to personality disorders and personality features)

Axis III: Organ inferiority/organ jargon (corresponds to physical disorders relevant to psychological treatment)

Axis IV: The shock (corresponds to psychosocial stressors)

Axis V: A barometer of life tasks (corresponds to 100-point scale for global assessment of functioning)

Let's break this down step-by-step. Adlerians would start by focusing on Axis II, which corresponds to a person's style of life. However, this does not mean that they believe that everyone has a personality disorder, nor does it imply that they frequently use these diagnosis codes. Instead, they look at a person's style of life that involves pervasive, patterned responses to life much like the personality "features" that can be listed on Axis II (American Psychiatric Association, 2000). In conjunction with Axis II, Adlerians consider Axis III physical disorders (i.e., organ inferiority) or physical expressions (i.e., organ jargon) that are related to the client's style of life. For example, a child who felt singled out as a child for not having good athletic ability may carry this sense of being ostracized or humiliated into adult areas of life, such as work and love relationships. Axis IV refers to the "shock" or challenge (i.e., such as a job loss, divorce, or breakup) that overwhelmed the client's coping mechanisms, triggering the symptoms and syndromes used on Axis I to somehow manage feelings of inferiority (i.e., depression, anxiety, or overeating). Axis V records the overall impact on the person's functioning. Although a bit awkward at first, this template provides a useful way to translate and integrate between the *DSM* and Adlerian theory.

Targeting Change: Goal Setting
Long-Term Goal: The Courage to Develop Social Interest
Adler defined *normal adjustment* as having "enough energy and courage to meet the problems and difficulties of life as they come along" (Ansbacher & Ansbacher, 1956, p. 154). Life difficulties can occur within any of the six life tasks: work, love, friendship, spirituality, self-acceptance, or parenting. Greater levels of social interest improve functioning in each of these areas (Dreikurs, 1989). Thus, Adlerian counseling requires clients to develop the *courage* they need to face their insecurities and go to the places and do the things that they fear most; the counselor's role is to encourage clients to take the risks needed to develop the social interest needed to fulfill their life tasks.

Wellness, Positive Psychology, and Social Interest
Modern Adlerians have explored the links between social interest and positive psychology wellness research (Carlson et al., 2006; Leak & Leak, 2006; Myers, 2009). Both Adlerian theory and positive psychology emphasize building on and developing strengths (rather than remedying weaknesses) as the preferred approach to addressing strengths. In addition, both approaches set long-term goals of *wellness* as opposed to health, wellness referring to a state of physical, emotional, and social well-being that is achieved through conscious effort and health referring to a more neutral state in which one is not ill and does not require effort (Myers, 2009). The Adlerian primary goal of developing social

interest correlates with the findings of positive psychologists that social connection, altruism, empathy, and social consciousness are highly correlated with happiness (Leak & Leak, 2006). Similarly, Adlerian theory's emphasis on developing social interest within the six life tasks aligns with positive psychology research that emphasizes that meaningful relationships, satisfying work, self-acceptance, and spirituality are all strongly linked to life satisfaction (Myers, 2009). Thus, when setting goals, Adlerian counselors can also draw on a wellness perspective that emphasizes personal choices and positive actions lead to a sense of sustainable wellness; simply reducing symptom frequency is only a first step in achieving this long-term goal. Furthermore, like Adlerian counseling, wellness counseling involves psychoeducation in positive psychology and the correlates of happiness.

Developing Adlerian Goal Statements

General Principles   Adlerian theory provides clear guidelines for how to develop early, working, and closing phase goals.

- *Early phase goals:* Address initial crisis symptoms.
- *Working phase goals:* Reduce symptoms related to presenting problem; increase social interest and functioning in life tasks most closely related to the problem.
- *Closing phase goals:* Increase social interest and functioning in other key areas of functioning.

Examples of Early and Working Phase Goals   Early and middle phase goals aim to reduce insecurities and basic mistakes that are fueling the presenting problem(s):

- Reduce insecurities that lead to depressive thinking.
- Reduce insecurities that fuel jealousy in relationship.
- Reduce insecurities that lead to underfunctioning at work
- Develop more realistic expectations of performance at work.
- Reduce the tendency to overgeneralize that leads to arguments with spouse.
- Increase ability to take risks in relationship to increase sense of intimacy.
- Reduce tendency to calculate self-worth based on work performance.

Examples of Closing Phase Goals   Late phase goals aim to take the client beyond basic health (lack of symptoms) and toward developing habits of living that promote wellness and social interest in all six areas of functioning: work, friendship, love, self-acceptance, spirituality, and parenting:

- Increase intimacy and connection with family of origin.
- Increase sense of connection with friends and local community.
- Increase sense of connection to divine by reconnecting with spiritual practice.
- Increase self-acceptance related to sexual orientation.
- Increase emotional connection and redefine relationships with adult children.
- Take steps to pursue line of work (or volunteering) that is personally satisfying.

The Doing: Interventions

Psychoeducation and Task Setting

Perhaps their predominant type of intervention, Adlerians use psychoeducation in all phases of counseling (Carlson et al., 2006). Psychoeducation involves providing clients with psychological information that they can use to change their thoughts, feelings, and/or behaviors. For psychoeducation to be practically useful, counselors need to follow up by setting up specific tasks based on the new information (Sweeney, 2009). In the case study at the end of this chapter, the counselor uses psychoeducation to help Budi understand his diagnosis of depression, the psychological impact of being diagnosed with a disabling condition, and how his role as eldest son in his family has affected his relationship with others.

Phase 1 Topics for Psychoeducation: Establish an Egalitarian Relationship
- Describing client's role and rights in the counseling process, including when setting goals and deciding what to discuss.

- Explaining how Adlerian counseling can address the presenting problem and how it works.
- Defining social interest and its role in the client's problem.

Phase 2 for Psychoeducation: Assess Lifestyle and Private Logic
- Providing a rationale for the assessment process.
- Defining lifestyle and describing how private logic develops and how it is related to the presenting problem.

Phase 3 for Psychoeducation: Encourage Insight and Self-Understanding
- Offering information and research results that counter the inaccurate and/or unrealistic private logic that fuels the problem.
- Providing an explanation of the style of life psychological processes based on Adlerian theory.

Phase 4 for Psychoeducation: Education and Reorientation
- Providing convincing research and theoretically based information to motivate clients to take new action related to a specific problem.
- Offer specific instructions on how to best approach changing behaviors or habits of thought.

Tips for Effectively Providing Psychoeducation and Task Setting

- *Practice!* Yes, I'm serious. There aren't too many counseling or psychotherapeutic skills I recommend that new counselors "practice" on family and friends, but psychoeducation is the major exception. Try explaining concepts and research outcome to people who haven't read books like this one. Notice the types of questions they ask after you explain a concept. That will help you learn what you might be leaving out, what type of jargon need defining, and what people actually find useful.

- *Ask first:* Perhaps the single greatest secret to making psychoeducation work is *timing*: providing information when the client is in a receptive state. How do you know when they are ready? Ask them, "Would you be open to learning more about X?" If you fail to ask, you risk disrupting the otherwise collaborative relationship.

- *Keep it very, very brief:* During a 50-minute session, I recommend keeping total psychoeducation time to 1 to 2 minutes—that's the max. Any other brilliant information you have to share should be saved for the following week because most clients cannot meaningfully integrate and act on more than this. This is one situation where extroversion becomes an Achilles' heel; so when you launch into a psychoeducational speech—stop yourself ASAP.

- *Make one point—and one point only:* Try to teach only one concept, point, or skill in a session—the role of social interest, for example. Anything else is too much to be *practically* useful.

- *Ensuring understanding and acceptance:* After briefly providing information, *directly ask* if clients understand and if they believe it is useful and realistic for their life.

- *Apply it immediately:* After you provide information, immediately identify how it can be practically applied in the client's life to address a problem that occurred in the past week or upcoming week.

- *Step-by-step tasks:* After offering 2 minutes of psychoeducation, the following 48 minutes involve step-by-step instructions on how to apply the information to solve a current problem. Get specific: who does what when and where and how often.

- *Follow up:* The next time you meet, ask the client if they used the information to any extent; if not, why; and, if so, what happened. Some clients benefit more than others from psychoeducation, and you will find that they often use it far differently than you anticipated.

Psychoeducation Example: Wellness Shandra was working with a 43-year-old business executive who complained of "losing his zest for life." He states that he "loves" his wife and two kids but works long hours during the week and constantly checks his email and phone on the weekend. During the lifestyle assessment, you learn that one of his basic mistake assumptions is that he believes his value as a person is tied to his work performance, resulting in a nagging sense that he always needs to be working to ensure his worth. He readily agrees to this interpretation in the insight stage and is ready to make changes in the reorientation phase. That's when Shandra believes that he is ready to learn more about *wellness:*

Shandra: "Last week, we began talking about creating greater balance between your work and home life. So, I thought it might be useful to share some information about *wellness.*" "Would you be interested in hearing what I have to say? [Ask permission]"

Ricardo: "Sure. That sounds like something I need to be thinking about."

Shandra: "When counselors and psychologists think of wellness, they put it on a continuum with illness/unhappiness and health." She draws this on the whiteboard:

Wellness ———————— Health ———————— Illness/Unhappiness

"We all know what illness and unhappiness is: something is "wrong": we feel sad, angry, unhappy; this is where you were at when you first came to see me. Then there is health; it's the absence of illness or problem. That's closer to where you are right now: you are starting to feel less sad about things in your life. But then there's wellness. Wellness refers to an overall sense of *well-being*—mind, body, spirit—and not just the absence of problems or illness. One of the major differences between wellness and health is that a person actually needs to take proactive steps [Ricardo is a professional and understands words like this, so it's okay to use; otherwise, say "make a choice to do things"] to achieve wellness, usually by adopting habits that lead to a sense of well-being. I want to pause here and see if you are following me or have any questions?" [She kept it brief; one major term defined; illustrated it on a board; and checked in to see if the client understood.]

Ricardo: "Yes, yes. It kind of puts words to what I think I need to do. I can see that I am going to have to do some things differently—and I don't like that—but I think I know what you are saying is true."

During the rest of the session—*for the next 48 minutes*—Shandra will help Ricardo identify one—and only one—way to implement this idea (task setting), such as how he is going to get through the weekend without checking email so that he can focus his energy on his family. Shandra will refrain from providing more psychoeducation (it's so easy to turn a session into a classroom) and will instead focus on applying the information. If he is able to apply this information, next week she can share another bit of research from positive psychology that he may benefit from.

Homework

Often as a follow-up to psychoeducation and task setting, Adlerian counselors assign "homework," tasks to be completed between sessions (Manaster & Corsini, 1982). Homework assignments can vary widely, depending on the phase of counseling and the particular issues a client is working on. Examples of homework include the following:

- Call an estranged relative.
- Go on a date with your wife (this week or once a week).
- Develop a detailed list of things you are afraid of that hold you back at work.
- The next time you begin to feel inferior, write a list of the evidence "for" and "against" this perception.
- Identify friends who you could reconnect with to extend your social circle.
- When you come home at night, begin the evening by thanking or appreciating your spouse for something that she did rather than complaining about something that didn't get done.

Interpretation of Symptoms

During the third phase of Adlerian counseling, counselors "interpret" the purpose of symptoms to provide client's insight into their situation. Distinct from psychoanalytic forms of interpretation, Adlerian interpretation attempts to identify *the purpose of the symptom* and its role in the client's style of life (Ansbacher & Ansbacher, 1956; Sweeney, 2009). For example, based on the lifestyle assessment, a counselor may interpret a person's procrastination as a way of avoiding taking a risk and possibly failing. General guidelines for offering Adlerian interpretations include the following:

- *Purpose focused:* The interpretation should focus on the *goal* or *purpose* of a *behavior* (e.g., procrastination) and avoid globally labeling the person (e.g., lazy, fearful, lacking drive).
- *Tentatively offered:* Interpretations should be offered *tentatively* rather than an unquestionable truth (e.g., could it be that you procrastinate to avoid taking the risk of failing?).
- *Open to revision:* Counselors should encourage and allow the client to rephrase or even correct the counselor (e.g., "It's not so much that I am avoiding risk as much as I am simply afraid to fail." or "No, I don't think that is my issue. I think I am saying yes to things I don't want to do.").
- *Strengths emphasis:* The overall tone of the interpretation process should be encouraging, highlighting potential strengths, hope, and resilience (e.g., "So in some ways the procrastination has served to create a sense of safety, but it seems that you may not need that as much as you did in the past.").

Self-Concept Statements

Adlerians listen for *self-concept statements*; these are statements that clients make that reveal how they see themselves. Carlson et al. (2006) identify three types of self statements that counselors target for intervention:

1. *Inferiority-based self statements:* The client's self-concept falls short of his or her *personal* self-ideal (e.g., "I am stupid, worthless).
2. *Inadequacy-based self statements:* The client's self-concept falls short of what the client believes is the "worldview" or cultural values (e.g., "I am incompetent, a fool, a loser").
3. *Guilt-based self statements:* The client's self-concept falls short of ethical or moral beliefs (e.g., I'm bad, evil, unforgivable).

When counselors hear these types of statement, they help the client explore the comparison process and how to develop more useful, fair, and accurate comparisons. In some cases, clients are making poor decisions of which they feel guilty; the counselor then helps them identify how this happened and how to remedy it. In other cases, clients rigidly try to apply unrealistic standards of superiority; counselors can help these clients explore how they developed these and replace them with more realistic and fair evaluations of themselves. In the case study at the end of this chapter, the counselor uses self statements to help Budi develop a sense of self that is not based on his ability to take care of others and instead learn to engage in more egalitarian relationships in which his needs are also considered.

Challenging and Reframing Basic Mistakes and Private Logic

Once clients have achieved sufficient insight, counselors may directly *challenge* the logic or realism of a person's private logic or more gently *reframe* belief so that it is more useful. An example of challenging basic mistakes, counselors may ask clients who believe they must be superior to others "what would happen if everyone had that belief?" (Carlson et al., 2006, p. 140). Counselors can then follow up with questions that highlight the impossibility of a world in which all people are better than everyone else and the ugliness of a world in which everyone lived by this belief. Similarly, in many cases, negative situations can be *reframed* in more positive ways. For example, "The upside of worrying is that you tend to be good with details." Counselors can use positive reframing to simultaneously encourage clients and undo basic mistakes.

Natural and Logical Consequences

Introduced by Dreikurs, consequences take two forms in Adlerian counseling—natural and logical—and are used primarily with children (Mosak & Maniacci, 1999; Sweeney,

2009). *Natural consequences* require no conscious human intervention; they occur as part of the physical or social environment. If a child does not do his homework, he loses points, he does not learn, and his grades suffer. If you say harsh words to your friend, you weaken or lose the friendship. Whenever possible, Adlerian counselors encourage parents use natural consequences to help children and others learn from experience. However, if natural consequences are not readily apparent or sufficient, then logical consequences are used instead to *encourage* children to make better decisions (e.g., if you are unable to keep your toys neat and tidy, then you have more toys than you can manage, and some will be taken away until you can manage what you have effectively). Such consequences and encouragement are preferred to behavioral systems of punishment and reward.

Antisuggestion

A classic Adlerian technique, the *antisuggestion* is a type of *paradoxical technique*. The antisuggestion involves the counselor taking the paradoxical position of discouraging change and/or encouraging the symptom, particularly when the client claims that a symptom is "uncontrollable" (e.g., worrying or getting nervous; Ansbacher & Ansbacher, 1956; Carlson et al., 2006; Sweeney, 2009). Antisuggestions can be used in session or out of session. For example, in situations where this is appropriate and safe, the counselor can suggest that the client practice exaggerating a symptom, such as spending extra time worrying every morning. If you haven't tried it, "making yourself" worry makes it very difficult to worry; thus, many clients find relief this way. Alternatively, in session, a counselor may make the antisuggestion that perhaps this much concern (carrying a first-aid kit to the playground, an extra set of clothes to the grocery store, etc.) about their child's safety is warranted; in most cases, the client will then *argue* for *not worrying* and then *convince themselves* that they need to change.

Spitting in the Soup

An attention-grabbing name for a counseling technique and more hygienic than it sounds, *spitting in the soup* refers to making overt the covert benefits and hidden power of having a symptom. Once the ulterior benefits of the symptoms are revealed, the symptom leaves a "bad taste." Here are some examples:

- The one benefit of depression is that you have gotten everyone in your family to pay more attention to you.
- You must have reached near rock-star status to have everyone in the subway looking at you.
- The nice part about panic is that you get your wife to end the shopping trip early—it even saves you money.
- It must be very rewarding to know that no other mother at the school worries this much about her children.
- The great part about temper tantrums is that it fills up your toy chest fast.

Interventions for Special Populations
Couples and Families

Numerous counselors and therapists have developed Adlerian approach for working with couples and families. Adler and Dreikurs developed the world's first child guidance clinics in Vienna before World War II, making the Adlerian approach perhaps the first family counseling approach. Dreikurs spent most of his career developing approaches for working with children. More recently, Dinkmeyer and McKay (2007) have developed an evidence-based parent education program using Adlerian principles (see "Snapshot: Research and The Evidence Base").

Carlson et al. (2006) describe a brief Adlerian approach to couples counseling that involves four steps:

Step 1: Relationship: The counselor begins by developing a relationship in which both members of the couple feel heard and understood and encourages each partner to access his or her resources and best parts of themselves.

Step 2: Assessment: Next, the counselor helps the couple to better understand their styles of lives, including the beliefs, feelings, motivations, and goals that underlie problem behaviors in the relationship. For example, a partner's apparent "lack of interest" or "distance" may be an expression of one partner's sense of inferiority; similarly, the other partner's "demands for attention and connection" may be an expression of the other partner's inferiority and/or need for belonging. The counselor would help both partners to better understand the dynamics that motivate the behavior of each and how these individual dynamics inform their couple interactions.

Step 3: Insight: Using information gathered from the assessment, counselors help couples to gain insight into each person's personal beliefs, feelings, and goals and how these translate to problematic couple dynamics. The counselor may use psychoeducation to facilitate this process.

Step 4: Reorientation: Once couples gain insight, they are ready to take action and find alternatives to the problem behavior. The counselor works with the couple to find strategies that help them change their behaviors and sustain these new relational skills.

Putting It All Together: Adlerian Treatment Plan Template

Use this treatment plan template for developing a plan for clients with depressive, anxious, or compulsive types of presenting problems. Depending on the specific client, presenting problem, and clinical context, the goals and interventions in this template may need to be modified only slightly or significantly; you are encouraged to significantly revise the plan as needed. For the plan to be useful, goals and techniques should be written to target specific beliefs, behaviors, and emotions that the client is experiencing. The more specific, the more useful it will be to you.

Treatment Plan

Initial Phase of Treatment (First One to Three Sessions)
Initial Phase Counseling Tasks

1. *Develop working counseling relationship. Diversity note:* Adapt for ethnicity, gender, age, and so on.
   Relationship building approach:
   a. Use **encouragement, empathy,** and **education** to create an **egalitarian relationship** in which the client has a sense of **free will.**

2. Assess *individual, systemic, and broader cultural dynamics. Diversity note:* Adapt for family structure, ethnic/religious norms, gender, age, ability, sexual/gender orientation, and so on.
   Assessment strategies:
   a. Assess **lifestyle, basic mistake, parenting style, family constellation, early recollections, organ inferiority,** and **dreams.**
   b. Use "the question" to help determine purpose of symptom and goals for treatment.

Initial Phase Client Goals *(One or Two Goals): Manage crisis issues and/or reduce most distressing symptoms*

1. *Decrease* **insecurities** and **basic mistake assumptions** that fuel crisis thinking and behaviors to reduce [specific crisis symptoms].
   a. **Psychoeducation** on how to manage [crisis behavior]; **encouragement** to follow through with new response to feelings that signal crisis.
   b. Challenge **basic mistake** and assumptions related to crisis thoughts and behaviors.

(continued)

Working Phase of Treatment (Three or More Sessions)

Working Phase Counseling Task

1. *Monitor quality of the working alliance. Diversity note*: Adapt for diversity issues.
    Assessment Interventions:
    a. Monitor for signs that client has a sense of equality and ownership in relationship.

Working Phase Client Goals (Two or Three Goals). Target individual and relational dynamics using theoretical language (e.g., decrease avoidance of intimacy, increase awareness of emotion, increase agency)

1. *Decrease* **insecurities** that lead to [specific dynamic or problem] to reduce [specific symptoms: depression, anxiety, etc.]
    Interventions:
    a. **Psychoeducation** to correct basic mistake belief: [specify].
    b. Challenge unrealistic **self-concept statements** and **basic mistake beliefs**: [specify].

2. *Decrease* avoidance of **life tasks** and/or **social connections** in [specify: work, relationship, communal, etc.] contexts to reduce [specific symptoms: depression, anxiety, etc.].
    Interventions:
    a. **Interpretation** of avoidance behaviors in terms of how they enable client to avoid misguided childhood fears, social contact, key life tasks, and so on.
    b. **Spitting in soup** and **antisuggestion** techniques to unmask how symptoms allow client to avoid feared life tasks.

3. *Decrease* tendency to **value self** based on external achievements and approval from others to reduce [specific symptoms: depression, anxiety, etc.].
    Interventions:
    a. Challenging **basic mistake belief** that self-worth is based on performance and approval from others.
    b. Alter **self-concept statements** to reflect a more realistic valuing of self that focuses on "what am I doing?" rather that "how am I doing?"

Closing Phase of Treatment (Last Four or More Sessions)

Closing Phase Counseling Tasks

1. *Develop aftercare plan and maintain gains. Diversity note*: Manage end of counseling by adjusting for sociocultural and gender expectations for handling loss.
    Intervention
    a. **Psychoeducation** on **wellness** and **positive psychology** to identify key components to maintaining happiness and well-being.

Closing Client Goals (One or Two Goals): Determined by theory's definition of health and normalcy

1. *Increase* **self-acceptance** and overall sense of wellness to reduce potential for relapse of symptoms.
    Interventions:
    a. **Psychoeducation** on **social interest** and **positive psychology** to develop habits of wellness, such as a strong social network, gratifying activities, and optimistic basic assumptions.
    b. Examine **natural consequences** of acting from **social interest versus basic mistake** assumptions.

2. *Increase* **social connections** in intimate relationships and work contexts [and/or parenting, spiritual contexts] to reduce potential for relapse of symptoms.
    Interventions:
    a. **Psychoeducation** on importance of functioning in all **life tasks** to achieve balance.
    b. Develop homework and life habits that support **social interest** in all areas of living.

Snapshot: Research and the Evidence Base

Quick Summary: Little research has been conducted on the general efficacy of Adlerian counseling; the majority of research has been on applications with children. In particular, *Systematic Training for Effective Parenting (STEP)* is a promising evidence-based treatment for parent training.

Like many other theories, Adlerian counseling has not been carefully examined with quantitative outcomes studies because of difficulties in operationalizing terms, such as social interest, as well as a general sense on the part of practitioners that their theory works, so they are less motivated to do research than practice (Sweeney, 2009). Research studies using Adlerian theory have focused on parent–child and teacher–child relations. For example, McVittie and Best (2009) conducted a study on the effectiveness of an Adlerian-based parenting program; their large-scale, self-report study indicated that parents reported setting clearer limits, increasing their sense of positive connection, and decreasing harshness. Similarly, Kelly and Daniels (1997) studied the effect of teachers using praise versus encouragement on children in grades 4 through 10; they found that teachers who used encouragement were viewed as more potent than those using praise. Pilkington, White, and Matheny (1997) studied the correlation of birth order on coping resources in school-aged children and found some support for differences between the oldest and middle children, with the former having the highest level of coping and the latter the lowest. Despite these initial studies, Adlerian theory and practice would benefit from more detailed research studies on the methods and effectiveness of this approach.

Evidence-Based Treatment: Systematic Training for Effective Parenting (STEP)

Systematic Training for Effective Parenting (STEP) is a promising evidence-based parenting program based on Adlerian principles (Dinkmeyer & McKay, 2007). The STEP program has been researched for almost four decades (Gibson, 1999) and is currently listed as a "promising practice" by state and federal agencies. Using Adlerian principles, the STEP program is an extremely positive parenting approach that uses encouragement, appreciation, and motivation to improve child behaviors and parent–child relations. At its heart, it helps parents develop social interest and cooperative behaviors and directly addresses the classic Adlerian concept of developing "courage to be imperfect." The programs include a specific program for children under 6 (Dinkmeyer & McKay, 2008) and one for teens (Dinkmeyer et al., 2007).

The program includes lessons on the following:

- Understanding yourself and your child
- Understanding beliefs and feelings
- Encouraging your child and yourself
- Listening and talking to your child
- Helping children learn to cooperate
- Discipline that makes sense
- Choosing your approach

Snapshot: Working With Diverse Populations

Quick Summary: Although one of the oldest approaches, Adlerian theory has had from its inception surprisingly modern feminist and multicultural values, thoughtfully integrating the impact of family and social networks and spirituality in their understanding of human behavior.

Adler defined mental health as having high levels of social interest, community feeling, and empathy for others, even those others who are quite unlike oneself (Ansbacher & Ansbacher, 1956). He clearly and frequently referred to the subjugation of women and their unfair treatment and considered this in his assessment and diagnosis; although such a practice seems common today, it was a radical stand for social justice in the 1910s. More recently, Adlerians have also been advocates for gay, lesbian, bisexual, and transgendered individuals (Mansager, 2008). Several elements make Adlerian counseling well suited for working with persons from a wide range of backgrounds:

- *Social interest:* The emphasis on social interest is particularly appropriate for cultures that value family and community over individuality. In addition, the primary goal of the approach is to help people develop a greater sense of "community feeling" and connection with one's broader community; this is particularly important for marginalized populations, whether marginalized because of their sexual orientation, language abilities, physical abilities, or ethnic origin. Furthermore, feminist approaches to human development emphasize that this emphasis of relationship over separateness is common in women and should not be pathologized (see Chapter 13).
- *Superiority, racism, and other "-isms":* Adler viewed any attempts to see oneself as superior to another human being as a sign of maladjustment, thus providing a strong antiracist, antisexist, and antiheterosexist foundation to his theory.
- *Spirituality:* Whereas many theories either ignore or are suspicious of religion and spirituality, the Adlerian theory views a person's relationship to something greater as an important relationship to cultivate. This emphasis on spirituality is consistent with values in many traditional cultures and ethnic groups.
- *Social factors impacting mental health:* Adler carefully assessed and considered the impact of broader social and family factors in the development of problems. Individuals and their symptoms were considered in the context of the *environment*, an important practice when working with persons from minority and marginalized groups.

Interestingly, Adler's emphasis on community feeling as a primary goal and measure of health may not fit or be equally valued by all clients, including highly driven immigrants, White males, and women. In addition, the assessment of lifestyle, with its emphasis on childhood experiences and memories, may not seem relevant to people who prefer a more pragmatic approach or who do not share the dominant Western assumption that these events shape a person's personality.

Adlerian Case Study

Budi, a 44-year-old Indonesian immigrant, reports that, although he has often been down before, the past 2 years have been very bad. The depression began (or got much worse) after his diagnosis with a debilitating nerve condition that has required him to be wheelchair bound; there is little hope of return to normal functioning. He still works and enjoys working. He is generally a quiet man who reads and is a serious chess player who enters amateur contests. He has married and has a 3-year-old daughter. He immigrated to the United States to pursue education as an engineer. The eldest of six children, he planned to return home after college but remained in the United States to help support his family back home. He grew up in a traditional Indonesian Muslim family; the family was close knit, a clear family hierarchy was observed, sensitive issues were not directly discussed, and shame was avoided at all costs. Children were expected to be obedient.

Adlerian Case Conceptualization

This case conceptualization was developed by selecting key concepts from "The Viewing: Case Conceptualization" section of the chapter. You can use any of the concepts in that section to develop a case conceptualization for this or other cases.

Lifestyle assessment to include the following:

- Social interest and inferiority
- Parenting style

- Family constellation and birth order
- Basic mistakes
- Organ inferiority or physical weak points
- Life tasks

Social Interest and Inferiority

Overall, AM (adult male; confidential notation for client in case) demonstrates is a "low social interest, successful person" who focuses more on *how* he is doing in life than what he is doing. His focus is on whether he is able to support and provide for others, and at this level he is socially engaged and demonstrates many positive elements of social interest. However, rather than building social connections that are personally rewarding and fulfilling, his social interactions are focused on gaining social approval; this lack of focus on himself has lead to his periods of feeling down and depressed.

Parenting Style

AM's parents raised him in traditional Indonesian family structure in which there were clear hierarchical lines, with father in charge, then mother, then AM (as the eldest), with grandparents having considerable influence over the family. His parents were relatively strict and made clear their expectations for him to be a role model and caretaker for the younger children. He was closest to his maternal grandmother, who often relaxed the rules for him. AM has tried to bring more warmth to his relationship with his young daughter, but by American standards, he maintains a cool, somewhat removed role in her life.

Family Constellation and Birth Order

AM aptly characterizes the typical eldest child in Indonesian culture. He has taken seriously his responsibility to his family, sending money home each month to support them. His childhood involved significant responsibility in caring for his siblings and pressure to serve as a good role model. He has continued to strive for superiority as an adult.

Basic Mistakes

AM's basic mistake assumptions are rooted in his early role in the family as a caretaker for his siblings, namely, the following:

- I must put my selfish desires second in order to care for others and to ensure that the family's basic needs are met.

Organ Inferiority or Physical Weak Points

AM's recent nerve degeneration that has resulted in his being wheelchair bound has created numerous and multilayered forms of stress. First, since his identity has been built around his ability to care for others, this new role is scary because it is unfamiliar and because it threatens his ability to do the very things from which he derives his fragile sense of connection and worth. In addition, it greatly limits his ability to live life as he is accustomed. Although he has continued to work and engage in most family activities, he is no longer able to engage in sports and avoids most social activities because of the hassle. Finally, because his diagnosis is not final, he still holds out hope that things may improve and cannot accept current circumstances.

Life Tasks

In many ways, AM has done well to address many key life tasks. He has a profession that he enjoys and a family he is connected too. However, he does not have an extensive friendship or community life in the United States, although he does have friends with whom he plays chess. Although raised a Muslim in Indonesia, he has not practiced much in the United States but still maintains a belief in God.

Treatment Plan

Initial Phase of Treatment (First One to Two Sessions)

Initial Phase Counseling Tasks

1. *Develop working counseling relationship. Diversity note*: Carefully approach issues that might cause shame or be too direct; maintain a more formal, respectful tone and approach.
   Relationship building approach:
   a. Use **encouragement, empathy,** and **education** to create an **egalitarian relationship** in which AM has a sense of **free will** and choice.

2. *Assess individual, systemic, and broader cultural dynamics. Diversity note:* Adapt for cultural norms and family roles.
   Assessment strategies:
   a. Assess **lifestyle, basic mistake, parenting style, family constellation, early recollections, organ inferiority,** and **dreams.**
   b. Use **"the question"** to help determine purpose of symptom and goals for treatment: If you were not depressed, what would be different? If you were not in a wheelchair, what would be different?

Initial Phase Client Goal

1. *Decrease* **insecurities** and **basic mistake assumptions** to reduce sense of hopelessness.
   Interventions:
   a. **Psychoeducation** on how to manage depressed mood related to disability; encouragement to follow through with new response to feelings that signal crisis.
   b. Challenge **basic mistake assumptions** related to depression and need to care for others.

Working Phase of Treatment (One or More Sessions)

Working Phase Counseling Task

1. *Monitor quality of the working alliance. Diversity note:* Maintain engaged but formal, respectful tone.
   Assessment Intervention:
   a. Monitor for signs that client has a sense of **equality** and **ownership** in relationship.

Working Phase Client Goals

1. *Decrease* **insecurities** that lead to need to support others to the point that his own dreams are not addressed to reduce depressed mood.
   Interventions:
   a. **Psychoeducation** to **correct basic mistake** belief that his value comes strictly from taking care of others at his own expense.
   b. Challenge unrealistic **self-concept statements** and **basic mistake beliefs**: If he can't care for others (because of his disability), others will abandon him.

2. *Decrease* avoidance of pursuing **personally fulfilling activities** and goals to reduce depression and increase **social network.**
   Interventions:
   a. **Interpretation** of **avoidance behaviors** in terms of how they enable client to avoid making decisions about his personal life and being responsible for his own happiness.
   b. Examine **birth order** and its effect on his life decisions and current life situation.

(continued)

3. *Decrease* tendency to **value self** on the basis of external achievements and approval from others to reduce depression.
   Interventions:
   a. Challenging **basic mistake belief** that self-worth is based on approval from others.
   b. Alter **self-concept statements** to reflect a more realistic valuing of self that focuses on "what am I doing?" rather that "how am I doing?"

Closing Phase of Treatment

Closing Phase Counseling Tasks

1. *Develop aftercare plan and maintain gains. Diversity note:* Develop plan that addresses personal, family, and cultural values and vision for living well.
   Intervention:
   a. **Psychoeducation** on **wellness** and positive psychology to identify key components to maintaining happiness and well-being.

Closing Phase Client Goals

1. *Increase* **self-acceptance**, acceptance of physical limitations, and overall sense of wellness to reduce potential for relapse of depression.
   Interventions:
   a. **Psychoeducation** on **social interest** and positive psychology to develop habits of wellness, such as a strong social network, gratifying activities, and optimistic basic assumptions.
   b. Examine **natural consequences** of acting from **social interest** versus basic mistake assumptions.

2. *Increase* **social connections** in local community to reduce potential for relapse of depression.
   Interventions:
   a. **Psychoeducation** on importance of functioning in all **life tasks** to achieve balance.
   b. Develop homework and life habits that support **social interest** in all areas of living.

ONLINE RESOURCES

Journal

Journal of Individual Psychology
www.utexas.edu/utpress/journals/jip.html

Associations and Societies

International Association of Individual Psychology
www.iaipwebsite.org/public/content.php?id_cont=9

North American Society of Alfred Adler
www.alfredadler.org

Select Training Institutes

Adler Graduate School (Minnesota)
www.alfredadler.edu

Adler School of Professional Psychology (Chicago)
www.adler.edu

Adlerian Training Institute
www.adleriantraining.com

Alfred Adler Institute of New York
www.alfredadler-ny.org

Alfred Adler Institute of San Francisco and Northwest Washington
www.pws.cablespeed.com/~htstein

Link to More Resources

Link to Additional Resources from the Adler Graduate School
www.alfredadler.edu/resources/adlerianlinks.htm

References

*Asterisk indicates recommended introductory readings.

Adler, A. (1924). *The practice and theory of individual psychology* (Trans. P. Radin). New York: Harcourt, Brace & Company.

Adler, A. (1959). *Understanding human nature* (Trans. C. Brett). New York: Hazeldon Press.

Adler, A. (1978). *The education of children*. Chicago: Regnery. (Original work published 1930)

American Psychiatric Association. (2000). *Diagnostic and statistical manual of mental disorders* (4th ed., text revision). Washington, DC: Author.

*Ansbacher, H. L., & Ansbacher, R. R. (Eds.). (1956). *The individual psychology of Alfred Adler* (5th ed.). New York: Basic Books.

*Ansbacher, H. L., & Ansbacher, R. R. (Eds.). (1964). *Superiority and social interest, a collection of later writings*. Evanston, IL: Northwestern University Press.

Bitter, J. R., Christensen, O. C., Hawes, C., & Nicoll, W. G. (1998). Adlerian brief therapy with individual, couples, and families. *Directions in Clinical and Counseling Psychology, 8*(8), 95–111.

Bitter, J., & Nicoll, W. (2000). Adlerian brief therapy with individuals: Process and practice. *Journal of Individual Psychology, 56*(1), 31–44.

Carlson, J. (n.d.). Jon Carlson home page. Retrieved May 18, 2010, from http://www.joncarlson.org

Carlson, J., Watts, R., & Maniacci, M. (2006). *Adlerian therapy: Theory and practice*. Washington, DC: American Psychological Association. doi:10.1037/11363-000

*Dinkmeyer, D. C., & McKay, G. D. (2007). *The parent's handbook: Systematic training for effective parenting*. Bowling Green, KY: Step Publishers.

*Dinkmeyer, D. C., & McKay, J. L. (2008). *Parenting young children: Systematic training for effective parenting (STEP) of children under six*. Bowling Green, KY: Step Publishers.

*Dinkmeyer, D. C., McKay, G. D., & McKay, J. L. (2007). *Parenting teenagers: Systematic training for effective parenting of teens*. Bowling Green, KY: Step Publishers.

Dreikurs, R. (1958). *The challenge of parenthood*. New York: Duell, Sloan and Pierce.

Dreikurs, R. (1968). *Psychology in the classroom*. New York: HarperCollins College.

*Dreikurs, R. (1989). *Fundamentals of Adlerian psychology*. Oxford: Greenberg. (Original work published 1933; Translated by Dreikurs from Adler's German)

Dreikurs, R., & Loren, G. (1968). *A new approach to discipline: Logical consequences*. New York: Meredith Press.

Dreikurs, R., & Mosak, H. H. (1967). The tasks of life: II. The fourth task. *The Individual Psychologist, 4*, 51–55.

Gibson, D. G. (1999). *A monograph: Summary of the research related to the use and efficacy of the systematic training for effectiveness program 1976–1999*. Circle Pines, MN: American Guidance Services, Inc.

Hartshorne, J., Salem-Hartshorne, N., & Hartshorne, T. (2009). Birth order effects in the formation of long-term relationships. *Journal of Individual Psychology, 65*(2), 156–176.

Kelly, F., & Daniels, J. (1997). The effects of praise versus encouragement on children's perceptions of teachers. *Journal of Individual Psychology, 53*(3), 331–341.

Leak, G. K., & Leak, K. C. (2006). Adlerian social interest and positive psychology: A conceptual and empirical integration. *Journal of Individual Psychology, 62*, 207–233.

Maniacci, M. (2002). The DSM and individual psychology: A general comparison. *Journal of Individual Psychology, 58*(4), 356–362.

Mansager, E. (2008). Affirming lesbian, gay, bisexual, and transgender individuals. *Journal of Individual Psychology, 64*(2), 124–136.

*Manaster, G. J., & Corsini, R. J. (1982). *Individual psychology: Theory and practice*. Chicago: Adler School of Professional Psychology.

McVittie, J., & Best, A. (2009). The impact of Adlerian-based parenting classes on self-reported parental behavior. *Journal of Individual Psychology, 65*(3), 264–285.

Mosak, H. H., & Di Pietro, R. (2006). *Early recollections: Interpretative method and application*. New York: Routledge.

Mosak, H. H., & Dreikurs, R. (1967). The tasks of life: III. The fifth task. *The Individual Psychologist, 5*, 16–22.

*Mosak, H. H., & Maniacci, M. P. (1999). *Primer of Adlerian psychology: The analytic-behavioural-cognitive psychology of Alfred Adler*. New York: Brunner/Routledge.

Mosak, H. H., & Sculman, B. H. (1988). *Lifestyle inventory*. Muncie, IN: Accelerated Development.

Myers, J. E. (2009). Wellness through social interest. In T. J. Sweeney (Ed.), *Adlerian counseling and psychotherapy: A practitioner's approach* (5th ed., pp. 33–44). New York: Routledge.

Pilkington, L., White, J., & Matheny, K. (1997). Perceived coping resources and psychological birth order in school-aged children. *Journal of Individual Psychology, 53*(1), 42–57.

*Sweeney, T. J. (2009). *Adlerian counseling and psychotherapy: A practitioner's approach* (5th ed.). New York: Routledge/Taylor & Francis Group.

CHAPTER

6

Person-Centered Counseling and Psychotherapy

The good life is a process, not a state of being. It is a direction not a destination.

—Carl Rogers

Lay of the Land

This is one chapter you will want to read while fully awake. Person-centered counseling is one of the most influential and widely used approaches. Regardless of which theory you intend to use when you are done with this book, the person-centered approach to build a counseling relationship with a client will be useful to you in one way or another. But before we get to your new friend Carl, it is important to understand the philosophical foundations of humanistic-existential theories, such as person centered.

Humanistic-existential counseling approaches are grounded in phenomenological philosophy, a philosophy approach that examines a person's subjective inner reality. These approaches are sometimes referred to as *experiential* approaches because of their focus on inner experience. Although contemporary practitioners typically draw from the full range of humanistic-existential approaches, these initially developed as three separate counseling approaches:

- *Person-centered counseling (Chapter 6):* Person-centered counseling—also known as client-centered or Rogerian counseling—is one of the quintessential counseling approaches. Developed by Carl Rogers (1942, 1951), this approach is based on the assertion that three core conditions—including accurate empathy, counselor genuineness, and unconditional regard—are sufficient to promote client change. The focus is on the emotional and relational processes that promote change rather than the use of specific techniques to achieve desired outcomes. This approach assumes that people tend *naturally* toward positive growth.

- *Existential counseling (Chapter 7):* Existential counseling is grounded in existential philosophy, which has more neutral assumptions about the human conditions in comparison to the more optimistic humanistic foundations of person-centered

(continued)

counseling. Existential counseling posits that clients experience symptoms and distress because they are avoiding or need to more effectively deal with broader existential issues, such as each human's ultimate separation from others, death, loss, and existential anxiety. This approach emphasizes insight and reflection on existential issues to more effectively resolve the underlying anxiety that fuels a client's presenting concern.

- *Gestalt counseling (Chapter 8):* Similar to person-centered counseling, Gestalt counseling is a humanistic approach that focuses on helping people to self-actualize or to become more fully themselves. However, the techniques are more emotionally provocative and confrontational than the person-centered approach.

Philosophical Foundations

Compared to the analytic chapters, traditional philosophy plays a much more central role in humanistic-existential therapies (similar to the postmodern therapies in Chapter 12, where you will also have to spend some clear-headed time with philosophers). So, here is a brief review of the threads of philosophical discourse that provided the foundation for person-centered as well as existential and Gestalt therapies.

Phenomenology

These three counseling approaches are grounded in the same general philosophical tradition: phenomenology. Phenomenology refers to the study of human consciousness: our *inner* lives, particularly our emotions. This is in contrast to approaches that are based on logical positivism, which focuses on external, objective reality (i.e., cognitive-behavioral approaches). In contrast, phenomenology focuses on *subjective,* inner reality that cannot be easily observed or measured. Thus, the counselor relies heavily on clients' *self-report* as to what they are experiencing, combined with a general understanding of how emotion and cognition work. Well-known philosophical phenomenologists include Edmund Husserl, Martin Heidegger, Paul Ricoeur, and Alfred Schutz.

Humanism

In broad—and therefore oversimplified terms—*humanists* tend to be the more optimistic phenomenologists. A specific expression of phenomenology, humanism is based on the premise that all people tend naturally toward positive growth, and thus humanists exude bountiful hope and enthusiasm and have faith in everyone's potential for growth. The role of the humanistic counselor is to *remove the blockages* to this natural tendency of self-actualization rather than remediate deficiencies. The counselor serves as a type of midwife who assists in fostering the natural growth and development process rather than as a technician who facilitates change. Activists in the humanistic tradition include Abraham Maslow, William James, Thomas Mann, Albert Einstein, and Kurt Vonnegut.

Existentialism

Existentialists are the realists in phenomenological circles. They view life not as inherently positive or negative but, rather, as inherently meaningless, or neutral, until a person creates meaning. Thus, the counselor's role in these approaches is somewhere between a midwife and a coach in that they encourage and point the client in the direction of creating meaning in his or her life. Unlike humanists, they do not believe there is some predetermined self that one needs to actualize; instead, one is free to choose who to become, and failing to consciously choose is nonetheless a choice, one that is not likely to have a happy ending. Clients are the ones responsible for finding and/or creating meaning in their lives; the counselor's role is simply to encourage them to engage in the difficult process of recognizing that existence is meaningless until one takes responsibility for one's life and creates meaning. Famous existential philosophers include Soren Kierkegaard, Friedrich Nietzsche, Jean-Paul Sartre, and Albert Camus.

Phenomenology in Action

Most practicing phenomenological counselors in the 21st century draw from both the humanistic and existential traditions when working with clients (Kirschenbaum & Jourdan, 2005); thus, these three approaches—person centered, Gestalt, and a counselor may identify more with either a humanistic or an existential view of human nature but generally will be drawn from both views and all three of the phenomenological theories presented in Chapters 6–8. In addition, there are family counseling approaches that are grounded in phenomenology, with Virginia Satir's Human Growth Model, Carl Whitaker's Symbolic-Experiential, and Sue Johnson's Emotionally Focused Couples Counseling (an empirically supported treatment; see Chapter 10) approaches being the most well-known (for a full discussion, see Gehart, 2010).

Commonalities Across Humanistic-Existential Theories

These therapies share several common assumptions and practices, discussed in the following sections.

Focus on Subjective Reality

All three approaches are grounded in the philosophical traditions of *phenomenology*, which focuses on *subjective, internal* reality (compared with the philosophical traditions of logical positivism that explore *objective, external* reality; Rogers, 1951). Simply put, this philosophical position directs counselor's attention, curiosity, and questions to the client's *subjective, internal reality* more so than the external "facts." For example, when a humanistic counselor hears a client state that she is angry, the counselor's focus and questions are directed to the client's internal experience of anger rather than examining the more logical (or illogical) reasons for why she is angry. Thus, the assessments and interventions of these approaches focus primarily on the client's inner experience and inner world more so than the outer world, based on the belief that change is best promoted by attending to the client's inner reality.

Warmth and Empathy

Another hallmark feature of most therapies grounded in phenomenology and humanism is the counselor's expression of genuine warmth and empathy. In the 21st century, most folks who walk into a counselor's office expect the counselor to be "nice" and understanding (Miller, Duncan, & Hubble, 1997, 2004). It wasn't always this way. This new expectation of counselors is directly due to the impact phenomenologically based approaches to counseling. As most people know, the early psychodynamic and psychoanalytic counselors were *not* warm and fuzzy: they asked patients to lie on couches while they sat behind silently taking notes with a periodic raise of the eyebrow and "veer-rie interezing" (or at least that is the Hollywood version, which is a bit of an exaggeration but makes the point). However, influenced by phenomenological counselors, later forms of psychodynamic counseling encouraged empathy. Additionally, although the first generation of behavioral, cognitive, and cognitive-behavioral counselors put little emphasis on empathy, later generations have also warmed up over the years. It was the humanists, most notably Carl Rogers, who championed the idea of counselors engaging their clients from a position of warmth and empathy.

Rogers didn't advocate these ideas because he thought counselors should be "nice" and because he thought being "sweet" would make clients feel better. No, there is actually a philosophical reason why he did this. He firmly believed that it was only in such a warm, genuinely empathetic environment that clients would feel safe enough to have the courage to (a) identify, (b) experience, and (c) critically reflect on their inner life, namely, their emotional inner experiences. Thus, in humanistic counseling, *empathy is the primary vehicle for therapeutic change*. This is quite different from any other approach that claims to encourage counselors to be empathetic, such as self psychology and new forms of cognitive-behavioral. For the humanist, empathy *is* the mechanism of change. For other counselors who use "empathy," they employ it to develop a relationship in which the client will feel safe enough to *engage in the other mechanisms that promote change*, such as analysis of interpersonal dynamics or thought stopping techniques.

Self of Counselor

Another key feature of phenomenologically based therapies is that the self of the counselor is used to promote change. What does that mean? Phenomenological counselors believe that the counselor relates to the patient as a whole, real, unedited person—not from the distant role of a professional. *How* this is done can differ across approaches. For example, person-centered counselors tend to maintain a softer style, while some Gestalt counselors maintain that the counselor needs to be real even with extremely difficult emotions, such as anger, frustration, and boredom as they relate to the client. Thus, both the characteristic softer style of person-centered counselors and the often highlighted dramatic and provocative style of Gestalt counselors come from the same working principle of using the genuine self of the counselor.

The self of the counselor is used to provide clients with both (a) a role model and (b) a genuine person with whom to have an authentic human encounter. By bringing one's full humanity into the counseling process, clients have the opportunity to experience real intimacy and human connection, often in a way that they have never experienced it before. This does not mean that the client and counselor are in a fully egalitarian relationship: the client is still the focus of the conversations and process. Counselors, however, listen and speak from the position of another human being who has known suffering and struggle, even if these are never discussed. For lack of a better word (I am from California after all), the "vibe" in the room is that "I feel your pain" even if the counselor's "pain" is never once mentioned or even referred to.

Self-Actualization and Maslow's Hierarchy of Needs

Maslow (1954) was an early humanist—not a therapist—who described human motivation in terms of a *hierarchy of needs*, including five areas of functioning:

- *Physiological needs:* Breathing, food, sex, freedom from pain
- *Safety needs:* Shelter, financial security, personal safety, health
- *Love and belonging:* Friends, family, community, social connectedness
- *Esteem:* Feeling valued by others and self
- *Self-actualization:* Realizing one's full potential; becoming more and more who one is

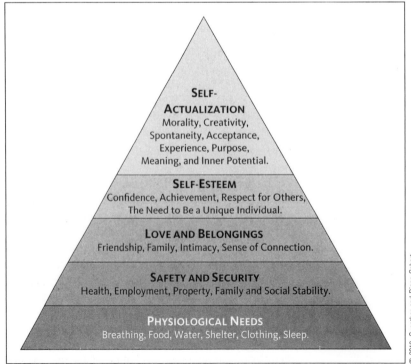

The first four areas are the most basic needs that must be in place in order for a person to self-actualize, which is the ultimate goal of all humanistic and existential forms of therapy; thus, his work is often cited by humanistic counselors. Self-actualization involves a humble acceptance of the positive and negative aspects of being human generally (existential realities) and of who one is individually (subjective reality) coupled with an unstoppable drive to become more fully human, more fully oneself, and more fully alive. Persons who have achieved a high level of self-actualization strive to contribute to the good of humanity, live by clear ethical and moral codes, and do not rely on acceptance from others to approve of themselves.

Person-Centered Counseling

In a Nutshell: The Least You Need to Know

Arguably, one of the most influential theories in the field of counseling (Kirschenbaum & Jourdan, 2005), person-centered counseling is a process-focused approach to helping people become more fully themselves. Developed by Carl Rogers (1942, 1951, 1961, 1980)—thus, it is often referred to as Rogerian counseling or its early term of client-centered counseling—person-centered counseling is based on the radical and startling proposition that the necessary and sufficient elements of therapeutic change are (a) counselor congruence or genuineness, (b) accurate empathetic understanding of the client, and (c) unconditional positive regard. Rogers asserted that if these three things were in place, over time clients would become more fully themselves and eventually the problems they came to counseling for would resolve. Person-centered counseling *does not* develop treatment plans to directly address the presenting problems that clients report, such as depression, conflict with a spouse, or indecision with career direction. Instead, the counseling focuses on helping clients to experience their in-the-moment internal experiences to expose the facades they live behind and the socially imposed shoulds that may be organizing their lives. As clients are able to more accurately and deeply experience themselves *while in relationship to the counselor*, they become better at making decisions that need to be made, experiencing themselves more fully and accurately, and relating to others, all of which works together to help them resolve the issues that brought them to counseling in the first place. Thus, techniques are avoided in favor of the counselor promoting a basic process of becoming more fully and accurately aware of the one's inner world.

Common Myths

Numerous myths and misunderstanding surround person-centered counseling. So, let's bust a few of those before we go any further:

> *Myth:* Person-centered counselors are "nice" and always work to make the client to "feel good."

> *Closer to the truth:* Person-centered counselors maintain an unconditional positive regard for people while still acknowledging that people make poor decisions, hurt others, and are capable of horrific acts.

Unconditional positive regard is often misunderstood to mean that the counselor never, ever, ever confronts the client on inconsistencies, dangerous decisions, or unrealistic thinking. New counselors further mistranslate unconditional positive regard to simply mean "being nice," in the typical social meaning of the word. Unfortunately, unconditional positive regard is only very loosely related to niceness as most of us think of it. Instead, it has a more spiritual quality: think Mother Teresa or Gandhi-like niceness. Unconditional positive regard is an attitude that focuses on the client's basic human worth at a fundamental level. It also recognizes that humans have free will and that they make bad decisions, have irrational fears, and are capable of hurting themselves and others. In essence, unconditional positive regard involves embracing the whole person—light and darker sides—rather than a Pollyanna "everyone is good; all feelings are good; it's all good" naive approach. Being able to meaningfully embrace clients with unconditional positive regard is an idealistic and lofty goal toward which you can spend a lifetime working.

> *Myth:* Person-centered counselors "validate" the client's feelings, always taking the client's side.
>
> *Closer to the truth:* Person-centered counselors honor and "validate" each person's subjective experience as his or her subjective experience, understanding that it may or may not be closely correlated with other people's experience of the same event.

Related to being nice, many new person-centered counselors hear about "validating" client feelings and translate this as having to always take the client's side on an issue. This is very dangerous because when you are working with an individual client, you are unable to assess or affect persons outside the session. Therefore, if you even give the impression that the other person is "wrong" and the client is "right and justified" in his or her feelings and perceptions, there is very little that is going to change as result of that session. Instead, there is a subtle yet important distinction to be made. Each person has his or her unique experience and emotional reaction to a situation—that much can be validated. However, that does not mean that our emotions are based on any type of accurate perception of others or are based on realistic expectations. I can be upset with my husband for not remembering how I take my tea; that does not mean that those feelings are "valid" in the sense that they are based on realistic expectations and interpretations of others. Instead, I may need to be validated in terms of "yes, this is how I feel," but the counselor's job in this situation would be to help explore where my expectations came from and to help me take responsibility for my half of the interaction.

> *Myth:* One of the most useful techniques is to ask clients, "How does that make you feel?"
>
> *Closer to the truth:* Asking "How does that make you feel?" implies that the counselor is interested in a person's emotional experience but is unable to accurately identify the client's subjective experience because of a *lack* of empathy.

Second only to traditional analysis on the couch, this is one of Hollywood's favorite ways to mock counselors and the strange things we do. The question "How does that make you feel?" is often used by new counselors trying to use a person-centered approach. The question has its place in this approach and others, but it is *not* a particularly good or key question. Since person-centered counseling posits that empathy is a core condition, *the counselor should have a fairly good idea about how that made the client feel and reflect it back to the client*—hence, the question is rarely needed in this approach. However, when starting out, many new counselors find that they don't have a good sense of how the client might be feeling and use this question to find out. Used too often, more than once per session, the question can quickly become annoying, *especially* because most clients have seen counselors mocked in movies and television for asking this question.

The Juice: Significant Contributions to the Field

If you remember one thing from this chapter, it should be ...

Core Conditions

The necessary and sufficient conditions of personality change boldly identified by Carl Rogers (1957) are arguably some of the most influential ideas put forth in the field of counseling and psychotherapy (Kirschenbaum, 2004; Kirschenbaum & Jourdan, 2005). Rogers (1957) identifies six conditions necessary for constructive personality change over a period of time:

1. Two persons are in psychological contact.
2. The first, whom we shall term the client, is in a state of incongruence, being vulnerable or anxious.
3. The second person, whom we shall term the therapist, is *congruent* or integrated in the relationship.
4. The therapist experiences *unconditional positive regard* for the client.

5. The therapist experiences *empathetic understanding* of the client's internal frame of reference and endeavors to communicate this experience to the client.

6. The communication to the client of the therapist's empathic understanding and unconditional positive regard is to a minimal degree achieved. (p. 241; emphasis added)

In later writings, these six conditions are boiled down into three conditions that the therapist must create in the counseling relationship:

1. Congruence or genuineness of the counselor
2. Unconditional positive regard
3. Accurate empathy

These three conditions are the heart of person-centered counseling. Rogers (1957) believed these to be necessary and sufficient for personality change regardless of the counselor's theory of choice or the client's presenting problem; he clearly states that this is his hypothesis until empirically proven otherwise. Rogers researched the hypothesis put forth in this article for the following three decades, and many after him have continued to test and refine his hypothesis (Kirschenbaum & Jourdan, 2005). Nonetheless, the debate rages on as to whether his hypothesis is correct (Brown, 2007; Hill, 2007; Kirschenbaum & Jourdan, 2005; Mahrer, 2007; Wachtel, 2007). At present, most would agree that the conditions outlined by Rogers in 1957 are *neither* sufficient *nor* necessary, but there is a substantial body of evidence to indicate that they are clearly *facilitative* and "crucial," meaning that they are *helpful* to *extremely helpful* in promoting change (Kirschenbaum & Jourdan, 2005). Translated even more simply, although there are some documented exceptions, in most cases the conditions identified by Rogers are highly correlated with positive counseling outcomes, *no research has identified a specific population or problem for which these conditions are counterindicated* (inappropriate). The common factors movement (see Chapter 2) is an outgrowth of the research that indicates that the qualities advocated by Rogers are highly correlated with positive therapeutic outcome, more so than the counselor's choice of theory. To boil it down even further, although they may not be necessary and sufficient for all clients in all cases, they are extremely important for positive outcomes regardless of the counseling theory you choose to work from—so read the following sections closely, as they probably make up the most important part of this book in terms of being a great counselor.

Genuineness or Congruence   The first condition is counselor *genuineness* (Rogers, 1957), later referred to as *congruence*, which refers to the counselor's outer expressions being "congruent" with his or her inner experience (Rogers, 1961). In 21st-century vernacular, we call this "being real." However, Rogers is referring to a humanistic, philosophical definition of what it means to be real, whole, and integrated, not what popular culture might define as real. Rogers's definition emphasizes being freely and deeply one's self while able to *accurately* "take in" what is experienced and simultaneously remaining aware of one's internal processing of that experience. Rogers explained congruence stating that "by this we mean that the feelings the therapist is experiencing are available to him [or her], available to his [or her] awareness, and he [or she] is able to live these feelings, be them, and able to communicate them if appropriate. No one fully achieves this condition, yet the more the therapist is able to listen acceptingly to what is going on within himself [herself], and the more he is able to be the complexity of his feelings, without fear, the higher the degree of his congruence" (Rogers, 1961, p. 61). Thus, congruence and genuineness is an idealized goal to which counselors continually aspire to more fully achieve. Far from an all-or-nothing state of affairs, it is a continually evolving and ever-deepening process.

Another way to understand Rogers's definition of genuineness is to approach it from its opposite, which is playing a role or having a facade (Rogers, 1957), including the role of "professional." Being congruent means that one does not try to "act" professional, "be" helpful, or otherwise take on a role or mask. This is a fine distinction because in some ways there are professional boundaries that need to be maintained: this is not a friendship but a helping relationship that has certain legal and ethical constraints. On the other hand, the typical slightly detached professional role, especially at the time Rogers was developing his ideas, is also not appropriate. Much like Goldilocks, there is a place in the middle that is just right—and the actual contours of this middle ground often vary from client to client.

Finally, I should mention that it is very difficult to be genuine in this way when first starting out simply because the new counselor has too many other things to think about: getting informed consent, conducting a mental status interview, assessing for danger, making a diagnosis, using new interventions, and so on. The more a counselor's mind is trying to remember these things, the less able the counselor is able to be genuine because too much focus is elsewhere. With time, these other tasks become second nature, and it becomes easier to be genuine. Perhaps one of the best indicators that a counselor is being genuine is a pervading sense of inner calm and centeredness, no matter what the client says or does.

Unconditional Positive Regard *Unconditional positive regard* is what it sounds like—valuing your clients no matter what they say or do (Rogers, 1957)—and has also been described as warm acceptance, nonpossessive warmth, prizing, affirmation, respect, support, and caring (Hill, 2007). This sounds a bit Pollyanna, so let's try to analyze what Rogers really meant by this. The underlying attitude here is not a one-dimensional belief that "all people are good" and that good counselors "love everybody." After all, counselors work with some of the most difficult, angry, and mean people in society: child molesters, criminals, divorcing spouses, gang members, negligent parents, substance abusers, and so on. If you have developed unconditional positive regard based on the Pollyanna notion that all people are good, it is going to fail you with these clients. Instead, unconditional positive regard needs to be built on a more subtle and reflected philosophical premise.

Unconditional positive regard is founded on the idea that we are all human and that we all suffer and therefore have the capacity for good and evil (or destructive behavior if you prefer). If you see yourself as far superior to the pedophile, vengeful divorcee, or gangbanger, you are probably unaware of the darker potentials that lie within each of us. Thus, unconditional positive regard is best motivated by a deep sense of compassion for how hard it is to be human—and for how easy it is to get off track and make bad decisions. When you view clients from this perspective, you can still hold them accountable for their past and current decisions and yet have compassion and hope for their current situation and future.

Accurate Empathy Rogers defines *empathy* as being able "to sense the client's private world as if it you're your own, but without ever losing the 'as if' quality" (Rogers, 2007, p. 243). In the practice of counseling, empathy involves not only the ability to accurately perceive the internal world of the client but also the ability to meaningfully share this understanding with the client. Rogers (1957) explains that "to sense the client's anger, fear, or confusion as if it were your own, yet without your own anger, fear, or confusion getting bound up in it, is the condition we are endeavoring to describe. When the client's world is this clear to the therapist, and he moves about in it freely, then he can both communicate his understanding of what is clearly known to the client and can also voice meanings in the client's experience of which the client is scarcely aware" (p. 243). Doing this requires that the counselor be keenly in tune with his or her internal world while having clear enough boundaries to perceive how another person's internal world hangs together.

Once the counselor has a sense of what the client *might* be feeling, the counselor then *reflects* (see below) this back to the client to (a) indicate that the counselor has understood, (b) check to make sure the counselor has understood correctly, and (c) provide the client with an opportunity to reflect on his or her internal experience in a slightly different context—namely, in external dialogue in the words of another person. Having one's intimate private world described by someone else is often a profoundly moving experience that often transforms one's experience, perception, and/or understanding of one's own experience. *That* is where the counseling comes in. For this reason, the question "How does that make you feel?" (see "Common Myths") is generally not as helpful as being able to convey accurate empathy.

Empathy should be conveyed tentatively, and the counselor should create space in the relationship for the client to say, "No, that is not how I feel," and not get into a tug-of-war over who's right about how the client feels. To be sure, there will be times when the counselor's reflection is accurate and yet the client disagrees for one reason or another. If this is the case, the counselor may want to rephrase it in a less dramatic version (e.g., rather than "You are angry at your mother" to say "You didn't like what your mother said yesterday") and then allow the client to further explore this *at her or her own pace.* The good news about empathy is that you don't have to get it right every time. If you have established a strong relationship and frequently seem to understand, the times when you don't the client feels safe enough to correct you. In fact, when working with clients who tend toward people pleasing, I do not believe a rapport has been established until a client feels safe enough to tell me that I got it wrong. Only then do I know that the client has dropped the people-pleasing facade and feel safe enough to be real with me. All that said, indeed, there are times, once you have a strong rapport, when it is effective to ask that oft-mocked question, "How does that make you feel?"

Cultural and Gender Considerations Although in theory it is simple enough, demonstrating appropriate empathy is far more difficult than it initially sounds because culture and gender greatly affect how one expresses empathy and what a person experiences as empathetic. For example, some people expect heartfelt, warm expressions of empathy: "You feel deeply betrayed by your daughter's choice," while others find such empathetic statements shameful and insensitive because they lose face or think that you are putting words into their mouth. Such persons may experience a subtle or even nonverbal expression of empathy more sincere and meaningful: a silent nod with a look of understanding. Thus, counselors need to become skilled in different ways of conveying empathy. In the case study at the end of this chapter, the counselor adapts the core conditions to work with May, a Taiwanese American woman who is struggling with panic and perfectionism, by using culturally appropriate expressions of emotion.

Measuring Empathy In your practicum class, you may learn about Carkhuff's (1969) 5-point scale for measuring empathy. This scale is used in training to help new counselors learn how to refine their empathy reflection skills. The scale is as follows:

Level 1: No empathy: Reflection focuses on content or intellectual part of client message. *Example: You think your daughter made the wrong decision.*

Level 2: Some empathy communicated: Some empathy expressed but some aspects of emotional experience ignored or missed. *Example: You don't like your daughter's decision.*

Level 3: Basic empathy: Reflects client emotion back at the same level that client expressed it. *Example: You are angered by your daughter's decision.*

Level 4: Deepened empathy: Reflects back client emotion at a slightly deeper level than client expressed, providing an enhanced understanding to further the client's exploration of internal process. *Example: It sounds like you are very disappointed and embarrassed by your daughter's decision.*

Level 5: Significantly deepened empathy: Counselor significantly expands and deepens the reflection, identifying subtle emotions that may not have been clearly expressed. *Example: It sounds like you feel betrayed yet also guilty about your daughter's decision.*

Let me be the first to tell you that every comment you make as a counselor cannot and should not be a level 5. It's impossible (because you need the other exchanges to work up to a level 5), but also you would at best sound loony and at worst be an incredibly annoying conversational partner. Nonetheless, being an eager student, when I trained using this scale, I had the sad misunderstanding that every response should be at a 5. The key thing to remember here is that trying to get to a level 5 statement once or a few times during a single session is an appropriate goal. In fact, all you really need is one level 5 reflection that is truly meaningful to the client—that is all that really needs to happen in a single session for it to be profoundly useful to the client.

Rumor Has It: The People and Their Stories

Carl Rogers

Carl Rogers is widely regarded as the most significant person in the history of psycho-therapy: in both 1982 and 2007, *Psychotherapy Networker* readers nominated him by a landslide as the most influential psychotherapist in the United States. He is beloved because he so consistently and unmistakably embodied the warm, caring spirit of which he spoke in writings and demonstrated in his work. He was a truly remarkable man whose influence continues to grow.

Born in 1902 outside of Chicago, he grew up in a conservative, Protestant midwestern family that did not value the expression of emotion (Kirschenbaum, 2004). He entered college, planning to follow in his father's footsteps as a farmer, but soon decided to pursue a career in religion. While studying at Union Theological Seminary in New York, he began taking classes in psychology and then decided to pursue a doctorate in clinical psychology, completing his fellowship at the Institute for Child Guidance. While finishing his dissertation in 1928, he took a position in Rochester, New York, where he spent the next 12 years as director of the Child Study Department at the Rochester Society for the Prevention of Cruelty to Children and then at the Rochester Guidance Center. During this period, he was influenced by students of Otto Rank, who used "relationship therapy" that emphasized patient self-insight and self-acceptance within a therapeutic relationship. In his last years in Rochester, Rogers (1939) wrote his first book, *The Clinical Treatment of the Problem Child*.

Based on the success of this book, he took a full-time professorship at Ohio State University and soon published what was to become a revolutionary book that many considered the launch of the counseling profession: *Counseling and Psychotherapy: New Concepts in Practice* (Rogers, 1942). After 4 years in Ohio, he took a position at the University of Chicago (1945–1957), where he was able to do more research on his theory, which he then called *client-centered therapy*. In 1957, he moved to the University of Wisconsin, where he had a joint position in the Departments of Psychology and Psychiatry and was able to conduct research on schizophrenia. In 1961, he published what was to be his most popular book, *On Becoming a Person: A Therapist's View of Psychotherapy*.

Wanting to further his research, in 1963 he moved to La Jolla, California, where he took a position at the Western Behavioral Sciences Institute. In 1973, he and others formed their own organization, the Center for Studies of the Person, where he remained for his last 15 years. In California, he expanded his ideas, now called *person-centered therapy*, for working in business, education, group leadership, and other health professions. His student-centered learning theories (Rogers, 1969) have been particularly influential in transforming modern education. In addition, in the last decades of his life, he used his person-centered approach to promote peace and reduce international conflict, working with Protestants and Catholics in Northern Ireland, Blacks and Whites in South Africa, and conflicting parties in South America. Rogers actively worked on the Carl Rogers Peace Project until his death in 1987.

Natalie Rogers

The daughter of Carl Rogers, Natalie Rogers (1997) carried on her father's work, applying his ideas primarily in the area of art and expressive therapies.

Robert Carkhuff

Carkhuff began his career studying the conditions that were correlated with positive outcomes in therapy, his findings largely in line with those of Rogers (Truax & Carkhuff, 1967). His later work integrated person-centered and behavioral methods to balance "insight" with "action." Carkhuff developed scales for measuring Rogers's core conditions as well as other core conditions that he identified through his research (Brazier, 1996). Because they are more behaviorally defined, Carkhuff's core conditions are frequently used to teach new counselors basic skills.

Big Picture: Overview of Counseling Process

Person-centered counseling is a *process-oriented* approach, meaning that the counselor's attention is on the *how* things happen (process) rather than *what* happens (content). As the name implies, the focus is on *persons*—most notably their inner processes—rather than their problems (Rogers, 1961). As a humanistic approach, counselors' primary aim is to help clients become more fully themselves, more authentic, and less attached to social roles and expectations. The person-centered counselor has a strong belief that symptoms will resolve themselves as clients becomes more self-actualized because they will view problems differently and take more responsibility for their emotions and life situations.

The process of self-actualization is not as easy or smooth as it initially sounds. In session, the counselor pays less attention to the content of the client's life—which is almost always less anxiety provoking to discuss—and instead focuses on *how* the client interacts with self, others, and life challenges: Does the client tend to blame others, or does the client take responsibility for his or her life? Does the client focus on details of external events, or is the client able to identify what is going on within himself or herself? Does the client have realistic expectations of self and others? The process is not always easy, as the counselor will gently "confront" attitudes, beliefs, and inconsistencies that keep the client from becoming more self-actualized. Throughout this process, the counselor gently and consistently redirects the client to more clearly articulate thoughts, feelings, and longings, especially those that may be difficult to admit to self or others, such as embarrassment, anger, shame, resentment, and so on. Through this process, the client begins to integrate contradictory and less-than-perfect parts of the self, reducing defensiveness and increasing his or her openness to experience. The counselor's primary role is to help the client remove the barriers—most of which the client has erected—to his or her own self-actualization.

Rogers (1961) describes seven stages of the change process a person typically experiences from the time of entering counseling to achieving—at least to some degree—self-actualization.

Seven Stages of the Change Process

1. *First stage:* In this stage, a person's personality seems fixed, personal problems are not acknowledged, there is a remoteness of experiencing, and there is little desire to change; the person is not likely to voluntarily enter counseling.
2. *Second stage:* If a person in the first stage is able to feel "received" by the counselor, he or she begins to loosen up and is more open to seeing problems, which are viewed as external to the self ("bad things happen to me"), with little sense of personal responsibility.
3. *Third stage:* If clients continue to feel accepted and understood by the counselor, they become better able to express past feelings and personal meanings.
4. *Fourth stage:* If clients continue to feel safe with the counselor, they begin to become more open to reconsidering their constructs about self and others and are increasingly able to verbalize deep emotions.
5. *Fifth stage:* As clients continue to explore themselves in the safety of the counseling relationship, they are increasingly able to verbalize in-the-moment emotions and experiences and an increasing desire to be the "real me."
6. *Sixth stage:* Rogers describes a distinct shift in the sixth stage, where the person is now able to experience difficult emotions as they arise in the present moment with

acceptance rather than fear, denial, or struggle.[1] Once this change happens, it tends to be irreversible, meaning that the client will continue to accept even the most difficult emotions rather than deny them.

7. *Seventh stage:* In this stage, it is no longer necessary for the client to be received by the counselor to self-actualize, although it is still helpful because the client has learned how to sustain the process of self-actualization without outside help. This stage generally occurs outside the counseling relationship.

Making Connection: Therapeutic Relationship

Relationship as Change Agent

Unlike most psychotherapies, person-centered counselors view the counseling relationship as the primary vehicle for change—*not* the counselor's interventions. They believe that it is through the authentic, human relationship between the counselor and client that the client is able to progress through the seven stages above and become more authentically themselves (Rogers, 1961). This is different than psychodynamic approaches in which the client is "working through" his or her issues in the therapeutic relationship and the counselor is interacting from a therapeutic role to "repair" and "correct." Instead, the person-centered counselor views the relationship as two authentic humans in relationship; when the client experiences being allowed to be fully himself or herself in relationship, one's inherent tendency to strive for positive growth is activated.

Therapeutic Presence and the Core Conditions

As discussed above—and as we will continue to repeat throughout this section—Carl Rogers (1961, 1980) based his person-centered approach on three counselor qualities used to promote change in clients, the core conditions being: (a) congruence or genuineness of the counselor, (b) accurate empathy, and (c) unconditional positive regard. These are the heart of the counseling relationship, but they are not an end in themselves. They are best thought of as the key ingredients in a chemical reaction that, when mixed together, create something far greater and more powerful than the inert ingredients alone. The result of this chemical experiment in this case is called *therapeutic presence* (Gehart & McCollum, 2008; Geller & Greenberg, 2002; McDonough-Means, Kreitzer, & Bell, 2004). Therapeutic presence is a quality of being, having intrapersonal, interpersonal, and transpersonal elements, including that of empathy, compassion, charisma, spirituality, transpersonal communication, client responsiveness, optimism, and expectancy, making it elusive and difficult to operationalize concept. That said, research indicates that clients know it when they feel it.

Clients tend to accurately sense how much and what type of information to share with counselors based on their quality of presence (Geller & Greenberg, 2002; McDonough-Means et al., 2004). If a counselor exudes even the slightest bit of anxiety while a person retells a tale of sexual abuse or trauma or judgment while sharing about a relationship or drinking episode, the client is likely to edit, recast, or simply cut short their relaying of experience. If the counselor is uncomfortable with sharing their emotions about what is going on in the present moment (i.e., immediacy), the client will be too. As counselors become more experienced in session while also practicing personal reflection and self-care, the quality of their therapeutic presence is likely to become more noticeable and facilitative.

The Viewing: Case Conceptualization

When Carl Rogers talked with people, he didn't just experience unconditional positive regard and empathy. He also carefully observed what they spoke about and how they

---

[1] This acceptance of immediate experience is the goal of mindfulness meditation, which has been most fully developed in cognitive-behavioral therapies discussed in Chapter 11; humanistic therapists also integrate mindfulness to cultivate the type of lived experience described by Rogers in this stage.

spoke to assess to what extent they were in touch with their authentic selves. He developed a seven-stage model (Rogers, 1961) that described how he saw people moving along a continuum from a rigid definition of self to a more flowing and ever-changing experience of self. Rather than simply change the definition of self—from one static identity to another—Rogers (1961) came to believe that self-actualization involves a process of letting go of static definitions of self and increasingly embracing a fluid experience of self in lieu of a singular identity.

In the early stages, people are unaware of their feelings, speak more about others than themselves, and often feel more like the victim than protagonist in their life stories. As people experience the effect of the core conditions in the counseling, these things change. People begin to experience their emotions as they are happening in the moment; they are able to readily identify what they are feeling, and they take greater responsibility for what happens in their life and how they emotionally respond. These stages are used to conceptualize where the client is along the continuum of self-actualization. Rogers maintained that people generally hovered around a single stage in all areas of functioning, although minor exceptions may be noted at a particular time or in a specific context. Table 6.1 illustrates the changes as people move through the stages.

TABLE **6.1**

Seven Stages of Rogers's Change Process

	Stage 1	Stage 2	Stage 3	Stage 4	Stage 5	Stage 6	Stage 7
Experience and communication of self	Communication about externals	Able to discuss nonself topics	Expression of self as object; self-experiences as objects	Increased awareness of self	Desire to be "real me"	Self as object tends to disappear	Self as process
Recognition of feeling	Unrecognized or not owned	Described as unwanted or past objects	Little acceptance of feelings	Feelings described as objects in present	Begin owning feelings	Feelings readily accepted	Feelings accepted and owned
Expression of feelings	Little to none	May be exhibited but not owned	Description of feelings	More intense description of past feeling	Expressed freely in present	Full; physical loosening	Full and flowing
Present moment experiencing	Little to none	Bound by structure of the past	Bound by past primarily	Less bound by past, less remote	More immediate but still somewhat surprising	Immediate and rich; process quality; physiological loosening	Immediate and rich in and out of session
Personal constructs	Extremely rigid; black/white	Considered "facts"	Rigid but recognized as constructs	Discovery of constructs	Critical examination of constructs	Dissolve in experiencing moments	Tentatively held
Complexity and contradiction	Unrecognized	Expressed but unrecognized	Recognition of contradictions	Concern about incongruence	Surprise and fright as feelings bubble through; more acceptance	Vividly experienced and dissolve in congruence	Acceptance and ownership of changing feelings
Perception of problems; responsibility for situation	Unrecognized	External to self. No sense of personal responsibility	Personal choices seen as ineffective	Some self-responsibility in relation to problems	Increased responsibility	No longer external or internal; problem not perceived as object	Full responsibility for self and emotions; confident about self as process

Experience and Communication of Self

As people become more self-actualized, *how* they experience themselves changes. The sense of self evolves from a static entity to one where the self is more of a process that is constantly unfolding and changing. Paradoxically, rather than "discovering" a constant self, a person discovers that the self is constantly in flux and unfolding.

Recognition of Feelings

Rogers theorized that the more self-actualized a person is, the better that person can identify and own emotion. In assessing clients, counselors look for whether clients can identify a range of emotions when they discuss the concerns they bring to counseling. Can they identify feelings of anger, hurt, joy, or fear? In most cases that warrant seeking counseling, a wide range of emotions is present to some degree or another. In some cases, a client has great difficulty identifying any emotion; in others, there is a particular favorite, such as anger or hurt, that is primarily felt. The more self-actualized a person is, the greater the range of emotion and the greater his or her ability to "own" that emotion as one that he or she feels without shame, fear, or embarrassment.

Expression of Emotion

In the process of self-actualization, people become better able and more comfortable with expressing their full range of emotions. Early in the process, people may not express any emotion: they appear almost emotionless and therefore at times appear to themselves and others as having "everything under control." However, that sense of control is extremely fragile. Through the counseling process, people become more aware of their feelings, initially describing them as if they were happening to someone else. As they continue, they become able to describe both past and present emotions fully and in a way that is flowing and natural.

Gender and ethnic background often significantly impact which emotions are expressed and how they are expressed. For example, in most cultures, women are allowed to more freely express emotion than men. All cultures have values related to emotional expression that define where, how, and with whom emotion is best expressed and also which emotions are socially acceptable in which situation. For example, Japanese culture values emotional restraint in most public settings, whereas Mediterranean cultures, such as the Greeks and Italians, value relatively bold expression of emotion in the same situations. Thus, counselors need to carefully consider gender and culture as well as age and socioeconomic status to fairly interpret a person's emotional expression. In the case study at the end of this chapter, the counselor carefully takes into account norms for emotional expression, the client's level of acculturation, and the client's symptoms when assessing her patterns of emotional expression.

Present Moment Experiencing

Present moment experiencing refers to the ability to mindfully experience emotions in the present moment. When experiencing emotions in the here and now, a person is able to (a) actually feel the emotion and (b) reflectively articulate the emotion (e.g., "I am feeling angry" rather than launch into an angry tirade that blames others). The more a person can experience intense, difficult emotions in the present while still being able to productively talk about them, the greater his or her level of self-actualization. Initially, most clients have little present moment experiencing; most of their experience is related to thoughts and worries about the past or future. Through the counseling process, clients become increasingly able to feel their feelings in the present moment *and be aware of this experience*, experiencing and witnessing their experience at the same time.

Personal Constructs and Facades

Rogers (1961) often described inauthentic living as living behind a "mask," or facade. These facades are the *personal constructs* we use to tell us who we are, how we should behave, and what we are worth. In contrast, authentic living refers to living in the process of being human, accepting the varied flow of experience that cannot be captured by a single construct or definition of who we are. For example, if a person maintains the construct that she is a "nice" person, she will have to suppress, ignore, or otherwise disregard the very real and normal human reactions, such as anger, disappointment, boredom, and dislike; she will have to disregard parts of herself, some vital, in order to maintain the facade. Initially, a person's personal constructs are rigid and black and white: *I am X, not Y.* As people become more self-actualized and begin to experience themselves more as an unfolding process than a static entity, these constructs become less and less important, and instead they simply experience themselves as a complex being having a series of unfolding life experiences that involve a fluid and adapting sense of self. In the case study at the end of this chapter, the counselor helps May become less identified with her perfectionist and high-achieving facades, allowing herself to increasingly experience herself as a constantly evolving process.

Complexity and Contradictions

Humanistic counselors also assess for a person's ability to engage the complexities and contradictions that characterize our internal lives and life more generally. We often believe that humans are "logical" creatures that make sense, having singular opinions and emotions that are rational. This is one myth that is quickly busted if you ever decide to practice mindfulness meditation for even 60 seconds. The Buddhists liken the mind to a monkey that jumps from tree to tree, up and down, here and there, in an erratic, unpredictable pattern. The mind similarly jumps from topic to topic, past to future, thought to feeling, without necessarily being consistent or coherent. In fact, the more complex the topic, the more likely a person has contradictory thoughts and emotions: both loving and resenting a significant other, both liking and hating one's career, and so on.

Early in the counseling process, most people are totally unaware of their own contradictory thoughts and feelings. As they become more aware, they become increasingly concerned about the lack of congruence. Rather than "pick a side" and end contradiction, the process of self-actualization moves toward greater acceptance of these contradictions as part of the complexity and "messiness" of being human. The greater a person's ability to accept these inherent contradictions in oneself, others, and life, the more resourceful one will be in managing life stressors.

Perception of Problems and Responsibility

In the early stages, problems are perceived as caused primarily by the outside world: others, circumstances, and so on. As people progress through the stages, there is an increasing awareness of one's responsibility and agency in every situation, and therefore problems are increasingly described with an emphasis on how one is contributing and/ or perpetuating the situation. For example, rather than complain that "my wife is always nagging me" or "my husband never helps out around the house," clients increasingly say that the problem is "I have a hard time motivating myself to get things done" or "my expectations are too high for myself and others."

Often in life, it feels like life happens "to us": people do things to make us angry, hurt us, or prevent us from getting what we want. It may be a lover who says something thoughtless, a boss who passes us up for a promotion, or a parent who doesn't have time for us. The more self-actualized a person becomes, the greater the awareness that life is a two-way street. In most cases, how we interact with another contributes to how they respond to us. In all cases, we have control in how we decided to respond in terms of actions, words, and even emotions. When clients described the problems in terms of being agents of their own lives, they take responsibility for their part in creating the problem situation and are quick to assume full responsibility for resolving the problem no matter the source. In contrast, clients with lower levels of agency tend to feel victimized and often are mystified about how to go about solving problems.

Peak Experience and Flow

Rogers describes the self-actualized self as "fluid" and "flowing." Recent positive psychology researchers also describe peak experience as a *flow* state, a unique quality of experience in which a person feels fully present, in sync, and immersed in a challenging activity for which one has sufficient skill. Typically during flow experiences, time seems to be moving more slowly, and activity seems to happen without effort or thought. A classic example is the football quarterback making a seemingly impossible pass to another player; often when interviewed afterward, the athlete will describe the event as though he, the ball, and the receiver were one. Other common flow experiences involve playing music, cooking, writing, running, dancing, and similar activities. Flow experiences typically are associated with activities that require effort and practice. After a certain level of mastery, the activity takes on an effortless, automatic, and fully alive quality for distinct periods of time. These are a type of peak experience associated with the humanistic view of being self-actualized. Counselors can ask about the frequency and quality of these flow experiences in assessing a client's level of functioning. For example, typically depression is an experience in which there are few if any experiences of flow; as people begin to recover, they often find that flow experiences return.

Targeting Change: Goal Setting

Self-Actualization: "Becoming That Self Which One Truly Is"

It's easy to write the final goal on a person-centered treatment plan because the overarching goal in person-centered counseling is consistent with most other humanistic approaches: to promote *self-actualization*. Self-actualization refers to fulfilling one's potential and living an authentic, meaningful life, or, as Rogers (1961) explains, "to be that self which one truly is" (p. 163). Self-actualization is correlated with Rogers's (1961) Stage 7 level of development. Unlike existentialists, Rogers firmly believed that humans *naturally* tend toward positive, prosocial growth; the counselor's primary job is to provide the correct environment that fosters this growth (i.e., the core conditions). Maslow (1954) also identified self-actualization as the highest order in his hierarchy of human needs, coming only after more basic physiological, safety, social, and self-esteem needs are met.

Self-actualization (Rogers, 1961) is characterized by the following:

- Openness to present moment experiencing of emotions
- Trust in self
- Internal locus of evaluation and control
- Living without roles, facades, shoulds, or social expectation
- Being a complex, dynamic, and unfolding process (rather than a static entity)
- Openness to experience
- Acceptance of others

Self-actualization is always a long-term, late phase goal: the broad, overarching direction for counseling. Unfortunately, it is a vague goal unless smaller goals that address impediments are used in the middle phase.

Process Goals

It's well established that self-actualization is a *big* goal. However, most of the work in counseling occurs in smaller goals along the way that address *process* issues: a person's internal process. Here is where your case conceptualization comes into play. You can identify areas of growth and turn these into middle phase goals. For example, if a woman describes her life as unfairly limited by all the things she *should do* to be a "good wife," counselors write a goal to "increase living by conscious choice rather than a list of shoulds." Similarly, if a man reports wanting to constantly please others to his own detriment, a process goal would be to "reduce attempts to please others in ways that are detrimental to personal needs."

Example of goals related to specific areas of functioning:

Emotional Expression and Here-and-Now Experiencing

- "Increase ability to identify emotions in present moment."

Victimization and Experience of Problems

- "Increase sense of responsibility for own problems and their resolution."

Agency

- "Increase sense of agency and proactive behavior in work life."

Facades and Masks

- "Reduce use of facades in personal relationships to increase experience of intimacy."

Peak Experience and Flow

- "Increase frequency of peak experience and flow in work life."

Perfectionism and Unrealistic Expectations

- "Increase ability to set realistic expectations for self and other to increase acceptance."

Trust Self

- "Increase ability to trust the evolving and changing nature of the self."

Interventions

Self of the Counselor and the Core Conditions

The fundamental "instrument" of intervention in person-centered counseling is the "self" of the counselor; the counselor's way of being in the world. It's hard to get more nebulous than that, so you will find a list of other "techniques" in the rest of this section that are all trying to cultivate this one essential instrument of change: the counselor. As a highly relational form of counseling, person-centered counseling relies on the person-hood of the counselor to bring a quality of presence that helps clients to transform and become more comfortable with experiencing their authentic selves. In a smaller nutshell, the self-of-the-counselor is the vehicle through which the core conditions are established. Thus, in many ways, the crux of change in person-centered counseling is the quality of the relationship between the counselor and counselee.

In practical terms, using the self of the counselor could involve a wide range of activities, including expressing empathy, using humor, and self-disclosure. What is demanded of the counselor changes depending on the client, the problem, the topic of conversation, and the goals for counseling. Ultimately, it is the clearly communicated authenticity of the counselor that sets the stage for clients to identify, explore, and freely express their authentic selves. Knowing how to use one's personhood to facilitate authenticity in others requires significant maturity, self-awareness, and reflection on the part of the counselor: you can't learn it from a book or by practicing deeper levels of empathy. It's a way of being that takes time—and an excellent supervisor—to cultivate.

Focused Listening or Attending

"Very early in my work as a therapist, I discovered that simply listening to my client, very attentively, was an important way of being helpful. So when I was in doubt as to what I should do in some active way, I listened" (Rogers, 1980, p. 137). This is an excellent piece of advice that is useful not just in counseling contexts but also in most every sphere of life: *when in doubt, listen*. Still not sure? Listen some more.

One of the first skills new counselors learn is listening. Listening in person-centered counseling has a very specific form based on its philosophical foundation in phenomenology. As you might remember from the beginning of the chapter, phenomenology encompasses the study of the internal, subjective world. Thus, when a person-centered counselor listens to clients share their stories, they are listening for and attending to descriptions of the persons' *internal world*, most notably their emotions and logic that connects this affective inner world. For example, if a woman begins to describe how she no longer feels loved by her husband, the counselor does not focus on what the husband is doing, what she can behaviorally do differently, or how she could reframe what is going on. Instead, the counselor is curious about the contours of her internal life. Does she feel betrayed, hopeless, rejected, ugly, angry, or sad? The counselor listens for a rich and nuanced description of her internal emotional experience and selects these descriptions to comment on or ask about.

Summarizing

For those of us who expect life to be hard and difficult and who may also assume that "great counseling" must be hard, summarizing as a counseling intervention can be difficult to understand. How can simply restating what a person has just said be helpful and worth paying for? Basically, most of us aren't listening carefully when we speak; even if we are, it sounds very different when someone else says it, especially if it is about a difficult topic. For example, many people frequently make fun of themselves or put themselves down. But when someone else says the same thing—or simply agrees with what was just said—they feel offended, hurt, or angry. That is the same principle at work when summarizing. When counselors paraphrase back the essence of what a client just said, it helps clients to hear what they said in a different way. In most cases, it hits home harder than when they said it themselves. When another person skillfully summarizes emotionally difficult material, clients often hear and feel things in a new way: the reality of a situation often comes into bold relief.

For summarizes to be effective, they need to be (a) well timed, (b) about emerging insights (not just anything the client says), (c) in the client's language, and (d) not biased by the counselor's values, assumptions, or desires. For example, if a woman is going on about all the ways she is not happy with her boyfriend whom she was planning to marry and states that she knows the relationship is doomed, she is likely to find a summarization from a counselor helpful in crystallizing her insight: "Even though you initially thought he was the one you would marry, you have begun to realize during the events of the past few months that this relationship will not work for you long term." If the client is struggling against this reality, it can help to recast the summary in the form of a question: "It sounds like you are beginning to question whether this relationship will work for you based on the events of the past few months?"

Clarifying

Similar to summarizing, clarifying statements and questions are not glamorous. They seem so simpleminded that you sometimes wonder if it is worth asking. Nonetheless, clarifying questions are some of the most important because often what seems simple and obvious is not. Just as the name implies, clarifying questions involve querying clients to provide more detail or explanation about what they are talking about. Clarifying questions can be categorized into two types, with each playing an important role. The first type of clarifying questions addresses factual issues: who, what, where, and how. These clarifying questions are not considered therapeutic in and of themselves in person-centered counseling and if overused actually distract from the counseling process. However, these can be important questions, especially when working with persons from diverse backgrounds. Counselors use fact-focused clarifying questions to ensure that they understand the basic information that makes up the client's experience. These questions help counselors avoid bias by ensuring that they don't project their assumptions onto clients. These questions help clients share their story: Who else was there? When did this happen? What happened next?

The other type of clarifying questions focus on the client's emotional process. These questions help the client more clearly articulate and conceptualize their internal process and are essential in promoting self-actualization. These clarifying questions are used to help the client more deeply probe and explore their internal emotional life. For example, "You say you are 'upset.' Can you say more about what you mean by this?" Or, "There is a lot to be sad about in this situation, can you share what saddens you the most?" These questions help clients to sharpen their ability to identify, name, and share their emotions and thereby better understand and accept their inner life.

Reflecting Feelings

One of the most readily identifiable things that a person-centered counselor does, *reflecting feelings* refers to identifying feelings that the client just described or that seem to underlie what the client just said. For example, if a client complains about an incident at work, rather than focusing on who did what to whom, the counselor listens for the client's emotional experience, which may be one of being betrayed, taken advantage of, or loss—or even all three. This technique highlights and amplifies clients' awareness of their emotions, reactions, and feelings so that they can more consciously experience them. This technique is especially useful in the earlier stages of actualization when emotions are more difficult to identify, access, and experience. Even with clients who are skilled at identifying their emotions, having another person describe your emotional state can be a powerful experience that provides new experiencing and insight into one's subjective experience.

Process Questions

Process questions refer to questions or comments that direct clients' focus toward their inner process rather than content. In everyday conversation, people tend to ask follow-up questions about the content of what happened: who said what to whom when. The conversation stays at a more factual-level description of what happened. Speculation as to why things happen distracts from a client's inner process. In contrast, counselors use process questions to help clients focus on the inner experience, emotions, and subjective reality—broadly speaking, to get them out of their heads and into their heart and bodies. Thus, the focus is on inner *emotional process* rather than factual description or rational analysis of what happened. Process questions can include the following:

- Can you describe what was going on inside of you when you heard the news?
- When you heard the door shut, what was going on inside for you?
- As you are telling me the story now, what types of feelings are coming up? Are these the same or different from what you experienced when things were happening?

Carkhuff's Core Conditions

Robert Carkhuff (1969, 2000; Truax & Carkhuff, 1976) extended Rogers's research by studying the observable and measurable behaviors that facilitated change in counseling. Researching a variety of facilitative conditions, Carkhuff identified several core conditions that are often used to help new counselors develop basic counseling skills. They include the following:

- Empathy (similar to Rogers's accurate empathy)
- Authenticity and genuineness (similar to Rogers's authenticity)
- Respect (similar to Rogers's unconditional positive regard)
- Concreteness and specificity
- Self-disclosure
- Confrontation
- Immediacy

As the first three have been discussed at length earlier, we will just focus on the last four here.

Concreteness and Specificity

Carkhuff identified concreteness and specificity as counselor behaviors that facilitate the counseling process. Counselors demonstrate concreteness and specificity with questions and statements that help clients to clarify what is vaguely expressed. For example, to describe oneself as "upset" is really not saying much. For some this means to feel angry, others sad, and yet others anxious. Similarly, to say that "my mother's death made me sad" is also quite vague if it isn't followed up with more; such a major loss can be sad in many different ways. Counselors can help clients increase their inner awareness by asking questions that help them to be more concrete and specific about their subjective experiences.

Self-Disclosure

Self-disclosure is a bit like saffron. One of the most valued spices, in large quantities or in the wrong dish, saffron is a culinary disaster that cannot be fixed. So too is self-disclosure in counseling. It is so difficult to get right that I often caution new counselors to not use it until after their first year of training. This is not always possible and in some senses is impossible if you take into account that wearing a wedding band, your style of clothes, and your choice of mobile phone are all forms of disclosure at some level. However, what person-centered counselors more generally refer to as self-disclosure involves sharing *relevant* personal experience—generally personal struggles that are similar to what the client is dealing with—with the client *for the sole purpose of helping the client achieve their goals.* Self-disclosures may serve several clinical purposes: providing a role model, offering hope, or normalizing the client's experience. All of these are valid uses of self-disclosure and are highly effective when used with the right person at the right time. *However*—and this is a big however—when used at the wrong time with the wrong client, the damage done to the therapeutic relationship is often irreparable because once you reveal personal information, it cannot be taken back or undone. If there is a miscommunication, that can be cleared up. But if your client begins to doubt your credibility, was offended in some way, or has any of an infinite number of interpretations, it may be difficult or impossible to repair the counseling relationship, greatly reducing the chance of a positive outcome. Thus, self-disclosure requires excellent judgment in determining what will be most helpful to clients.

Confrontation

One of the more often misunderstood techniques, affective confrontation—especially when done in person-centered counseling—is not a harsh, critical confrontation but rather the counselor's effort to address discrepancies in verbalizations, perception, and/or body language. In the first case, the counselor points out that what the client just said does not jive with what was said earlier, either in this or another conversation: "you are saying now that you don't care, but earlier you said you were angry." The counselor may also point out discrepancies in terms of how another person is "all to blame" and the client an innocent victim in a situation where each played a part: "you say you don't like how your husband spoke to you; can you also describe how you spoke to him?" Alternatively, the counselor can comment on how the client's body language (e.g., on the edge of tears) is not congruent with what the client is saying (e.g., "I'm fine"). The spirit of these confrontations, unlike Gestalt, is generally one of curiosity and support rather than challenge.

Immediacy

"Immediacy" refers to the condition whereby counselor and client are able to discuss the client's immediate emotional state, which can be related to (a) an outside topic, (b) in-session behaviors, or (c) the counselor–client relationship. The ability to feel and immediately reflect on and discuss the emotion-of-the-moment is considered a higher-ordered level of emotional expression and a sign of increasing levels of self-actualization, the ultimate goal of counseling. Counselors can facilitate immediacy in several ways. One is to comment on an emotion that the counselor can clearly observe: "It seems as though you were offended by the comment I just made." Alternatively, counselors can prompt clients to try to identify what they are feeling in the moment: "What emotions are you feeling as you tell me about the car accident you saw on the way to the appointment *or* as we discuss your thoughts about ending the marriage?" Immediacy is intense and intimate and thus must be used with caution. The client can feel put on the spot, attacked, or belittled if the counseling alliance isn't strong enough. It is not a technique to use frequently in most cases—even once a session can be too much for some clients. Additionally, it must be well timed, in a moment where the client is open to feeling vulnerable and exposed. In the case study at the end of this chapter, the counselor uses immediacy often with May to create opportunities for her to experience her authentic self in relation to another.

Focusing

Gendlin (1984; see also Gendlin, Beebes, Cassens, Klein, & Oberlander, 1968) developed a technique called *focusing* to help clients more quickly access their emotions. The technique involves directing clients to identify *preverbalized* experience, which may be in the body or otherwise brought into awareness. Then clients are encouraged to carry it forward by bringing close attention to it, describing the experience with words, and then moving into action.

What Person-Centered Counselors Do Not Do

Often effective counseling is more about what you don't do than what you do do. In person-centered counseling, it is particularly important that counselors avoid doing the following, as each of these prevents clients from engaging their inner process:

- *Using reassuring clichés:* "In the end, it will all be okay" or "There are people in far worse situations" rarely make anyone feel better. As you probably know from first-hand experience, having someone offer such clichés usually incites ire rather than comfort. However, even worse for the person-centered counseling process, this externally offered reassurance cuts short the internal process that a client needs to master to self-actualize.

- *Giving advice:* Another tempting but unhelpful response in person-centered counseling is advice giving. Most clients want advice. In some cases, that is all they want and are frustrated if you don't offer it. However, person-centered counselors are resolute in not giving it but rather encouraging clients to look inward to find their own inner advice and answers. That said, when working with culturally diverse or immigrant clients, counselors may need to consider whether certain forms of advice or education might be appropriate given their expectations and needs.

- *Requesting an explanation:* Phenomenology is at its core descriptive: seeking a description of a person's subjective, internal experience. The counselor's attention is on getting a better, richer description of the emotional terrain of this inner world rather than a logical explanation for how the pieces fit together. The dogged focus on describing the emotional terrain, which requires a particular state of mind, is quickly derailed by requests for information. To use pop-psychology lingo, person-centered counseling is a "right-brain" activity; asking for explanations is a "left-brain" intrusion into this process.

- *Agreeing with the client:* Ahh! This is one of the most common traps for new counselors. Don't clients need their counselors to "support" them by agreeing with their perspective? I could do a whole chapter on the dangers of agreeing with clients—although there are some rare instances where it does help—but much like counselor self-disclosure, it is more likely to backfire.

  So, let's review some of the many ways this seemingly friendly, kind, and benign act can halt progress or worse. First, when counselors agree with clients, they end the clients' internal dialogue and struggle to answer their own questions and quickly derail the clients' ability to develop their internal locus of control, which is correlated with both self-actualization and long-term happiness. Second, clients often change their opinion and feelings over the course of treatment, if not mid-session, because, in fact, most of us have conflicting emotions about most everything (see "Complexity and Contradictions" earlier). This problem is most apparent when working with women who are being abused by their partners; part of the logic of these relationships is that a person has extreme variability in their feelings toward the abusive partner; thus, one week she wants to stay, and the next she wants to leave. If a counselor takes a side, then the client is less likely to speak up when feelings change. Third, when describing another person or situation, clients—like all of us—see the situation from their perspective. However, by subtly or directly "agreeing" with your clients about how "unfair" a situation is or how wrongly they were treated, you undermine the process of self-actualization that involves taking greater responsibility and accepting others. In short, agreeing with clients is a slippery slope that gets you farther away from the desired goal.

- *Disagreeing with the client:* It is perhaps easier to understand why you don't want to disagree with clients. On one level, it generally does not help convey a sense of empathy. But, more important, counselors avoid disagreeing for the same reason they avoid agreeing: it circumvents the more critical inner process of self-reflection that is ultimately the goal of person-centered counseling.

- *Giving approval:* Giving approval is another tricky situation in counseling. Often you will hear counselors say, "I gave her permission to have her feelings" or "I validated her feelings." *Validation* and *giving permission* can involve a variety of subtle but important differences. Obviously, counselors should not be in the business of "giving approval" for actions or feelings. They have no special sanction from God, the president, or anyone else to determine what is acceptable and what is not. Similarly, if a counselor "validates" a client's emotion or "gives a client permission" to have an emotion, this too can undermine the process of self-actualization if the client uses the counselor to "be okay with" his or her emotions, behaviors, and/or decisions. Instead, counselors want to be careful to encourage clients to validate their own emotions and to give themselves permission to feel what they feel rather than rely on an external source to do that. That is the goal. However, in certain circumstances, particularly early in treatment, clients might need a counselor to help them with this process. However, the goal should always be to encourage clients to determine the value and appropriateness of their own emotions rather than look to the counselor for approval.

- *Expressing disapproval:* Similar to disagreement, counselors avoid expressing disapproval because it undermines the client's autonomy in the same way that offering approval undermines it. Even in circumstances—or especially in circumstances—where a client is not engaging in socially expected behaviors, such as an affair, physical violence, or abusing substances, and the counselor refrains from expressing disapproval, the client will be more likely to express disapproval and a desire to change. If the counselor is the first to propose that change is necessary, clients tend to resist more even if they agree because they do not have ownership of that idea.

Interventions for Special Populations
Nondirective Play Therapy

One of the more popular forms of play therapy, Virginia Axline's (1989) nondirective play therapy is based on Rogerian counseling principles. Axline's play therapy is ideally conducted in a dedicated play therapy room that has possibilities for playing with art media, dollhouses, puppets, dress up, games, sand tray, and other play therapy equipment. In this setting, the counselor allows the *child to lead the play* by choosing activities. The counselor interacts with the child throughout the play to reflect feelings and inner processes.

Eight Principles of Axline's Play Therapy Using humanistic principles, Axline (1989) identifies eight principles of nondirective play therapy:

1. The therapist must develop a warm, friendly relationship with the child in which good rapport is established as soon as possible.
2. The therapist accepts the child exactly as he is.

3. The therapist establishes a feeling of permissiveness in the relationship so that the child feels free to express his feelings completely.
4. The therapist is alert to recognise the *feelings* the child is expressing and reflects those feelings back to him in such a manner that he gains insight into his behaviour.
5. The therapist maintains a deep respect for the child's ability to resolve his own problems if given an opportunity to do so. The responsibility to make choices and to institute changes is the child's.
6. The therapist does not attempt to direct the child's actions or conversation in any manner. The child leads the way; the therapist follows.
7. The therapist does not attempt to hurry the therapy along. It is a gradual process and is recognised as such by the therapist.
8. The therapist establishes only those limitations that are necessary to anchor the therapy to the world of reality and to make the child aware of his responsibility in the relationship. (pp. 73–74; emphasis in the original)

Axline readily admits that this approach is not a panacea that will work with all children all the time. Moreover, effectively establishing such a relationship is not an easy task, and counselors will need to work hard to be successful. Nonetheless, Axline's methods are still widely used, particularly with kids who have experienced trauma, abuse, or loss and/or are experiencing internalizing symptoms, such as depression, grief, or anxiety. Gary Landreth and his colleagues (Bratton, Ray, Edwards, & Landreth, 2009) have continued the development of humanistic therapies with children in their model of *child-centered play therapy*.

Expressive Arts Therapy

Natalie Rogers (1997), Carl Rogers's daughter, applies the principles of person-centered counseling to artistic expression with children and adults. Her methods help people access deep emotions that may be difficult to put into words, either because they are not fully in consciousness or because they are too multifaceted to capture in language. She builds on her father's work by creating (a) a psychologically safe environment and (b) a psychologically free environment, namely, the counseling relationship. Natalie believes that a third element is also necessary to foster personal growth: stimulating and challenging experiences, which she provides through opportunities for spontaneous creative expression. Her work is based on some of the following principles:

- All people have an innate ability to be creative.
- The creative process is healing. The expressive product supplies important messages to the individual. However, it is the process of creation that is profoundly transformative.
- Personal growth and higher states of consciousness are achieved through self-awareness, self-understanding, and insight.
- Self-awareness, understanding, and insight are achieved by delving into our emotions. The feelings of grief, anger, pain, fear, joy, and ecstasy are the tunnel through which we must pass to get to the other side—to self-awareness, understanding, and wholeness.
- Our feelings and emotions are an energy source. That energy can be channeled into the expressive arts to be released and transformed.
- The expressive arts—movement, art, writing, sounding, music, meditation, and imagery—lead us into the unconscious. This often allows us to express previously unknown facets of ourselves, thus bringing to light new information and awareness.
- Art modes interrelate in what I call the Creative Connection. When we move, it affects how we write or paint. When we write or paint, it affects how we feel and think. The Creative Connection is a process that brings us to an inner core or essence that is our life force energy.
- A connection exists between our life force—our inner core, or soul—and the essence of all beings.
- Therefore, as we journey inward to discover our essence or wholeness, we discover our relatedness to the outer world. The inner and outer become one (N. Rogers, 1993, p. 30).

Putting It All Together: Person-Centered Treatment Plan Template

Use this treatment plan template for developing a plan for clients with depressive, anxious, or compulsive types of presenting problems. Depending on the specific client, presenting problem, and clinical context, the goals and interventions in this template may need to be modified only slightly or significantly; you are encouraged to significantly revise the plan as needed. For the plan to be useful, goals and techniques should be written to target specific beliefs, behaviors, and emotions that the client is experiencing. The more specific, the more useful it will be to you.

Treatment Plan

Initial Phase of Treatment (First One to Three Sessions)
Initial Phase Counseling Tasks

1. *Develop working counseling relationship. Diversity note*: Adapt counselor's emotional expression for ethnicity, gender, age, and so on.
   Relationship building approach:
   a. Use **unconditional positive regard**, **accurate empathy**, and **genuineness** to establish the necessary conditions for change.

2. *Assess individual, systemic, and broader cultural dynamics. Diversity note*: Carefully adapt assessment for cultural and gender norms for expression of emotion and self-constructs.
   Assessment strategies:
   a. Assess for ability to identify, express, and experience **emotions** in **present moment**.
   b. Assess for ability to experience self as an **unfolding process**, accept proactive **responsibility** for problems, embrace **complexity** and **contradictions**, and experience **flow**.

Initial Phase Client Goals (One or Two Goals): Manage crisis issues and/or reduce most distressing symptoms

1. *Decrease* experience of overwhelming **emotions** and sense of helplessness to reduce [specific crisis symptoms].
   Interventions:
   a. Help client **identify**, **own**, and **accept emotions** underlying crisis behaviors.
   b. Help client develop a proactive and **competent sense of self** in relation to **complexity** and challenge that underlie crisis.

Working Phase of Treatment (Three or More Sessions)
Working Phase Counseling Tasks

1. *Monitor quality of the working alliance. Diversity note*: Adapt relationship to be responsive to gender and cultural forms of emotional expression, independence, and communal values.
   Assessment Intervention:
   a. Assess for client's ability to **express self genuinely** and constructively disagree with counselor; Session Rating Scale.

Working Phase Client Goals (Two or Three Goals): Target individual and relational dynamics using theoretical language (e.g., decrease avoidance of intimacy, increase awareness of emotion, increase agency)

1. *Increase* ability to **recognize** and constructively **expression emotions** to reduce [specific symptom: depression, anxiety, etc.].

(continued)

Interventions:

a. **Empathetically reflect** unacknowledged feelings that are difficult for the client to express.

b. Assist client experiencing emotions in the present moment using **immediacy**.

2. *Increase* ability to recognize **authentic self** without **facades** to reduce [specific symptom: depression, anxiety, etc.].
Interventions:

a. **Process questions** to enable client to clarify inner experience of self.

b. **Immediacy** to help client experience self in relationship to counselor.

3. *Increase* ability to view self as **responsible** for problem situations and **active agent** in making changes to reduce [specific symptom: depression, anxiety, etc.].
Interventions:

a. **Confront contradictions** related to powerlessness and victim thinking.

b. **Immediacy** to help client experience sense of agency in counseling relationship and present experiences.

Closing Phase of Treatment (Last Four or More Sessions)
Closing Phase Counseling Task

1. *Develop aftercare plan and maintain gains. Diversity note*: Attend to gender and cultural norms for community, interconnection, and emotional expression.
Intervention:

a. **Process questions** to help client identify how best to manage potential future challenges; terminate only after client has developed ability to reflect on self without assistance.

Closing Phase Client Goals (One or Two Goals): Determined by theory's definition of health and normalcy

1. *Increase* ability to experience **self as an unfolding, evolving,** and **complex process** without holding on to **personal constructs** to reduce potential for relapse in [specific symptom: depression, anxiety, etc.].
Interventions:

a. **Unconditional positive regard** to enable to client to also accept all elements of self.

b. **Process questions** with **immediacy** to facilitate experience of self in the here and now.

2. *Increase* ability to **authentically communicate self** with others while simultaneously respecting and enabling the other to also be fully themselves to reduce potential for relapse in [specific symptom: depression, anxiety, etc.].
Interventions:

a. Relate to client using **genuineness** and **authenticity** to create context in which it is safe for client to do the same.

b. **Immediacy** of how client is experienced by counselor in session to enhance ability to effectively relate to others as an authentic self.

Snapshot: Research and the Evidence Base

Quick Summary: Carl Rogers developed person-centered counseling based on extensive and ongoing research, but over time the humanistic counseling culture has been less enthusiastic about empirical study (McLeod, 2002). The most robust findings have been that the qualities of the counseling relationship espoused by person-centered counselors have been found to be one of the most significant common factors that predict positive outcome in all forms of counseling (see Chapter 2).

In his article "The Necessary and Sufficient Conditions of Therapeutic Change," Carl Rogers (1957) set forth a research hypothesis that would define his career and redefine the landscape of psychotherapy for generations to come. In the decades that followed this publication, he pursued a meticulous research agenda that attempted to determine whether his core conditions were (a) necessary and/or (b) sufficient. In his search for answers, Rogers was the first researcher to record counseling sessions (Brazier, 1996), providing the technological and ethical foundation for *process research*, the study of in-session counseling processes that promote or hinder change. Consistently, the vast majority of studies over the past four decades have found that the *client's* perception of the core conditions—more so than the counselor's or neutral third party's—is correlated with positive outcome (Kirschenbaum & Jourdan, 2005). However, although there is strong support for importance of empathy, positive regard, and congruence, most concede that the core conditions may be neither necessary nor sufficient (Kirschenbaum & Jourdan, 2005). Nonetheless, they are considered "extremely helpful" with virtually all clients.

As discussed in Chapter 2, common factors research has reintroduced and recontextualized the importance of Rogers's core conditions. Rather than particular models accounting for change, the common factors movement posits that similarities rather than differences across models are more closely correlated with successful counseling outcomes, with the counseling relationship accounting for 30% of outcome variance (Miller et al., 1997). These findings continue to be replicated in large-scale studies that compare person centered with cognitive-behavioral and psychodynamic counseling (Stiles, Barkham, Mellor-Clark, & Connell, 2008). Thus, although there has been a revival of Rogers's work, it is likely that the person-centered model will be practiced in combination with other humanistic, experiential, and/or existential approaches (Kirschenbaum & Jourdan, 2005).

Snapshot: Working With Diverse Populations

Quick Summary: Because they focus on the individual's subjective lived experience, the person-centered approaches tend to be easily adapted to various diverse populations; however, when working with clients who prefer a more structured, practical approach (e.g., the impoverished, men, and immigrants), the nondirective style and emphasis on affective expression may be a poor match.

A pioneer in cross-cultural exchange, Carl Rogers expanded the use of his approach to foster intergroup and international dialogue beginning in the 1970s, including Irish Catholics and Protestants and South African Blacks and Whites (Kirschenbaum, 2004). He used the same core conditions used in counseling to facilitate understanding of human differences in larger social settings. Thus, the ethos and legacy of person-centered counseling enthusiastically embraces diversity and advocacy work.

Despite using theories that are generally well suited for work with diverse clients, in day-to-day counseling practitioners must be extremely careful to not inadvertently force humanistic values and assumptions on clients, such as valuing emotional expression, preferring particular forms of "congruent" communication, or expecting different levels of emotional expression from women versus men (Gehart & Lyle, 2001). In particular, humanistic counselors should consider the following issues when working with diverse clients.

- *Nondirective versus directive:* Do I need to adapt my style to be more *directive* and *informative* to best meet this client's culturally based expectation of my role?
- *Valuing emotional expression:* Am I imposing a value of emotional expression that is not part of this client's existing value system? Does the client agree that they would like to increase, decrease, or change their forms of emotional expression, or am I imposing it on the basis of my theoretical lens? How sure am I and the client that increased emotional expression is necessary to address the presenting problem?
- *Expression of empathy:* What forms of expressing empathy are meaningful to the client? Does the client prefer expressions of empathy that are heartfelt, nonverbal, face-saving, or subtle?
- *Valuing self-actualization and autonomy:* Are self-actualization and autonomy a culturally and personally consistent goal for the client? Does the client believe that an

internal locus of control and evaluation is a desired outcome? Are relational and community connections equally or more valued?

- *Meaning seeking:* To what extent does the client believe that determining one's life purpose and meaning is an individual decision? Do religion, cultural expectations, or family play a greater role than the individual's wishes?

For example, empathy and congruent expression of emotion look different in one culture than another; furthermore, women and men and different personality types within the culture are likely to express emotion and empathy differently and interpret the emotions and empathetic expressions of others differently as well. Thus, very quickly, multiple elements of diversity make it difficult to fairly apply these ideas when intervening with clients, and thus humanistic counselors must proceed with caution because many of the embedded values and assumptions must be carefully translated across cultures.

Person-Centered Case Study

May, a 24-year-old, second-generation Taiwanese American, reports having panic attacks during her first year of veterinary school. She states, "Out of the blue, I just feel like the world is collapsing in on me; my heart races and I can hardly speak." She lives in a dorm on campus, her parents and younger brother living 3 hours away. She has always excelled academically, having enjoyed subjects such as art, history, and literature more than science and math. Her parents insisted that she choose a realistic and lucrative career, such as medicine, and they compromised on veterinary school because May loves animals. She says that she is happy with her choice to pursue veterinary medicine. Although highly acculturated in many ways, May is low key and cautious when expressing her emotions or discussing issues that may be shameful to her or her family. She always conducts herself with poise and grace. She has not told her parents that she is seeking counseling at the university health center.

Person-Centered Case Conceptualization

This case conceptualization was developed by selecting key concepts from the "Viewing: Case Conceptualization" section of this chapter. You can use any of the concepts in that section to develop a case conceptualization for this or other cases.

Stages of the Change Process

AF (adult female) is in the second stage of the change process and is beginning to see that there are problems, which are still seen as external to the self.

Experience and Communication of Self

AF very much experiences herself and others as static entities, and her description of herself is fixed: "I have always been X." At this time, it is hard for her to make sense of parts of herself that do not fit her image of herself.

Recognition of Feelings

AF is able to recognize some of her emotions but does so in a removed and nonexpressive manner that is common in Chinese culture, especially when discussing intimate or shameful topics.

Expression of Emotion

Even in session when discussing her panic attacks, AF tries to make it appear as if "everything under control." She describes her emotions almost as if they were happening to someone else or happened a long time ago, even positive emotions. Her expression of emotion is fairly typical of Taiwanese/Chinese culture; even so, this tendency may be playing a role in trying to manage her stress in graduate school.

Present Moment Experiencing

AF struggles to identify her present moment thoughts and emotions in session.

Personal Constructs and Facades

AF has developed a personal construct that entails being highly intelligent, as evidenced by her academic success, and always in control of her emotions; there is a general pursuit of perfection. The pressures of graduate school may be challenging this facade and social/family role and thereby contributing to her panic episodes.

Complexity and Contradictions

As is typical for someone of her age, AF has not embraced many of her inner contradictions and life's complexities. The new challenges of graduate school may be raising some of these issues for her, such as encountering failure and fear of the future. She has also abandoned her artistic and literary pursuits to focus on her chosen career, which may be creating anxiety by denying an essential and key part of her true self.

Perception of Problems and Responsibility

At this point, AF perceives the problem to be coming from the outside, almost out of nowhere. She suspects some of the stresses of graduate school "might" be contributing but is not convinced.

Peak Experience and Flow

AF does not describe having peak or flow experiences nearly as often; she associates these primarily with her former interest in art.

Person-Centered Treatment Plan

Initial Phase of Treatment (First One to Two Sessions)
Initial Phase Counseling Tasks

1. *Develop working counseling relationship. Diversity note*: Maintain a more low-key emotional tone and careful approach to potentially shameful topics.
   Relationship building approach:
   a. Use **unconditional positive regard**, **accurate empathy**, and **genuineness** to establish the necessary conditions for change.

2. *Assess individual, systemic, and broader cultural dynamics. Diversity note*: Carefully adapt assessment for Taiwanese American norms for expression of emotion and self-constructs, considering overall high level of acculturation.
   Assessment strategies:
   a. Assess for ability to identify, express, and experience **emotions** in **present moment**.
   b. Assess for ability to experience self as an **unfolding process**, accept proactive **responsibility** for problems, embrace **complexity** and **contradictions**, and experience **flow**.

Initial Phase Client Goal
1. *Decrease* overall sense of stress and anxiety to reduce panic episodes.
   Interventions:
   a. Help client **identify, own**, and **accept emotions** underlying panic; instruct client to do so on a daily basis with journal.
   b. Help client develop a proactive and **competent sense of self** in relation to **complexity** and challenge that are part of beginning graduate school.

Working Phase of Treatment (One or More Sessions)
Working Phase Counseling Tasks

1. *Monitor quality of the working alliance. Diversity note*: Attend to relationship and conflict patterns related to diversity factors.

(continued)

Assessment Intervention:
  a. Assess for client's ability to **express self genuinely** and constructively disagree with counselor; Session Rating Scale.

Working Phase Client Goals

1. *Increase* ability to **recognize** and constructively **express full range of emotions in culturally appropriate ways** to reduce panic.
   Interventions:
   a. **Empathetically reflect** unacknowledged feelings that are difficult for the client to express; address cultural and family rules related to emotional expression.
   b. Assist client experiencing emotions in the present moment using **immediacy** in session.

2. *Increase* ability to recognize **authentic self** without **facades** to reduce tendency for high achieving perfectionism.
   Interventions:
   a. **Process questions** that address less desirable aspects of self to enable client to clarify inner experience of self.
   b. **Immediacy** to help client experience self in relationship to counselor.

3. *Increase* ability to view self as **responsible** for her life situation and **active agent** in making changes to reduce the helplessness associated with her "out-of-the-blue" panic episodes.
   Interventions:
   a. **Confront contradictions** related to perfectionism and powerlessness as they relate to both family and school contexts.
   b. **Immediacy** to help client experience sense of agency in counseling relationship and present experiences.

Closing Phase of Treatment
Closing Phase Counseling Tasks

1. *Develop aftercare plan and maintain gains. Diversity note*: Plan should address continuing stress of remaining in graduate school.
   Intervention:
   a. **Process questions** to help client identify how best to manage potential future challenges; terminate only after client has developed ability to reflect on self without assistance.

Closing Phase Client Goals

1. *Increase* ability to experience **self as an unfolding, evolving, and complex process** without holding on to **personal constructs** and a need for perfection to reduce potential for relapse in panic symptoms.
   Interventions:
   a. **Unconditional positive regard** to enable client to also accept all elements of self.
   b. **Process questions** with immediacy to facilitate experience of self in the here and now.

2. *Increase* ability to **authentically communicate self** with families while simultaneously respecting and enabling the other to also be fully themselves to reduce potential for relapse in panic or perfectionism.
   Interventions:
   a. Relate to client using **genuineness** and **authenticity** to create context in which it is safe for client to do the same.
   b. **Immediacy** of how client is experienced by counselor in session to enhance ability to effectively relate to others, especially family, as an authentic self.

ONLINE RESOURCES

Associations and Training Institutes

Association for the Development of the Person-Centered Approach
www.adpca.org

Association for Humanistic Psychology
www.ahpweb.org

American Psychological Association, Division 32: Humanistic Psychology
www.apa.org/divisions/div32

Carl Rogers Website
www.carlrogers.info

Natalie Rogers: Expressive Arts Therapy
www.nrogers.com

World Association for Person-Centered and Experiential Psychotherapy and Counseling
www.pce-world.org

Journals

Journal of Humanistic Psychology
www.ahpweb.org/pub/journal/menu.html

Journal of the World Association for Person-Centered and Experiential Psychotherapy and Counseling
www.pce-world.org/pcep-journal.html

Person-Centered Journal
www.adpca.org/Journal/journalindex.htm

References

*Asterisk indicates recommended introductory readings.

Axline, V. (1989). *Play therapy.* London: Ballantine Books. (Original work published 1947)

Bratton, S. C., Ray, D. C., Edwards, N. A., & Landreth, G. (2009). Child-centered play therapy (CCPT): Theory, research, and practice. *Person-Centered and Experiential Psychotherapies, 8*(4), 266–281.

Brazier, D. D. (1996). The post-Rogerian therapy of Robert Carkhuff. *Amida Trust.* Available: http://www.amidatrust.com/article_carkhuff.html

Brown, L. S. (2007). Empathy, genuineness—and the dynamics of power: A feminist responds to Rogers. *Psychotherapy: Theory, Research, Practice, Training, 44*(3), 257–259. doi:10.1037/0033-3204.44.3.257

Carkhuff, R. R. (1969). *Helping and human relations: A primer for lay and professional helpers.* New York: Holt, Rinehart and Winston.

Carkhuff, R. R. (2000). *The art of helping* (8th ed.). Amherst, MA: Human Resource Development Press.

Gehart, D. (2010). *Mastering competencies in family therapy: A practical approach to theory and clinical case documentation.* Pacific Grove, CA: Brooks/Cole.

Gehart, D. R., & Lyle, R. R. (2001). Client experience of gender in therapeutic relationships: An interpretive ethnography. *Family Process, 40,* 443–458.

Gehart, D., & McCollum, E. (2008). Teaching therapeutic presence: A mindfulness-based approach. In S. Hick & T. Bien (Eds.), *Mindfulness and the therapeutic relationship* (pp. 176–194). New York: Guilford.

Geller, S. M., & Greenberg, L. S. (2002). Therapeutic presence: Therapists' experience of presence in the psychotherapy encounter. *Person-Centered and Experiential Psychotherapies, 1,* 71–86.

Gendlin, E. T. (1984). The client's client: The edge of awareness. In R. F. Levant & J. M. Shlien (Eds.), *Client-centered therapy and the person-centered approach: New directions in theory, research, and practice* (pp. 76–107). Westport, CT: Praeger/Greenwood Publishing Group.

Gendlin, E. T., Beebe, J., Cassens, J., Klein, M., & Oberlander, M. (1968). Focusing ability in psychotherapy personality, and creativity. In J. M. Shlien (Ed.), *Research in psychotherapy* (Vol. 1, pp. 217–241). Washington, DC: American Psychological Association. doi:10.1037/10546-012

Hill, C. (2007). My personal reactions to Rogers (1957): The facilitative but neither necessary nor sufficient conditions of therapeutic personality change. *Psychotherapy: Theory, Research, Practice, Training, 44,* 260–264. doi:10.1037/0033-3204.44.3.260

Kirschenbaum, H. (2004). Carl Rogers's life and work: An assessment on the 100th anniversary of his birth. *Journal of Counseling and Development, 82,* 116–124.

Kirschenbaum, H., & Jourdan, A. (2005). The current status of Carl Rogers and the person-centered approach. *Psychotherapy: Theory, Research, Practice, Training, 42,* 37–51.

Mahrer, A. (2007). To a large extent, the field got it wrong: New learnings from a new look at an old classic. *Psychotherapy: Theory, Research, Practice, Training, 44,* 274–278. doi:0.1037/0033-3204.44.3.274

Maslow, A. (1954). *Motivation and personality.* New York: Harper.

McDonough, S. I., Kreitzer, M. J., & Bell, I. R. (2004). Fostering a healing presence and investigating its mediators. *Journal of Alternative and Complementary Medicine, 10,* S25–S41.

McLeod, J. (2002). Research policy and practice in person-centered and experiential therapy: Restoring coherence. *Person-Centered and Experiential Psychotherapies, 1*(1–2), 87–101.

Miller, S. D., Duncan, B. L., & Hubble, M. (1997). *Escape from Babel: Toward a unifying language for psychotherapy practice.* New York: Norton.

Miller, S. D., Duncan, B. L., & Hubble, M. A. (2004). Beyond integration: The triumph of outcome over process in clinical practice. *Psychotherapy in Australia, 10*(2), 2–19.

Rogers, C. (1939). *The clinical treatment of the problem child.* Boston: Houghton Mifflin.

Rogers, C. (1942). *Counseling and psychotherapy: Newer concepts in practice.* New York: Houghton Mifflin.

Rogers, C. (1951). *Client-centered counseling.* Cambridge, MA: Riverside Press.

*Rogers, C. (1957). The necessary and sufficient conditions of personality change. *Journal of Consulting Psychology, 21*[2], 95–103.

*Rogers, C. (1961). *On becoming a person: A counselor's view of psychocounseling.* London: Constable.

Rogers, C. (1969). *Freedom to learn: A view of what education might become.* Columbus, OH: Merrill.

Rogers, C. (1980). *Way of being.* Boston: Houghton Mifflin.

*Rogers, C. (2007). The necessary and sufficient conditions of personality change. *Psychotherapy: Theory, Research, Practice, Training, 44,* 240–248. doi:10.1037/0033-3204.44.3.240 (Reprint of 1957 article).

Rogers, N. (1993). Person-centered expressive arts thearpy. *Creation Spirituality,* March/April, 28–30.

Rogers, N. (1997). *The creative connection: Expressive arts as healing.* Palo Alto, CA: Science and Behavior Books.

Stiles, W., Barkham, M., Mellor-Clark, J., & Connell, J. (2008). Effectiveness of cognitive-behavioural, person-centred, and psychodynamic therapies in UK primary-care routine practice: Replication in a larger sample. *Psychological Medicine: A Journal of Research in Psychiatry and the Allied Sciences, 38*(5), 677–688. doi:10.1017/S0033291707001511

Truax, C. B., & Carkhuff R. R. (1967). *Towards effective counseling and psychotherapy.* Chicago: Aldine.

Wachtel, P. L. (2007). Carl Rogers and the larger context of therapeutic thought. *Psychotherapy: Theory, Research, Practice, Training, 44*(3), 279–284. doi:10.1037/0033-3204.44.3.279

CHAPTER
7

Existential Counseling and Psychotherapy

Those who have a "why" to live, can bear with almost any "how."

—Viktor Frankl

Lay of the Land

Existential counseling is grounded in existential philosophy, which addresses questions related to "existence": What is the purpose and meaning of life? Why do we suffer? What is death? Having much in common, there are several distinct strands of existential counseling (Cooper, 2003):

- *Daseinanalysis:* Daseinanalysis (pronounced "da-zine-analysis") employs a more analytic approach to help clients open up to their world and to explore how their way-of-being in the world contributes to their suffering.
- *Logotherapy:* Singular in the existential approaches, logotherapy is based on the belief that life is inherently meaningful.
- *American existential-humanistic approach:* In contrast to Daseinanalysis, which emphasizes the in-the-world nature of being human, the American existential-humanistic approach focuses on the individual's need to be true to his or her own subjective experience, having a more inward focus.
- *British School of Existential Analysis:* Representing a diverse group of practitioners, the more recently developed British School of Existential Analysis includes practices that explore four dimensions of existence, including physical, social, personal, and spiritual.

Because these existential approaches share most of their basic premises and techniques, they will be presented together in this chapter.

In a Nutshell: The Least You Need to Know

Existential counseling and psychotherapy is not for the faint of heart or those who prefer simple, black-and-white life answers. As the name suggests, existential counseling and psychotherapy specifically focuses on helping people to deal with *existential* issues, such as finding life meaning, dealing with crises in identity, confronting our ultimate aloneness, and managing the "big picture" anxieties: What should I do with my life?

What have I done with my life? Why on earth didn't I do that with my life? Is there really a God/god/Goddess or someone—besides me—who is responsible for all of this? In short, existential counseling "involves assisting people to come to terms with the dilemmas of living" (Van Deurzen, 2002, p. xiiv).

Existential counselors contend that most of the issues for which people come to counseling have an existential root. By addressing these as well as the symptoms, the presenting problem as well as deeper life issues of meaning and significance are also addressed, resulting in longer-lasting effects of counseling. The existential approach is more of a philosophical stance than a concrete set of techniques for how to conduct a session. This philosophy emphasizes that humans are free and responsible for their choices and actions. Through the existential counseling process, clients learn to consciously define themselves and their life rather than feel the victim of circumstance. Rather than "cure" mental illness or psychological conditions, existential counseling helps people to live more authentic lives that have meaning and purpose.

The Juice: Significant Contributions to the Field

If you remember one thing from this chapter, it should be ...

I-Thou Relationship

> If *Thou* is said, the *I* of the combination *I-Thou* is said along with it.
> If *It* is said, the *I* of the combination *I-It* is said along with it.
> The primary word *I-Thou* can only be spoken with the whole being.
> The primary word *I-It* can never be spoken with the whole being. (Buber, 1958, p. 1)

When studying to become a counselor—if you are lucky—a handful of readings will strike like dynamite and shatter the foundation of what you think you know. I have come to believe this is due as much to reader readiness and timing as it is to the wisdom of the text. Martin Buber's (1958) *I and Thou* was one of these cataclysmic readings for me. When I first read it, I carried it everywhere and read it whenever I had a free moment, whether at the gym, filling my gas tank, eating a snack, or waiting for a class. Much to the annoyance of everyone in my life, I was so excited I couldn't stop talking about it. Therefore, years later as a new professor, I wanted my students to read it and have the same rock-your-life experience. Instead, they hated it. They revolted, saying it was indecipherable poetry that had no bearing on counseling or the modern world for that matter. I am sure they sold their books back to the bookstore before the end of the semester. Taking a hint, I never assigned it again. However, being crafty and persistent, I developed a related experiential assignment that students have come to love using the same I-Thou principles. But, before I share it with you, we need to define some terms.

Buber viewed existence as a *relational encounter*. Humans can be in relation in one of two ways: I-Thou (*Ich-Du* in the original German) or *I-It* (*Ich-Es* in German). In the I-Thou encounter, a person experiences the other as a fully independent subject (person or agent); each is fully authentic and receptive to the other's authenticity in this moment. This encounter is not characterized by communication of information but rather is a profound moment of witnessing and beholding the other, generally without words, as it is a state of being. Common experiences of I-Thou encounters include two lovers, an observer and a nature scene, a mother and an infant, or a religious seeker and God. In contrast, during an I-It encounter, the person engages the other as an object, more of a mental representation or class of person than an independent, authentic entity. In an I-It relationship, a person essentially relates to his or her conceptualization of the other rather than the actual other. Most of human life is spent in I-It encounters, whether ordering lunch at restaurant, diagnosing a client, or planning a wedding.

Buber maintained that human existence oscillates between these two modes of being, with I-Thou moments increasingly rare and devalued in modern cultures that emphasize efficiency, productivity, and social class. Furthermore, Buber emphasized that humans experience their humanity, purpose, and deepest joy only in the I-Thou moments. Humanistic and existential counselors and psychotherapists use Buber's distinction of I-Thou to conceptualize the counselor–client relationship as an I-Thou encounter in which each encounters the other as a separate, authentic self.

After my students told me that Buber's writings were too esoteric, I asked them to instead engage in mini "experiments" with I-Thou encounters. Over the course of the week, I asked them to choose three people—a stranger, an acquaintance, and an intimate other—and to strive to have an I-Thou and I-It encounter with each (for the stranger, they may need to do it with two different people). Granted this is a bit staged, but surprisingly almost all students returned the next week reporting that it was easiest to have an I-Thou encounter with a stranger, such as a store clerk or a person on the street. Friends and family members often didn't pick up on the students' attempts or were guarded because they feared that a "heavy topic" was being raised. In contrast, a stranger, although often caught off guard and not expecting a gesture of genuineness, tended to be more willing to be seen and more receptive. Perhaps this explains why counseling and psychotherapy have developed a strong tradition of privacy and confidentiality.

Rumor Has It: The People and Their Stories

Viktor Frankl

Born in Vienna to a Jewish family, Frankl, his wife, and his parents were sent to concentration camps, including Auschwitz and Türkeim. He was the only person to survive the camps besides a sister who escaped to Australia. As a trained psychiatrist, he was asked to assist newcomers in coping with shock and grief and eventually set up a suicide watch program in the camps. He worked to help fellow prisoners overcome despondency and hopelessness. His extraordinary experiences in concentration camps led him to develop *logotherapy*, therapy through meaning. He believed that even in the most dehumanizing, painful, and absurd circumstances, humans can find purpose, meaning, and the will to live. It was this sense of meaning that made the difference between life and death for many in the camps, determining who had the will to survive. After the war, he wrote *Trotzdem Ja zu Leben Sagen* (Saying Yes to Life Despite It All), which was translated into English as *Man's Search for Meaning* (Frankl, 1963). His later works included *The Doctor and the Soul* (1965) and *The Unheard Cry for Meaning* (1978).

Martin Buber

An Austrian-born Jewish philosopher, Martin Buber (1958) is most famous for his 1923 work *I and Thou*. He held a position at the University of Frankfurt am Main when Hitler came to power in 1938 and fled to Israel and settled in Jerusalem, where he continued his work on religious existential philosophy.

Rollo May

Born in Ohio, Rollo May (1961, 1969, 1973, 1981, 1983) had a difficult childhood; his parents divorced, and his sister was treated for schizophrenia. May was a key figure for bringing existentialism to the United States and applying the ideas in psychotherapy. His work emphasized that resisting anxiety takes courage and that our choices determine and shape the type of person we become. May founded the Saybrook Graduate School in San Francisco.

Irvin Yalom

Born in Washington, D.C., to a poor Jewish family, Irvin Yalom pursued a career in psychiatry, serving on the faculty at Stanford University. His existential approach (Yalom, 1980) identifies "four givens" of existence: death, freedom, existential isolation, and meaninglessness. In addition, his *Theory and Practice of Group Psychotherapy* (Yalom, 1970) is a highly influential text used by group therapy practitioners from virtually all theoretical approaches.

Big Picture: Overview of Counseling Process

The purpose of existential counseling is to help clients take responsibility for the circumstances in their lives and to make conscious choices that enable them to live more meaningful, authentic lives. Yalom (1980) further clarifies that existential counseling helps clients address the following four areas: (a) death and anxiety, (b) freedom and responsibility, (c) isolation and relationship, and (d) meaninglessness. Through an I-Thou, authentic connection (Buber, 1958) with their counselor, clients are encouraged to identify and confront the existential anxieties that underlie the problems and concerns they bring to counseling. More so than other humanistic-phenomenological approaches, existential counseling emphasizes insight in a style reminiscent of psychodynamic counseling theories (Yalom, 1980). Although existential counselors do not define progressive stages of counseling, in general there are three phases, which clients may move between many times while in counseling:

- *Phase 1:* Identify how the presenting problems related to the client's existential assumptions and beliefs.
- *Phase 2:* Clients examine and redefine attitudes regarding death, freedom, anxiety, responsibility, choice, meaning, meaninglessness, isolation, and so on.
- *Phase 3:* Clients take specific action to lead a more fulfilling, meaningful, and self-actualized life.

Making Connection: Counseling Relationship
I-Thou Relationship Between Counselor and Client

Although much of the counseling relationship will involve I-It encounters (Buber, 1958; see the "I and Thou Relationship" section under "Juice"), the counseling relationship involves cultivating the type of presence that characterizes I-Thou connections. In counseling, the I-Thou encounter generally takes the form of the counselor bearing witness to the client's humanity and struggle with the human condition. These are often silent moments in which the client feels "seen" and "heard" at a profound level. In taking an I-Thou stance, the counselor presupposes that clients have the ability to cope with life's difficult realities without overreliance on the counselor for encouragement and support. The counselor demonstrates empathy and concern but also, above all, trust in the client's ability to engage life in increasingly authentic ways.

Here-and-Now Presence

Existential counselors use their quality of presence (Bugental 1987; Krug, 2009) to help clients increase self-awareness, develop insight, take responsibility, and make choices. They believe that focusing clients on present moment, here-and-now experiences is the most effective way to help people change how they relate to themselves and others. Existential counselors focus on both *intrapersonal* (e.g., preverbal, kinesthetic, and tacit dimensions of experience) and *interpersonal* (e.g., safe and intimate relationships) forms of presence. Counselors encourage clients to identify what they are feeling and experiencing in the present moment and to examine their fears, anxieties, and yearnings that may underlie these feelings.

Promoting Responsibility and Independence

Existential counselors relate to clients in such a way as to maximize their sense of responsibility and independence, often by way of having them confront their ultimate *existential isolation* and separateness from others, including the counselor (Yalom, 1980). Although existential counselors may empathize with clients, they are careful to never imply that "I'm right there with you" because, ultimately, no one is. Existential counselors are more willing to allow their clients to experience the fullness and reality of this isolation—not to be cruel and uncaring—so that clients can live more authentically and will be motivated to make better choices. Thus, existential counselors avoid being overly reassuring, overly supportive, or overly helpful so that clients feel a stronger pull to take responsibility for their own lives.

The Viewing: Case Conceptualization

Existential counselors do not use formal methods for case conceptualization and instead explore the following universal and existential concerns in clients' lives:

- Meaning, meaninglessness, and purpose
- Freedom and responsibility
- Existential anxiety and guilt

- Death anxiety
- Existential angst
- Purpose of neuroses

Meaning, Meaninglessness, and Life Purpose

Most existentialists believe life is inherently *meaningless* (Yalom, 1980). They do not believe that there is a grand design to life or that we are each here with a specific purpose, thus differing with humanistic counselors who believe that all people share the general life purpose of self-actualization (Rogers, 1961). *Christian existentialists*, who draw primarily on the work of Kierkegaard (an existential philosopher who was also a devout Christian), believe that each person has free will and must *choose* to take a "leap of faith" in the face of life's apparent meaninglessness (Bretherton, 2006). Nonetheless, existentialists recognize that without meaning and purpose, a person is adrift in life. Thus, they believe that each person must consciously choose sources of meaning and purpose: "The meaning of life differs from man to man, from day to day and from hour to hour. What matters, therefore, is not the meaning of life in general but rather the specific meaning of a person's life at a given moment" (Frankl, 1963 p. 113). Frankl maintained that this *will to meaning* is the primary drive in a person's life.

Existential therapists focus their work on helping clients find life *Meaning*—that's "meaning" with a capital "M." They help people step back and look at the big picture of their life and ask difficult questions, such as the following: Is this *really* what I want for my life? Am I living a life that has meaning for me? Is this the life I dreamed of? If not, why not and how do I get where I want to go? If you are new to the practice of counseling, these may seem like obvious question that all counselors address. However, most clients come in crisis—such as a pending divorce, lost job, or psychotic break—or because of significant problems getting through the day—such as too depressed to get up, go to work, and have a conversation with the spouse and child over dinner. Much of the work in counseling addresses struggles in daily living—micro-level problems—and it can be hard to shift focus to the macro-level, existential issues.

Recent research on happiness by positive psychologists as well as the mental health recovery movement emphasize the importance of living a life with meaning and significance. In researching people who seem happier than the average, these people report that they feel their life has meaning and greater purpose (Seligman, 2002). Similarly, in recovery-oriented work with persons diagnosed with severe and persistent mental illness, the primary goal is to restore a sense of meaning and purpose more so than reduce symptom frequency; once a person has meaning and purpose, he or she is more likely to move toward recovery (Davidson, Tondora, O'Connell, Lawless, & Rowe, 2009).

Working with people on life meaning can involve several steps and stages. First, counselors need to help clients identify sources of meaning and purpose. For some, this is easy; they can quickly articulate these even if they are taking little action in the present. These clients may have abandoned life dreams and goals when settled for a more practical career or started a family earlier than planned. For others, identifying significant and sincere sources of meaning is an extremely difficult task. In some cases, they never clearly articulated any type of purpose, dream, or other meaning in childhood and adolescence, perhaps because they or their parents were more focused with following what was socially expected rather than relying on an internally generated life direction. For these clients, counselors need to move more slowly and creatively to help them discover what inspires and moves them, which may be a new life experience.

Once potential sources of life meaning are identified, clarified, and owned by the client, the next step is to determine how best to translate these into real-world action. In most cases, wholeheartedly pursuing these dreams would be destructive on many levels: quitting a high-paying job that supports a family of four to pursue life as a painter or to sail the globe may create more distress than joy. Thus, in many cases, the task becomes identifying ways to create that meaning within the fabric of the current life, perhaps through hobbies, a shift in career, a new relationship, or daily practices. In other cases, creating a life with purpose means reengaging in one's existing relationships, career, and pastimes from a new perspective and openness that is meaningful. The classic example of this is the father and husband who is overinvested in his work life and underinvested in his family; a shift of perspective and scheduling priorities often creates a dramatic shift in sense of connection and life purpose. Similarly, in the case study at the end of this chapter, the counselor helps Ben, a 34-year-old gay man struggling with alcohol issues, find more effective and substantial sources of meaning in his life, which had become narrowly defined by partying and recovering from partying on the weekends.

Freedom and Responsibility

Frankl's (1963) advice for living responsibly is as follows: "Live life as if you were living already for the second time and as if you had acted the first time as wrongly as you are about to act now!" (p. 114). Existentialists maintain that even though humans have certain limits to their freedom (e.g., they cannot control externals), they always have the freedom to choose how they *respond* to a situation. Frankl's role model for how one can choose to respond with dignity and integrity even in the most horrific life experiences—he survived four concentration camps—quickly quells quibbling on the subject. Ultimately, a person's greatest freedom is how he or she chooses to interpret (make meaning) and respond to life circumstances. Yalom (1980) further explains that humans aren't just free; they are "doomed" to freedom in that freedom implies responsibility. The freedom to make meaning and respond also implies responsibility for how one shapes and directs one's life. A person is responsible not only for actions taken but also for actions *not* taken: one's failure to act. May (2009) further explains, "Freedom does not come automatically; it is achieved. And it is not gained at a single bound; it must be achieved each day.... The basic step in achieving inward freedom is 'choosing one's self'" (p. 125).

When initially developing a case conceptualization, counselors listen for how clients describe their life circumstances: Are they victims of life, or are they the creator of their realities? When life gets off course, whom do they blame, and to whom do they turn to get back on course? Do they feel like they have control and freedom over how they respond, or do others "make them" respond badly? Do they feel that they have freedom without responsibility? It doesn't take long to get a sense of how fully a person has embraced his or her existential sense of freedom and the associated responsibility.

Capacity for Self-Awareness and Consciousness

May (2009) identifies the capacity for self-awareness as the hallmark quality of being human. Relatively early in life, humans are able to distinguish between "I" and the rest of the world. This awareness of self enables people to be aware of others and their desires, time, and its implications for the self; to examine history and its implications; and even to reflect on the self and awareness itself. In working with clients, counselors assess the extent to which a client is self-aware of thoughts, feelings, choices, desires, and actions and how these affect others. Promoting awareness of all aspects of being becomes a central goal in existential counseling.

Death Anxiety

Existentialists maintain that a person's fear of death—an undeniable and unalterable aspect of human existence—plays a major role in their psychopathology (Yalom, 1980). Virtually all humans are in denial about death to one extent or another and erect defenses to avoid this reality. The type of defense against death shapes a person's character structure, such as attempting to delay it by living healthfully, focusing on religious practices designed to transcend death, worrying about safety and health, living as though one is immune, or keeping oneself so busy that there is no time to think about it. Generally, one of these or similar strategies work to keep the death anxiety at bay. However, in cases of psychopathology, the person has not found an effective approach for managing this fear. When assessing clients, existential counselors consider the following questions:

- How does the client's presenting symptoms serve to manage his or her existential death anxiety?
- What are the beliefs—and sources of the beliefs—that fuel the client's particular fears of death?
- Is the client able to speak about death, fear of death, or his or her view of death?

Although existential counselors don't necessarily rush to the topic in the early phases, they use clients' description of their problems and how they handle them to identify how the fear of death shapes the presenting problem. However, they encourage clients to muster the courage to embrace the fact that they—and those they love—will die. The more deeply one acknowledges this fact, the more likely the person is to take responsibility for life, make better choices, and create a meaningful life. Living without awareness of life limits is more likely to lead to irresponsible and more regrettable life decisions.

Existential Angst

Existentialists posit that all people experience *existential angst* or *existential anxiety*, which should never be confused with garden-variety neurotic anxiety you read about in your diagnosis class (May, 2009). The existential versions are part of the package of human existence and refer to anxieties that often underlie and fuel other concerns and issues: the stress that comes from engaging freedom, choice, isolation, meaninglessness, death, and so on. The more aware one is of these existential realities—particularly the fact that each of us is free to make choices and are responsible then for who we become, how we affect others, and the quality of life we live—the *more* one experiences existential angst. When experiencing moments of existential angst, a person experiences intense awareness of how each decision irrevocably shapes one's life—and yet one cannot avoid choice and the heavy burden of freedom. In general, existential anxiety is not considered pathological—like the anxieties listed in the *Diagnostic and Statistical Manual of Mental Disorders*—but are considered *normal anxieties* (Reeves, 1977) and an essential part of conscious living. In fact, for most clients, existential angst is a sign that a person is becoming more aware of choices, freedoms, and responsibilities that are inherent to the human condition; by facing these existential anxieties, a person develops a stronger sense of being and affirms the self in the world.

Purpose of Neuroses

May (1961) asserts that every person (plant and animal for that matter) is "centered in herself [or himself] and an attack on this center is an attack on her or his existence itself" (p. 74). Therefore, he views presenting problems, anxieties, and neuroses as serving the purpose of preserving a person's centeredness, sense of self, and, ultimately, his or her own existence. For example, fears and neurotic anxieties are a person's response to avoid a perceived threat, anger and aggression are an attempt to protect the self by attacking a threat, and depression is an attempt to retreat from a threat. By viewing symptoms as a strategy for preserving the self against the perceived threat of harm or annihilation, existential counselors can quickly identify where pivotal choices need to be made and responsibility needs to be taken. For example, in the case study at the end of this chapter, the counselor helps Ben see how he uses alcohol to create an artificial and precarious sense of meaning and avoid directly confronting more critical existential realities, such as giving up early on two of his greatest life dreams.

Targeting Change: Goal Setting

The goals in existential counseling focus on encouraging clients to live more authentic lives by changing how they relate to broader existential anxieties and generate life meaning. The approach focuses on long-term changes at an existential level rather than the everyday symptoms with which the client may have presented. For example, if a woman reports feeling depressed after losing a relationship, the goals of treatment would target changing how she experiences being alone and/or how being in a romantic relationship affects her identity rather than focusing simply on reducing her depressed mood. Existential counselors maintain that it is the underlying meaning of the problem that needs to change more so than the person's life circumstances. Thus, early and middle phase goals are smaller steps along the way to achieving broader life goals.

The goals often address issues such as the following:

- Increasing a person's sense of meaning and purpose
- Reducing existential anxiety and/or fear of being alone

- Creating greater acceptance of death, loss, or change
- Developing a sense of identity that is less dependent on externals, such as a job, financial status, relationship status, and so on

Examples of working or closing phase client goals include the following:

- Increase ability to generate a sense of meaning and purpose in his or her life that is less dependent on the opinion of others
- Increase ability to manage existential anxieties about being single
- Increase acceptance of the process of aging

The Doing: Interventions

Similar to person-centered counselors, existential counselors do not use a standard set of interventions but instead rely more heavily on the person of the counselor to promote change. That said, there are several areas of particular focus in which they use their presence to help clients become more authentic and self-aware. These are discussed next.

Search for Meaning and Promoting Choice

"We must never forget that we may also find meaning in life even when confronted with a hopeless situation…. When we are no longer able to change a situation—just think of an incurable disease such as inoperable cancer—we are challenged to change ourselves" (Frankl, 1963, p. 116). Existential counselors help clients find meaning and purpose when facing life difficulties by redirecting their energies to changing how they *choose* to view and respond rather than lamenting an unchangeable situation. Counselors may do this by focusing on the spiritual dimension, existential elements, or any available source of reinterpretation. For example, when a client is diagnosed with terminal cancer, an existential counselor may shift the client's attention to *living* the last months with dignity.

Common strategies for choosing meanings that focus on changing oneself when the situation is unchangeable include the following:

- *Spiritual perspective:* Using religious and spiritual beliefs to view and recontextualize the situation so that there is more hope and meaning (e.g., there is life after death)
- *Existential philosophical perspective:* Offering existential philosophical views of death, isolation, responsibility, and freedom to promote greater agency (e.g., I am responsible for how I approach and free to choose how that will be)
- *Relational perspective:* Generating purpose and meaning by examining how one's choice affects significant others (e.g., I will live these last 3 months with courage because my children and husband need me to)
- *Identity preservation:* Deciding to take action that is congruent with one's view of self (e.g., I have lived my life with dignity and courage, and I shall approach death in the same way)

Acknowledging Existential Isolation

Although isolation comes in many forms, *existential isolation* refers to "an unbridgeable gulf between oneself and any other being" (Yalom, 1980, p. 355). Existentialists maintain that acknowledging this isolation is critical for creating life meaning and taking responsibility for one's life. "Deep loneliness is inherent in the act of self-creation" (p. 357), and thus a person isn't motivated to take active responsibility for who he or she is and becomes until he or she accepts the gravity of separateness. Early in the counseling process, counselors find appropriate moments to point out how ignoring existential isolation is contributing to problems in a client's life. Common examples include not consciously acknowledging one's own desires because a loved one (e.g., spouse, parent, or friend) would disapprove, making poor decisions to avoid feeling lonely, and staying in abusive relationships.

Defining and Affirming Self: Achieving Freedom

May (1961) discourages counselors from focusing on the *whys* and *hows* of the presenting problem and instead to focus on the intricacies of the "living, existing person here in the room with me" (p. 74). Viewing symptoms as perceived threats to the self, the counselor's attention is directed to gaining an understanding of the client's *subjective* awareness of self and the perceived threats to the self. The counselor encourages *self-affirmation* in those contexts in which the client feels threatened. For example, if a client is experiencing "stress" at work, the counselor would help the client identify the ways in which he or she perceives threats to the self, sort out existential from garden-variety neurotic anxieties, and encourage him or her to make decisions to take responsibility for preserving his or her sense of self and centeredness in the work context.

Courage and Encouragement

Much of what an existential counselor does is promote the *courage* required to be fully aware of one's own humanity (Frankl, 1963; May, 2009). Facing the reality of death, loneliness, and responsibility for one's life is no picnic. It's almost human nature to run from such truths. Yet being human demands that one face these realities at some point in life. To do so, we all need encouragement; that is exactly what the existential counselor offers: the encouragement to go to the places that scare you most. Ultimately, that's all the counselor can offer because simple, easy answers aren't available for existential questions, such as why are we here, who am I, and how should I live my life? Much of the encouragement is communicated nonverbally by the counselor demonstrating courage to substantively explore these issues. In the case study at the end of this chapter, the counselor uses encouragement throughout treatment to help Ben examine the unpleasant effects alcohol is having on his life and to have him revisit life dreams he had long given up on.

Love and Belongingness

Aware of the ultimate reality of isolation, existential counselors are all the more aware of the importance of human connection. May (2009; Reeves, 1977) identifies love as an important element of being human. Requiring a fair degree of self-actualization, May's specific definition of love is to delight in the presence of another, affirming the other's value and development as much as one's own. As experienced by the self-actualized person, love involves conscious will, freedom, self-awareness, empathy, choice, and courage. He warns that "when 'love' is engaged in for the purpose of vanquishing loneliness, it accomplishes its purpose only at the price of increased emptiness for both persons" (May, 2009, p. 183). Such love is simply a form of dependence. Instead, May claims that "you can only love in proportion to your capacity for independence" (p. 183). In session, existential counselors use this definition of love to help clients develop loving relationships that reflect a conscious choice to delight in being with the other while minimizing demands and dependency.

Paradoxical Intention

Frankl (1963) made a distinction between existential (normal) fear and neurotic fears and used different techniques for both: "A realistic fear, like the fear of death, cannot be tranquilized away by its psychodynamic interpretation; on the other hand, a neurotic fear, such as agoraphobia, cannot be cured by philosophical understanding" (p. 124). For neurotic and phobic fears, he recommends *paradoxical intention*, in which the client is invited to imagine and/or intend to have happen that which is feared. Frankl emphasized that this technique must be used in a playful, humorous spirit that promotes self-detachment. For example, if a person tends to panic in public places, the client would be asked to put together a detailed plan for going to a public place and doubling the intensity of the panic attack—the client is explicitly asked to make it bigger, more dramatic, and more outrageous than before. This assignment has the paradoxical effect of enabling the client to realize control over what seemed uncontrollable. This technique is also used in cognitive-behavioral and systemic family approaches.

Putting It All Together: Existential Treatment Plan Template

Use this treatment plan template for developing a plan for clients with depressive, anxious, or compulsive types of presenting problems. Depending on the specific client, presenting problem, and clinical context, the goals and interventions in this template may need to be modified only slightly or significantly; you are encouraged to significantly revise the plan as needed. For the plan to be useful, goals and techniques should be written to target specific beliefs, behaviors, and emotions that the client is experiencing. The more specific, the more useful it will be to you.

Treatment Plan

Initial Phase of Treatment (First One to Three Sessions)
Initial Phase Counseling Tasks

1. *Develop working counseling relationship. Diversity note:* Adapt expectations of independence and responsibility based on cultural, gender, and sexual orientation norms. *Relationship building intervention*:
   a. Create opportunities for **I-Thou** encounters and experiencing; promote **independence** and **responsibility**.

2. *Assess individual, systemic, and broader cultural dynamics. Diversity note:* Assess freedom and responsibility for gender and cultural expectations for collectivism versus individualism.
   Assessment strategies:
   a. Identify sources of **life meaning, purpose,** and **sense of freedom/ responsibility**.
   b. Assess for coping related to **death anxiety** and **existential angst** as well as capacity for **self-awareness**.

Initial Phase Client Goals (*One or Two Goals*): Manage crisis issues and/or reduce most distressing symptoms

1. *Decrease* client's attempts to avoid **existential angst** and **responsibility** to reduce [specific crisis symptoms].
   Interventions:
   a. Identify perceived threats to self and affirm self in relation to those threats.
   b. **Encourage** client to fully experience and acknowledge the fears and angst that client has been trying to escape through crisis behaviors.

Working Phase of Treatment (Three or More Sessions)
Working Phase Counseling Task

1. *Monitor quality of the working alliance. Diversity note:* Attend to relational and conflict resolution patterns based on diversity factors.
   Assessment Interventions:
   a. Assess for increasing capacity for ability to readily and comfortably experience **I-Thou** connection in session.

Working Phase Client Goals (*Two or Three Goals*). Target individual and relational dynamics using theoretical language (e.g., decrease avoidance of intimacy, increase awareness of emotion, increase agency)

1. *Increase* ability to identify significant sources of **purpose** and **life meaning** to reduce [specific symptom: depression, anxiety, etc.].
   Interventions:
   a. **Encourage** client to find sources of meaning that are worth living and struggling for.
   b. Affirm client's **sense of self** in relation to perceived threats as well as perceived life **purpose**.

(continued)

2. *Increase* capacity to take **responsibility** for daily choices and overarching life direction to reduce [specific symptom: depression, anxiety, etc.].
   Interventions:
   a. **Encourage** client to assume **responsibility** for self in situations that cannot be otherwise significantly changed or fixed by the client.
   b. Acknowledge **existential isolation** and the forms of **responsibility** derived from this insight.

3. *Increase* capacity to tolerate **anxiety** and **existential angst** to reduce [specific symptom: depression, anxiety, etc.].
   Interventions:
   a. **Encourage** client to acknowledge and take **responsible** action in relation to existential anxieties related to **death, freedom, isolation,** and **responsibility**.
   b. **Encourage** client to find relationships and/or communities in which he or she can feel a sense of **belonging** and **responsibility**.

Closing Phase of Treatment (Last Four or More Sessions)
Closing Phase Counseling Task

1. *Develop aftercare plan and maintain gains. Diversity note:* Manage end of counseling by adjusting for sociocultural and gender expectations for handling loss.
   Intervention:
   a. Help client identify ways to continue balancing **freedom** and **responsibility** in the face of existential challenges.

Closing Phase Client Goals *(One or Two Goals):* Determined by theory's definition of health and normalcy

1. *Increase* capacity to **authentically experience** and **express self** by living a life of **purpose** and **meaning** to reduce potential for relapse in [specific symptom: depression, anxiety, etc.].
   Interventions:
   a. **Encourage** clients to fully embrace life, life purpose, and self by authentic connection and self-expression.
   b. **Paradoxical interventions** to have client experiment with authenticity and facades to decrease tolerance of facades.

2. *Increase* ability to engage in meaningful relationships and communities to reduce potential for relapse in [specific symptom: depression, anxiety, etc.].
   Interventions:
   a. **Encourage** client to develop the ability to readily have **I-Thou encounters** with significant others, friends, families, and others in the community.
   b. **Encourage** client to take interpersonal risk to be **authentic self** in relation to others.

Snapshot: Research and the Evidence Base

Quick Summary: Although existentialists have documented numerous detailed case studies, little systematic research has been conducted on this approach (Mendelowitz & Schneider, 2008; Yalom, 1980). The most robust findings have been that the qualities of the counseling relationship espoused by humanistic counselors have been found to be one of the most significant common factors that predict positive outcome in all forms of counseling (see Chapter 2).

As you can imagine, as a highly philosophical approach, operationalizing existential concepts into discrete, measurable units is challenging, and this accounts for one reason why there is little rigorous study of this approach (Lantz, 2004). In addition, most counselors who are enthusiastic about this approach are typically more interested in philosophical than scientific implications (Mendelowitz & Schneider, 2008). Similar to the person-centered approach, the most significant research foundations for the existential model are found in the common factors literature that has identified an engaged, emotionally supportive counseling relationship as one of the best predictors of counseling outcome (Schneider & Krug, 2010). Nonetheless, some researchers have examined existential counseling in greater depth. For example, Goldner-Vukov, Moore, and Cupina (2007) found that psychoeducation combined with existential group sessions significantly improved outcomes with bipolar clients. In a study that considered physiological affects, van der Pompe, Duivenvoorden, Antoni, and Visser (1997) found that after 13 weeks of existential group counseling, woman diagnosed with breast cancer had improved immune and endocrine functioning.

Snapshot: Working With Diverse Populations

Quick Summary: Similar to the person-centered counselors, existential practitioners focus on the individual's subjective lived experience, making it relatively easy to adapt to various cultural value systems; however, if a client prefers a more structured, practical approach (e.g., the impoverished, men, or immigrants), the emphasis on existential issues may be a poor match.

Because it seeks to address issues at the heart of the human condition, such as death, greater meaning, and purpose, existential counseling has applications with clients from a diverse range of backgrounds (Hoffman, Yang, Kaklauskas, & Chan, 2009); however, the specific style, form, and timing of discussing existential issues vary greatly across cultures, and thus existentially oriented counselors must thoughtfully adapt the approach. Of particular interest, the existential approach has unique applications when addressing spiritual issues in counseling, providing counselors with clear conceptual guidelines and techniques for addressing the subtle and often highly emotional issues related to spirituality and religion (Hoffman, 2008). Similar to person-centered counselors, existentialists should be careful to avoid inadvertently forcing existential or humanistic values on clients from communal cultures, such as valuing individualism and direct emotional expression over community-focused values.

Existential Case Study

Adam, a 34-year-old plumber, says he is coming to counseling because his partner, Ben, said he would leave him if he didn't "deal with the drinking issue." Adam states that he likes to party on the weekends, hanging out at clubs and bars with his partner. He admits that he drinks to get drunk but quickly adds that he never drinks and drives and does not use illegal drugs. His partner, who works as an accountant, finds Adam's behavior "out of control," as he flirts with other men, is quick to anger, and is nonfunctional the next day. Although he rarely misses work because of drinking, he admits that sometimes it affects his performance. The youngest son and a second-generation Polish Jew, Adam also states that he never lived up to his parents' expectations of him in terms of either his career or having a family, although they have been generally supportive of his being gay. Although raised Reform Jew, he says that he does not attend services regularly because it does not fit with his current lifestyle. He also states that his original life goal was to be lawyer but that he partied too much in college and did not get good enough grades to go to law school. He chose plumbing because he is good at it and can make a decent living. He sometimes wonders if he wants to have children but doesn't think it is a good idea for a gay couple to adopt.

Existential Case Conceptualization

This case conceptualization was developed by selecting key concepts from "The Viewing: Case Conceptualization" section of this chapter. You can use any of the concepts in that section to develop a case conceptualization for this or other cases.

Meaning, Meaninglessness, and Life Purpose

AM's (adult male) alcohol abuse seems to be rooted in his sense of not having fulfilled life dreams to become a lawyer and have a family. The alcohol and partying create a sense of excitement that distracts him from his underlying sense of meaninglessness in his life. It is unclear if and in what ways being gay may affect his sense of life purpose and meaning, but he likely needs to explore the existential issues related to being gay and part of a marginalized group. Although he is not currently practicing, his Jewish faith is a resource he can draw on to help him find greater meaning and purpose.

Freedom and Responsibility

Although AM does not describe himself as victimized by life, he certainly is not taking responsibility for its direction or experiencing a sense of freedom that comes from having a sense of agency in life. In many ways, his alcohol use helps him to avoid responsibility for the important decisions in his life and allows him to maintain minimal levels of satisfaction that keep him from striving for what he really wants.

Capacity for Self-Awareness and Consciousness

Although AM is capable of meaningful self-reflection, he avoids it by partying and overindulging on the weekends.

Death Anxiety

Although AM does not discuss anxiety related to death, such anxiety is inherently related to one's sense of purpose and meaning. By not drinking and driving, he clearly values life and is not taking unnecessary risks.

Existential Angst

AM's alcohol use can also be seen as a tool for managing existential angst, which is likely heightened by being gay and part of a marginalized group. Having not pursued two major goals in life, including not having a family, is likely exacerbating his sense of being alone and without a clear purpose or answer for the question "What is this all for?"

Purpose of Neuroses

Whether consciously intended or not, one of the effects of being intoxicated and hung over every weekend is that it serves to avoid emotionally intimate connection with others. AM will need to work on developing the capacity to engage in I-Thou encounters.

Existential Treatment Plan

Initial Phase of Treatment

Initial Phase Therapeutic Tasks

1. *Develop working counseling relationship. Diversity note:* Adapt expectations of independence and responsibility based on cultural, gender, and sexual orientation norms. *Relationship building intervention*:
   a. Create opportunities for **I-Thou** encounters and experiencing; promote **independence** and **responsibility**.

2. *Assess individual, systemic, and broader cultural dynamics. Diversity note:* Assess freedom and responsibility considering gay and Jewish family norms. *Assessment strategies*:
   a. Identify sources of **life meaning, purpose,** and **sense of freedom/responsibility,** with careful attention to his experience of being gay and Jewish.
   b. Assess for coping related to **death anxiety** and **existential angst** as well as capacity for **self-awareness,** including his awareness related to alcohol use.

(continued)

Initial Phase Client Goals

1. *Decrease* client's attempts to avoid **existential angst** and **responsibility** to reduce problem drinking on the weekends.
   Interventions:
   a. Identify what **purpose** his heavy drinking is playing in his life and how it helps to avoid existential angst.
   b. **Encourage** client to fully experience and acknowledge the fears and angst that client has been trying to escape through drinking.

Working Phase of Treatment

Working Phase Counseling Task

1. *Monitor quality of the working alliance. Diversity note:* Ensure working alliance with client rather than side with his partner on the drinking issue.
   Assessment Intervention:
   a. Assess for increasing capacity for ability to readily and comfortably experience **I-Thou** connection in session.

Working Phase Client Goals

1. *Increase* ability to identify significant sources of **purpose** and **life meaning** as well as ways he has "settled" to reduce sense of meaninglessness and drinking.
   Interventions:
   a. **Encourage** client to find sources of meaning that are worth living and struggling for and revisit abandoned dreams of being a lawyer and having a family.
   b. Affirm client's **sense of self** in relation to perceived threats as well as perceived life **purpose**.

2. *Increase* capacity to take **responsibility** for daily choices and overarching life direction to reduce drinking.
   Interventions:
   a. **Encourage** client to assume **responsibility** for drinking and its effects on his relationship and work life and how he allowed it to derail his dream of becoming a lawyer.
   b. Acknowledge **existential isolation** and the forms of **responsibility** derived from this insight.

3. *Increase* capacity to tolerate **anxiety** and **existential angst** to reduce avoidance of life goals and dreams.
   Interventions:
   a. **Encourage** client to acknowledge and take **responsible** action in relation to existential anxieties related to his **life direction**.
   b. **Encourage** client to find relationships and/or communities in which he can feel a sense of **belonging** and **responsibility**.

Closing Phase of Treatment

Closing Phase Counseling Task

1. *Develop aftercare plan and maintain gains. Diversity note:* Set clear, measurable goals for alcohol use and/or abstinence with means for identifying early warning signs of relapse.
   Intervention:
   a. Help client identify ways to continue balancing **freedom** and **responsibility** in the face of existential challenges.

(continued)

Closing Phase Client Goals

1. *Increase* capacity to **authentically experience and express self** by living a life of **purpose** and **meaning** to reduce potential for relapse in drinking.
   Interventions:
   a. **Encourage** clients to make choices that enable him to embrace life, life purpose, and self by authentic connection and self-expression.
   b. **Paradoxical interventions** to have client experiment with authenticity and facades to decrease tolerance of facades.

2. *Increase* ability to engage in meaningful, intimate relationships to reduce potential for relapse in conflict with partner.
   Interventions:
   a. **Encourage** client to develop the ability to readily have **I-Thou encounters** with significant others, friends, families, and others in the community.
   b. **Encourage** client to take interpersonal risk to be **authentic self** in relation to others.

ONLINE RESOURCES

Associations and Training Institutes

Association for Humanistic Psychology
www.ahpweb.org

American Psychological Association, Division 32: Humanistic Psychology
www.apa.org/divisions/div32

International Society for Existential Psychotherapy and Counseling
www.existentialpsychotherapy.net

World Association for Person-Centered and Experiential Psychotherapy and Counseling
www.pce-world.org

Journals

International Journal of Existential Psychology and Psychotherapy
www.meaning.ca/ijepp.htm

Journal of Humanistic Psychology
www.ahpweb.org/pub/journal/menu.html

References

*Asterisk indicates recommended introductory readings.

Bretherton, R. (2006). Can existential psychotherapy be good news? Reflections on existential psychotherapy from a Christian perspective. *Mental Health, Religion, and Culture, 9*(3), 265–275. doi:10.1080/13694670600615490

Buber, M. (1958). *I and Thou* (R. G. Smith, Trans.). New York: Collier Books. (Original work published 1923)

Bugental, J. F. T. (1987). *The art of the psychotherapist*, New York: Norton.

*Cooper, M. (2003). *Existential therapies*. Thousand Oaks, CA: Sage.

Davidson, L., Tondora, J., O'Connell, M. J., Lawless, M. S., & Rowe, M. (2009). *A practical guide to recovery-oriented practice: Tools for transforming mental health care*. New York: Oxford University Press.

Frankl, V. (1963). *Man's search for meaning*. Boston: Beacon.

Frankl, V. (1965). *The doctor and the soul*. New York: Bantam.

Frankl, V. (1978). *The unheard cry for meaning*. New York: Simon & Schuster.

Goldner-Vukov, M., Moore, L., & Cupina, D. (2007). Bipolar disorder: From psychoeducational to existential group therapy. *Australasian Psychiatry, 15*(1), 30–34. doi:10.1080/10398560601083100

Hoffman, L. (2008). An EI approach to working with religious and spiritual clients. In K. J. Schneider (Ed.), *Existential-integrative psychotherapy: Guideposts to the core of* practice (pp. 187–201). New York: Routledge/Taylor & Francis Group.

Hoffman, L., Yang, M., Kaklauskas, F., & Chan, A. (2009). *Existential psychology East-West.* Colorado Springs, CO: University of the Rockies Press.

Krug, O. T. (2009). James Bugental and Irvin Yalom: Two masters of existential therapy cultivate presence in the therapeutic encounter. *Journal of Humanistic Psychology, 49,* 329–354.

Lantz, J. (2004). Research and evaluation issues in existential psychotherapy. *Journal of Contemporary Psychotherapy, 34*(4), 331–340. doi:10.1007/s10879-004-2527-5

May, R. (Ed.). (1961). *Existential psychology.* New York: Random House.

May, R. (1969). *Love and will.* New York: Norton.

May, R. (1973). *The courage to create.* New York: Norton.

May, R. (1981). *Freedom and destiny.* New York: Norton.

May, R. (1983). *The discovery of being: Writings from existential psychology.* New York: Norton.

May, R. (2009). *Man's search for himself.* New York: Dell. (Original work published 1953)

Mendelowitz, E., Schneider, K. (2008). Existential psychotherapy. In R. J. Corsini & D. Wedding (Eds.), *Current psychotherapies* (8th ed., pp. 295–327). Pacific Grove, CA: Brooks/Cole.

Reeves, C. (1977). *The psychology of Rollo May: A study in existential theory and psychotherapy.* San Francisco: Jossey-Bass.

Rogers, C. (1961). *On becoming a person: A counselor's view of psychocounseling.* London: Constable.

Schneider, K. J., & Krug, O. T. (2010). Evaluation. In K. J. Schneider & O. T. Krug (Eds.), *Existential–humanistic therapy* (pp. 89–99). Washington, DC: American Psychological Association.

Seligman, M. (2002). *Authentic happiness: Using the new positive psychology to realize your potential for lasting fulfillment.* New York: Free Press.

van der Pompe, G., Duivenvoorden, H. J., Antoni, M. H., & Visser, A. (1997). Effectiveness of a short-term group psychotherapy program on endocrine and immune function in breast cancer patients: An exploratory study. *Journal of Psychosomatic Research, 42*(5), 453–466. doi:10.1016/S0022-3999(96)00393-5

Van Deurzen, E. (2002). *Existential counseling and psychotherapy in practice* (2nd ed.). Thousand Oaks, CA: Sage.

Yalom, I. (1970). *The theory and practice of group psychotherapy.* New York: Basic Books.

Yalom, I. (1980). *Existential psychtherapy.* New York: Basic Books.

CHAPTER
8

Gestalt Counseling
and Psychotherapy

Learning is the discovery that something is possible.

—Fritz Perls

Lay of the Land

In a Nutshell: The Least You Need to Know

Pioneered by Fritz Perls—a dynamic therapist who is known for his often flamboyant and controversial style—and further developed by numerous others (Woldt & Toman, 2005; Yontef, 1993), Gestalt counseling is a phenomenological approach that emphasizes that people must be understood holistically and contextually—or, in Perls's native German, as a *Gestalt*. Similar to person-centered counselors, Gestalt counselors help people become more of who they really are by helping them to stop trying to be what they are not. Gestalt counselors achieve this end by enabling clients to develop present moment awareness of and direct contact with their internal world (including parts of the self that have been cut off) and the environment (significant others, society, etc.). Gestalt counselors believe neuroses and other problems develop when a person avoids direct contact with the environment or parts of the self. The in-session, present moment experiences facilitated by counselors enable people to reintegrate these cutoff parts of the self to create increasingly greater sense of *wholeness*.

Gestalt counseling methods are active, provocative, and experiential. Counselors in this approach interact as a whole person, using their emotional responses to clients as part of the process. Some Gestalt counselors use a more theatrical, cathartic style, while others use a more person-to-person approach (Yontef, 1993). Somewhat paradoxically, Gestalt theory encourages an "atheoretical" approach to counseling, meaning that rather than rigidly adhering to theory, practitioners focus more on the moment-by-moment flow of experience in the counseling relationship.

Through the Gestalt process of reintegrating cutoff parts of the self and increasingly making authentic contact with the environment, a person becomes a more vibrant and self-actualized person who is fully aware of and responsive to what is going on in his or her emotions, body, and relationships, resulting in a *natural flow of being*. Gestalt practitioners went through a more extreme "anything goes," antitheoretical phase in the 1960s but "sobered up" in the 1970s with a greater focus on a more supportive, dialogical engagement with clients (Yontef, 1993).

Gestalt counseling and psychotherapy should not be confused with *Gestalt psychology*, which is a specific line of psychological research. Gestalt psychologists study how the brain organizes incoming sensory information into Gestalts to find and/or create wholeness, coherence, and patterns from the vast amount of incoming perceptual data. For example, in the line below, you are likely to see six boxes rather than 24 dots based on the *principle of proximity* (four dots near each other are perceived as one Gestalt) and *principle of closure* (four dots that outline a square are connected in the mind to form one):

.. ..
.. ..

Similarly, you are probably familiar with Rubin's vase, in which one can perceive either a vase or two faces looking at each other. Because of the ambiguity in this scenario, the mind can alternately perceive either the vase or the faces, depending on what it takes to be the *figure* and what it takes to be the *background*. Perls used these terms metaphorically to describe inner psychological processes. For example, needs, feelings, or desires can rise to the foreground of the mind (e.g., anxiety about an exam) and then recede (e.g., be superseded by a family crisis). Additionally, Perls adapted the principle of closure to refer to intrapsychic events, describing the need to have psychological closure to conflict, scenarios, relationships, and so on, as *unfinished business*. Laura Perls, Fritz Perls's wife, a Gestalt psychologist, objected to the metaphorical use of the term "Gestalt" as it applied to psychotherapy, but Fritz nonetheless used it to describe his work—and the name stuck.

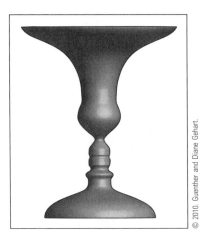

© 2010. Guenther and Diane Gehart.

The Juice: Significant Contributions to the Field

If you remember one thing from this chapter, it should be ...

Body Awareness

Gestalt counselors believe that every emotion has a physiological component (Perls, 1973; Polster & Poltser, 1973). When a person is cut off from the awareness of an emotion or part of the self, this becomes expressed in the body, usually as a tightening or dysfunction somewhere. Gestalt counselors are masters at picking up information from a person's body posture, fidgeting, tone of voice, and movements: "how a person sits ... tells so much about the contact he is willing to make" (Polster & Polster, 1973, p. 161). For example, a tight jaw may indicate holding back something a person wants to say and wringing of hands the suppression of what a person might want to do. Similarly, covering the abdomen may signal a sense of vulnerability, while stiff movements may be part of an attempt to hold oneself together. In the Gestalt view, the repressed and suppressed emotions that become expressed in the body is similar to Freud's; however, Perls believed that awareness of the *process of repression* was the key to integration, whereas psychoanalysts believed that interpretation of the *content of repression* was the primary goal.

Gestalt counselors help clients increase their awareness of their bodies and the emotions expressed through the body. Bringing a person's attention to body movements that are expressing repressed emotion is risky business: the mind has put a lot of energy into remaining unaware of the emotions, so you should proceed with caution and gentleness—or you may encounter quite a bit of resistance. Typically, Gestalt counselors approach bodily awareness by creating a *safe emergency*, which involves increasing the client's affective intensity while still supporting the client with affirmation (Yontef & Jacobs, 2000). In the case study at the end of this chapter, the counselor uses body awareness to help Monica more effectively manage trauma symptoms, such as flashbacks and nightmares.

Specific techniques for this include the following:

- *Where do you feel X in your body?* When a person is talking about a difficult emotion or situation, the counselor can ask, "Where do you feel the sadness [anger, hurt, disappointment, etc.] in your body?"
- *What would [body part/movement] say if it had a voice?* If the counselor has noticed a particular movement or body part that seems to be holding repressed emotion, the counselor could ask, "If that clenched fist could speak, what would it say?"
- *Exaggerate a movement:* If clients are having a difficult time understanding a particular body movement or expression, the counselor may direct them to exaggerate the movement to increase awareness: "Can you try to make yourself as stiff as you can? Exaggerate the stiffness. Feel and notice what emotions, memories, or thoughts emerge as you do this."

Rumor Has It: The People and Their Stories
Fritz Perls

Born in Berlin in 1893 to a Jewish middle-class family, Fritz Perls is the inspiration behind Gestalt counseling. He served as a psychiatrist in World War I in the German army, which later led to his introduction to Gestalt psychology and Laura Posner, whom he then married. He and Laura moved to Vienna to further study psychoanalysis, where he underwent analysis with Wilhelm Reich. As World War II loomed, he fled to the Netherlands and then South Africa, where he wrote his first book, *Ego, Hunger, and Aggression*. Soon after, he and Laura moved to New York, where, along with Paul Goodman, they opened the New York Institute for Gestalt Therapy in 1952. He left Laura and their two children to promote his therapy approach, eventually becoming affiliated with the Esalen Institute in California. Fritz was known for his highly provocative, controversial style in which he "provoked" clients to "grow up," offering a less supportive counseling relationship than most Gestalt counselors currently advocate.

Laura Posner Perls

An accomplished musician and artist and Gestalt psychologist by training, Laura Posner Perls spearheaded the development of Gestalt practices at the New York Institute of Gestalt Therapy. In contrast to her husband, Laura emphasized a supportive counseling relationship that emphasized interpersonal connection.

Erving and Miriam Polster

Well known for their book *Gestalt Therapy Integrated*, Erving and Mirian Polster (1973) were influential developers of Gestalt counseling, particularly the concept of contact boundaries.

Big Picture: Overview of Counseling Process
Layers of Neurosis

The Gestalt counseling process aims to help people achieve a greater sense of wholeness, awareness, and aliveness. Perls (1973) describes the process of becoming more authentic as a five-part process that he likens to the peeling of an onion:

1. *Phony layer:* At this point, a person lives according to "shoulds" and habit, living an inauthentic life (e.g., an engaged woman who becomes fixated on having the perfect wedding, perfect dress, and perfect partner).

2. *Phobic layer:* In the phobic layer or stage, a person begins to become worried and fearful that something is amiss; he or she may feel helpless but work hard to keep his or her feelings hidden (e.g., the soon-to-be bride starts having second thoughts and doubts).

3. *Impasse layer:* At the point of impasse, a person begins to feel stuck, not knowing which way to go and thus becoming more open to seeking help, preferably from someone who will tell him or her the "right" answer (e.g., the bride-to-be begins asking for advice from family, friends, religious support persons, and/or a counselor).

4. *Implosive layer:* In this next phase, the phony layer begins to collapse, and the person feels empty inside and lost, which makes him or her more open to present moment awareness and experiences (e.g., the soon-to-be bride loses touch with why she wanted to get married and have a wedding in the first place and begins to ask herself and her fiancé some difficult and discerning questions).

5. *Explosive layer:* In this final period, the person lets go of old pretenses, releasing bursts of new energy for authentic action (e.g., the young woman decides with a new sense of clarity that she wants to be married and designs a wedding that uniquely expresses who she and her partner are without relying on empty traditions or the latest fads).

Integration Sequence

The Polsters describe a similar change process that they call the *integration sequence* (Roberts, 1999):

1. *Discovery:* In the discovery phase, the client comes to new realizations about the self in which new "figures" emerge from the ground. Often the counselor is instrumental in helping the client make discoveries through interventions and experiments.

2. *Accommodation:* In the next phase, the client begins to accommodate this new perception and to behave in the world based on the discovery; the client may feel awkward and clumsy in his or her interactions.

3. *Assimilation:* In this third phase, the once novel realization becomes more representative of who the client is: "feels like me."

4. *Integration:* In the final phase, the new behavior fits seamlessly with the person's sense of self and seems effortless.

Making Connection: Therapeutic Relationship
Person of Counselor: Being Fully Human

The person of the counselor is the primary vehicle for change in Gestalt counseling (Perls, Hefferline, & Goodman 1951; Yontef, 1993). The counselor uses their whole personhood to make a real and authentic contact with the counselor. More so than most of the forms of counseling, the counselor engages the client without professional pretense or role. Thus, counselors freely share their thoughts, perceptions, and feelings as they occur in session to rattle and awaken the client's authentic self. In short, the counselor is fully human, expressing a full range of emotion and openly admitting to mistakes and failings.

Here and Now, Presence, and Spontaneity

One of the primary experiences Gestalt counselors offer clients is their *presence* in *here-and-now* experiences (Polster & Polster, 1973). The counselor is fully in the present moment with the client, living in the *now*, where past and future fade away: "Since neurotic living is basically anachronistic living, any return to present experience is in itself a part of the antidote to neurosis" (Polster & Polster, 1973, p. 11). Polster and Polster further define the counseling process as "an exercise in unhampered living *now*," and therefore the counselor's primary role is to help clients more fully experience themselves—all aspects of themselves—as they arise moment to moment in session. Thus, counselors encourage clients to explore the tightness in their breathing, the spontaneous feelings that arise as they share what is on their mind, and whatever seems to bubble up during the counseling hour. The counselor does not try to "make sense of it all" or even connect early comments in session with contradictory latter ones; instead, the focus is on becoming aware and fully experiencing and expressing the client's flow of consciousness.

Imperfect Role Model

Many people (including counselors) expect counselors to be near perfect, rarely getting angry, and having happily-ever-after relationships and everlasting good hair days. Many of us enter the field with the secret hope that maybe, just maybe, by reading enough books and learning how to help others through their problems, we won't have any of our own. It's tempting to hope for such bliss. Arguably, through popular books and media, the field frequently implies that such happiness and bliss are possible if you do enough positive self-talk, creative visualization, and feeling of emotion. But Gestalt counselors would argue that such problem-free living is a dangerous myth—so dangerous, in fact, that they are willing to be a role model for imperfection and thus a role model for the processes of integrating polarities. Thus, they do not hide behind a professional veneer, and instead they boldly go where many counselors will not. For example, they will freely comment on how a person's weight or grooming may be part of the reason that getting a date is difficult or confront a person who was victimized as a child and copes by feeling victimized by everyone and everything.

Dialogic Engagement

Drawing on the work of Buber (see Chapter 7), more recent Gestalt applications include *dialogic engagement*: "the dialogic view of reality is that all reality is relating" (Yontef, 1993, p. 33). Thus, growth happens "between" people and is best promoted in relationship rather through than individual awareness. The counselor's role is to engage the client fully, genuinely, and openly, willing to explore despair, love, anger, joy, humor, and sensuality. This dialogic openness requires discrimination on the part of the counselor to appropriately share personal feelings and information.

In dialogic approaches, the counselor uses the relationship as the primary context for making contact (Hycner & Jacobs, 1995). In the encounters between counselor and client, clients are able to develop awareness and differentiate self from nonself. Counselors use their authentic selves to help clients more clearly and safely experience what is self and nonself so that they can more freely experience here-and-now experiences.

Confirmation and Inclusion

Gestalt counselors believe "people become unique selves by the confirmation of other people" (Yontef, 1993, p. 36). *Inclusion* is considered the highest form of confirmation, when a person "feels into" the other's worldview while still maintaining a clear sense of self. The client practicing inclusion sees the world, life, and the client's situation as much as possible through the eyes of the client (Hycner, 1995). Since I know you'd ask, Yontef (1993) distinguishes inclusion from empathy by emphasizing that inclusion moves farther on the pole of really "feeling" another's world while simultaneously demanding greater awareness of self than empathy typically does. Generally, Gestalt counselors criticize empathy because it often leads to a confluence or blurring between self and other.

The Viewing: Case Conceptualization
Assessing the Field

Contemporary Gestalt counselors used Kurt Lewin's *field theory* as a primary tool for viewing clients and their lives (Parlett & Lee, 2005; Yontef, 1993). Similar to Gestalt psychology, field theory shares the view that a figure is intimately connected with its background. Field theory further posits greater and more dynamic interrelationships between figure and background than traditional Gestalt psychology. In field theory, the figure/ ground are viewed as a systematic web of relationships that forms a unitary whole: "everything affects everything else in the field" (Yontef, 1993, p. 297). Field theory can be applied to a variety of counseling phenomena: the client as a whole, the counseling relationship, and how clients perceive their situations. In every case, the counselor is part of the field, affecting what is being observed; simply asking clients about their situations affects their situations (Parlett & Lee, 2005). Thus, counselors remain cognizant for how their questions and presence shape and affect clients' lived experience.

Assessing the field requires investigation of the ever-fluctuating dynamics of the field and invites nondichotomous thinking, examining how each part affects the others (Lobb & Lichtenberg, 2005). For example, if a client complains that her partner has hurt her, the counselor explores not only how the client feels hurt but also how she may have contributed to her partner hurting her and how the client may have contributed to hurting her partner.

Questions for Assessing the Field

- What was your experience?
- How did you contribute to creating your experience?
- What were the experiences of others? How did you contribute to their experience?
- What other factors may have contributed to your experience? How might have you affected these factors?
- How is the sharing of this situation in the counseling encounter affecting your experience of this situation?

Contact Boundaries and Encounters

Gestalt counselors view each moment of lived experience primarily in terms of a form of *contact* between the self (organism) and outside world (others and environment; Perls, 1951; Yontef, 1993). If a person is able to make direct contact and authentically *encounter* the outside world, the person is living a full and authentic life. However, for a variety of reasons—such as early life lessons, fears, or social dictates—people avoid genuine contact to protect themselves. These *contact boundary disturbances* refer to distortions in perceptions of self or others.

An encounter involves a continuum of seven phases, beginning with initial perception, moving toward direct encounter, and ending in withdrawal. The human experience involves an endless ebb and flow of making contact with one person/object/ idea and then withdrawing and then making contact and withdrawing from another in an endless series of connections and disconnections. A person can avoid contact at any of the seven phases using specific resistance processes at each stage (Woldt & Toman, 2005):

Continuum Phase	Resistance Process	Example of Resistance
1. *Sensation/perception:* Organism perceives input from environment.	*Desensitization:* Failing to notice problems.	Ignoring increasing violence by partner in fights.
2. *Awareness:* One's lived experience becomes focused on the environmental sensation.	*Introjection:* Take in others' views whole and unedited.	Becoming what your parents wanted you to be.
3. *Excitement/mobilization:* The organism mobilizes to prepare for contact.	*Projection:* Assign undesired parts of self to others.	Rejecting sexual aspects of self and then perceiving others as "oversexed."
4. *Encounter/action:* The organism takes action to engage the other.	*Retroflection:* Direct action to self rather than other.	Rather than creating conflict with others, focus criticism on self.
5. *Interaction/full contact:* A back-and-forth exchange happens; the self becomes part of "we."	*Deflection:* Avoid direct contact with another or self.	Working long hours to avoid spouse or avoiding own emotions.
6. *Assimilation/integration:* The organism takes in and integrates new information, behavior, etc.	*Egotism:* Not allowing outside to influence self.	Claiming to be "in love" but not being open to changing self to meet needs of relationship.

(continued)

Continuum Phase	Resistance Process	Example of Resistance
7. *Differentiation/withdrawal:* The organism withdraws from contact and returns to its individual state.	*Confluence:* Agree with another to the extent that boundary is blurred.	Agreeing with spouse to extent that one no longer allows self to have a divergent opinion.

When assessing clients, Gestalt counselors look for where their clients are "stuck" in the cycle of making contact and direct their interventions to encourage clients make contact and complete the encounter cycle. In the case study at the end of this chapter, the counselor helps Monica address her avoidance of contact that stems from her childhood sexual abuse.

Polarities and Disowned Parts

Gestalt counselors view people as never-ending sequence of *polarities* or complementary parts, as adult versus child, strong versus weak, loving versus hateful, and so on (Polster & Polster, 1973). When a person is rigidly polarized—always acts like an adult, always strong, always loving, and so on—they typically have disowned the opposite quality, such as childishness, weakness, or hatefulness. On the surface, this may not seem like much of a problem. The problem is that we are talking about members of the human species, who are human after all. Being human, each person experiences, at some level, the full range of human emotion. Thus, although a person may be very responsible in their day job, the ability to be playful like a child is an important counterbalance. A person may do extensive personal growth to feel emotionally strong but will still encounter difficult moments, loss, tragedy, and trauma and during these times will need to allow himself or herself to feel his or her weakness. Similarly, a person may engage in religious and spiritual practices to become more loving but may also experience loss, victimization, or trauma that elicits feelings of animosity and hate; that is part of the human experience. One doesn't need to *act* on this hate, but it is important to be accepting of having such feelings. When such feelings are *disowned*, the person must develop elaborate avoidance strategies that impede a person's ability to be fully who he or she is. Thus, the Gestalt counselors try to identify the polarities within a person that may be contributing to the presenting problem. Common problematic polarities include the following:

- Social self versus natural self
- Adult versus child
- Perfect versus failure
- Emotional versus logical
- Shallow versus deep
- Responsible versus carefree

In the case study at the end of this chapter, the counselor helps Monica, a grocery clerk who has recently begun reexperiencing trauma symptoms related to her childhood sexual abuse. One of the ways Monica had coped with the abuse was to be responsible, take care of herself, and avoid all risk, creating polarization. Healing for her will involve integrating carefree and trusting parts of herself.

"Shoulds"

Gestalt counselors carefully listen for a person's use of "shoulds" to justify and explain their behavior and choices (Yontef, 1993). They believe that people who routinely organize their lives by doing what they "should" do rather than what they want to do, value, and so on are not living authentically and are in fact *avoiding* taking existential responsibility for their lives (e.g., "I am doing what others have told me to do rather than decide for myself what I want to be doing, believe in"). They view "shoulds" as a form of *neurotic self-regulation*, meaning that the person is regulating emotions in unhealthy ways. Gestalt counselors confront persons living by "shoulds" and encourage them to make more authentic choices that are not fear based or based on social pressure.

Unfinished Business

Like it sounds, *unfinished business* refers to any incompletely expressed feeling, which most often takes the form of resentment (Yontef, 1993). Gestalt counselors help clients identify unfinished business by playing the following game:

Unfinished Business Assessment Game

"For the next 2 (choose a time) minutes, I want you to list out as many things that you are feeling resentful about as you can. You can do this by starting your statements with: 'I resent …' Just keep going and try to identify as many as you can, no matter how silly they may seem. Have fun with it, and we will talk about it when you are done. Any questions? Ready? Go."

Targeting Change: Goal Setting

Awareness

"In Gestalt, the only *goal* is *awareness*" (Yontef, 1993, p. 150). The counselor's primary goal is to help clients increase their awareness of their experiences so that they can make direct contact with the environment without resistance. The ability to be aware and in contact requires (a) organismic self-regulation, (b) acceptance of what is, and (c) the integration of polarities.

Organismic Self-Regulation

Perls (1973) described the long-term goal of counseling as helping clients to become *organismically self regulating* rather than *shouldistic*, meaning ruled by cognition and lists of "shoulds." Yontef (1993) defines organismic self-regulation (and, yes, it is hard not to slip up and say orgasmic) as "choosing and learning happening holistically, with a natural integration of mind and body, thought and feeling, spontaneity and deliberateness" (p. 143). Vibrant and alive, such a person lives in a dynamic, responsive relationship with the environment, embracing the ebb and flow of life, including the more difficult moments, while responding authentically. An organismically self-regulated person has the courage to make "contact" with people and situations without having to rely on resistance processes to protect the self, trusting the self and life itself. This type of person takes responsibility for his or her relationship with others and the world and is able to *creatively adapt* to situations (Yontef, 1993). Furthermore, an organismically self-regulated person is *self-supporting*, meaning that this person can provide basic support for the self and does not need to manipulate others to meet personal needs.

Accepting "What Is": Paradoxical Theory of Change

Beisser (1970) posited a paradoxical theory of change that has been adopted by contemporary Gestalt counselors: the more one tries to change (and be who one is not), the more one stays the same. Thus, paradoxically, the long-term goals in Gestalt are less about correcting personal defects than about removing barriers to experiencing who one already is. Alternatively stated, the goal is to accept that what is "*is*" and to make peace with who and what one is. When a person is able to make contact with "what is," change spontaneously happens (Yontef, 1993). For example, many clients refuse to "make contact" with the "what is" of their body: they may believe they are not pretty or thin enough, be afraid of their sexuality or impulses, or be frustrated by pain or a debilitating condition. If the counselor can help clients make direct contact with "what is" by removing resistance barriers, clients' relationships with their bodies automatically transform to be more accepting, less fearful, and less judgmental. This paradoxical theory has been compared with Taoist and Buddhist "nondoing" and mindfulness practices (Smith, 1976).

Integration of Polarities

Another long-term goal in Gestalt counseling is *integrating polarities*, which involves accepting differences within the self and between self and the environment. In practice, integration takes the form of being less dogmatic, less rigid, and, quite simply, more complex as a human being because the person has accepted and integrated more aspects of the self. For example, if a man enters counseling defining his value in terms of his career achievements, the process of integration will involve accepting the "relaxed," "less-than-ideal," and less dominant parts of himself. Through this process, he may continue to excel at work but now also create time for a romantic relationship, hobbies, and "wasting time" with chitchat.

Initial and Working Phases

Early and middle phase goals in Gestalt counseling address the blockages to experiencing this integrated sense of self and generally address the presenting symptoms more directly. Examples are the following:

- Increase awareness of suppressed anger that fuels depression
- Decrease avoidance of difficult interpersonal exchanges and increase expression of feelings in situations where client fears negative rejection from others (or increase assertiveness with others)
- Decrease angry outbursts and hurtful comments with wife and children and increase ability to express more vulnerable emotions
- Increase ability to identify and separate own feelings from that of others and ability to act on these feelings

Closing Phase Client Goals

The closing phase client goals address the longer-term issues of (a) organismic self-regulation, (b) making contact with what is, and (c) integrating polarities. Examples are the following:

- Increase organismic self-regulation in marriage to increase emotional intimacy
- Increase acceptance of "driven" versus "relaxed" polarities to create better work–home balance
- Increase capacity to make direct contact with family of origin
- Increase ability to accept "what is" related to loss of mother

Interventions

Body Awareness (see "The Juice")

Gestalt Experiment and Empty Chair

A Hollywood favorite for mocking counselors, the Gestalt empty chair involves having clients pour out their hearts to an empty chair and then turn around and respond from the empty chair, having a conversation with themselves. Although this technique looks strange and even silly from the outside, when you are the one speaking, it is rarely a joke—it is challenging and powerful. This technique enables clients to have conversations with people and parts of themselves that they would otherwise never be able to have.

Gestalt counselors use the empty chair and similar Gestalt experiments because they prefer action over talk. Thus, their characteristic technique is the *Gestalt experiment*, which involves inviting the client to take action in the room by creating a "safe emergency" (Polster & Polster, 1973). An experiment may involve having an empty-chair conversation by speaking aloud to an imagined person in an empty chair, sharing things the person is too afraid to say to the imagined person directly. For example, if a person is angry with his boss but afraid to speak to her, the counselor may ask him to speak aloud what he has been too afraid to say to this person. The purpose of this empty-chair encounter is *not* to rehearse for an actual confrontation or to "vent" feelings but rather "to relate to reality out there by expressing his needs at that moment in time" and experience "in the present what it is like for him to flow from awareness to experimental action" (Polster & Polster, 1973, p. 235). This safe opportunity to experience acting and speaking from one's immediate lived experience makes it easier and more likely that the client will do so outside the session. In most cases, the person's actions outside the session will not be a replica of what occurred in counseling (most of us tone it down in the real world). The Gestalt experiment is *not* an "acting out" of emotion but rather a safe context for experimenting with authentic expression.

Gestalt experiments can take many forms (Polster & Polster, 1973):

- Enactment of unfinished business situation from the distant past
- Enactment of contemporary unfinished business situation
- Enactment of a characteristic (desired or undesired)
- Enactment of a polarity (both sides)

Yontef (1993) lists the purposes of experiments, including:

- To expand a person's repertoire of behaviors outside the session and stimulate experiential learning
- To create conditions in which the client can see life as his or her own creation and also take ownership of the counseling process
- To complete unfinished business, overcome blockages in awareness, and integrate polarities
- To stimulate a sense of strength, competency, self-support, and responsibility

---

Steps to Successfully Stage an Experiment

1. **Identify Focus:** Through dialogue, the counselor and client identify areas of unfinished business, polarities, resistance, and so on (e.g., unexpressed anger at mother).
2. **Initiate Experiment:** The counselor then invites the client into the experiment by specifically *directing* the client to experiment by speaking to an empty chair, saying something aloud, or taking physical action of some form (e.g., "I want you to pretend for a moment that your mother is in the chair next to you. Go ahead and speak to her, saying those things you wish you would have said the last time you saw her").
3. **Focus Experiment:** During the experiment, the counselor may encourage the client to address specific areas or take certain actions (e.g., "Why don't you address what happened during the divorce too").
4. **Experience the Experiment:** After the experiment, the counselor focuses on helping the client identify the here-and-now experiencing of the experiment (e.g., "What were you feeling inside when you were talking to your mother? Did any particular part of your body react? What are you feeling like now that you said that aloud?").

Semantics and Language Modification

Gestalt counselors direct clients to modify the language to highlight their autonomy, choice, and responsibility. Common examples include the following:

- *Questions to statements:* Gestalt counselors ask clients to change questions to statements because often questions are disguised statements or demands for support from others (Yontef, 1993).
- *"I" Versus "You" or "It" statements:* Rather than describing someone else as the agent in a situation ("*you* made me do X") or in a passive voice ("*it* just makes me feel X"), Gestalt counselors have clients rephrase a statement beginning with "I": "I decided to do X," or "I chose to feel X."
- *"Choose" Versus "Can't":* When a client says I "can't" but there is an element of choice, the counselor has the client restate his or her position acknowledging his or her choice: "I choose to spend time at work to make a deadline rather than come home on time."
- *"Want" Versus "Have To":* Similarly, Gestalt counselors have clients clearly distinguish between "having to do something" (which is ultimately extremely rare) and wanting to do something: "I want to pay taxes to avoid being pursued by the IRS" rather than "I have to pay taxes." By constantly highlighting that we all have free choice in most all life circumstances, *choose* increases a person's sense of freedom, will, and responsibility even if the life choices remain the same ("I am going to choose to keep paying taxes").
- *"But":* Another word Gestalt counselors watch for is "but," which is typically followed by excuses, polarity, or a double message. Instead, clients are encouraged to develop integration by replacing "but" with "and."

Staying With Feelings

To increase awareness, Gestalt counselors often encourage clients to "stay with" difficult feelings, coaching them through the continuum of contact: sensation, awareness, excitement, encounter, integration, assimilation, and withdrawal (see the section "Contact Boundaries and Encounters"). The counselor encourages the client in each phase to move through resistances to have direct experiences. Much like the experiment, encouraging clients to stay with feelings helps them to develop the skills and courage to do this outside of session.

Dream Work

Gestalt counselors use a unique approach to dreams. They see them as attempts to integrate parts of the self and/or as an existential message, and the counselor is not assumed to know the true interpretation better than the client (Yontef, 1993). Gestalt counselors view each character in the dream as a part of the self. For example, if a person is being chased in the dream, both the pursuer and the one fleeing are viewed as different aspects of the self. The counselor and client can explore how these parts interact, what each might represent, and how they have been neglected or emphasized in the person's life.

Putting It All Together: Gestalt Treatment Plan Template

Use this treatment plan template for developing a plan for clients with depressive, anxious, or compulsive types of presenting problems. Depending on the specific client, presenting problem, and clinical context, the goals and interventions in this template may need to be modified only slightly or significantly; you are encouraged to significantly revise the plan as needed. For the plan to be useful, goals and techniques should be written to target specific beliefs, behaviors, and emotions that the client is experiencing. The more specific, the more useful it will be to you.

Initial Phase of Treatment (First One to Three Sessions)
Initial Phase Counseling Tasks

1. *Develop working counseling relationship. Diversity note:* Adapt emotional expression for ethnicity, gender, age, and so on.
   Relationship building intervention:
   a. Confirmation of client's **unique self** while counselor is also expressing authentic self.

2. *Assess individual, systemic, and broader cultural dynamics. Diversity note:* Adapt assessment of emotions, emotional expression, and authenticity to gender and cultural norms.
   Assessment strategies:
   a. Assess client's ability to make **authentic contact** with others and environment.
   b. Identify **polarities, disowned parts,** "**shoulds,**" and **unfinished business.**

Initial Phase Client Goals *(One or Two Goals):* Manage crisis issues and/or reduce most distressing symptoms

1. *Increase* tolerance of difficult emotions and **unwanted parts of self** that fuel crisis to reduce [specific crisis symptoms].
   Interventions:
   a. **Body awareness** exercises to help client identify and more effectively manage crisis emotions.

(continued)

    b.   Encourage client to "stay with" difficult feelings that fuel crisis and coach client through experiencing these emotions to defuse crisis.

Working Phase of Treatment (Three or More Sessions)
Working Phase Counseling Tasks

1. *Monitor quality of the working alliance. Diversity note:* Adapt relationship to be responsive to gender and cultural forms of **emotional expression** and **contact norms**.
    Assessment Intervention:
    a.   Monitor frequency of **here-and-now experiencing**, willingness to tolerate differences between self and other, and **authentic expression of self**; use Session Rating Scale.

Working Phase Client Goals *(Two or Three Goals)*. Target individual and relational dynamics using theoretical language (e.g., decrease avoidance of intimacy, increase awareness of emotion, increase agency)

1. *Increase* **integration of polarities** between [X] and [Y] to reduce [specific symptom: depression, anxiety, etc.].
    Interventions:
    a.   **Gestalt experiments** and **empty-chair** exercises to facilitate awareness and integration of polarities.
    b.   **Modify language** to allow for both acceptance of polarities.

2. *Increase* ability to **self-regulate** in [X: specific context, relationship, problem, etc.] to reduce [specific symptom: depression, anxiety, etc.].
    Interventions:
    a.   Coach client on **staying with difficult feelings** to increase ability to self-regulate.
    b.   **Gestalt experiments** with alternative behaviors to increase self-regulation skills.

3. *Increase* ability to **accept "what is"** in relation to [unchangeable situation] to reduce [specific symptom: depression, anxiety, etc.].
    Interventions:
    a.   **Dream analysis** to better understand resistance to and rejection of what is.
    b.   **Language modification** to reduce "shoulds" in relation to "what is."

Closing Phase of Treatment (Last Four or More Sessions)
Closing Phase Counseling Task

1. *Develop aftercare plan and maintain gains. Diversity note:* Adapt for diversity factors.
    Intervention:
    a.   Increase capacity for **organismic self-regulation** in relation to potential future stressors.

Closing Phase Client Goals *(One or Two Goals):* Determined by theory's definition of health and normalcy

1. *Increase* capacity to **self-regulate** and expand **here-and-now experiencing** to be primary mode for daily living in all contexts to reduce potential for relapse in [specific symptom: depression, anxiety, etc.].
    Interventions:
    a.   Increasingly challenging **Gestalt experiments** to integrate spontaneity into all aspects of daily living.
    b.   **Dream work** to identify more subtle resistance and **polarities** that impeded full authenticity in daily living.

(continued)

2. *Increase* **self-regulation** and **authentic expression of self** in intimate relationships while simultaneously allowing for another's authenticity to reduce potential for relapse in [specific symptom: depression, anxiety, etc.].
   Interventions:
   a. **Empty-chair** experiments to develop awareness and skills for authentic relating.
   b. **Gestalt experiments** in significant relationships that help to build capacity for authentic intimacy.

Snapshot: Research and the Evidence Base

Quick Summary: Similar to person-centered (Chapter 6) and existential (Chapter 7) counseling, little systematic research has been conducted on Gestalt counseling outcomes aside from the effectiveness of the empty-chair technique (Wagner-Moore, 2004). Again, the most robust findings have been that the qualities of the counseling relationship espoused by humanistic counselors have been found to be one of the most significant common factors that predict positive outcome in all forms of counseling (see Chapter 2).

Attributed as much to the personal style of Perls as to the philosophical foundations of humanism, little research has been conducted on the process or outcomes of Gestalt counseling, with one significant exception: the empty-chair, or "two-chair," technique (Wagner-Moore, 2004). Greenberg and colleagues (Clarke & Greenberg, 1986; Greenberg, Elliott, & Lietaer, 1994; Greenberg & Rice, 1981) have specifically studied the two-chair technique separately from the Gestalt approach. In a series of studies comparing the two-chair technique to person-centered empathetic responding, participants in both studies reported a greater depth of experiencing and more shifts in awareness (Greenberg & Dompierre, 1981; Greenberg & Rice, 1981). Furthermore, another study that compared the two-chair technique to the cognitive-behavioral problem solving and a no-treatment control group found that the two-chair technique was superior to both. Several other studies have provided preliminary support for the two-chair technique with anger and unfinished business. Much more work needs to be done to explore the change mechanisms and outcomes of Gestalt work.

Snapshot: Working With Diverse Populations

Quick Summary: Similar to other phenomenological approaches, Gestalt's emphasis on the individual's subjective lived experience enables practitioners to adapt the approach to diverse populations; however, counselors need to be careful to carefully consider the embedded values and assumptions about emotional expression and individuality to ensure that these are not inadvertently forced onto clients.

Like other humanists, contemporary Gestalt counselors integrate cultural considerations as part of their assessment of the figure/ground and "field" in which the client lives and work to increase a person's awareness of how culture is a part of their daily experience of self and environment (Fernbacher & Plummer, 2005). Emphasis is placed on awareness of the counselor's personal positioning as human in a diverse and multi-faceted culture and considering how these factors affect how the client experiences the counselor. Additionally, the Polsters were some of the earliest advocates for women, identifying the processes through which society demands that they disown parts of the self for the sake of others and politeness (Roberts, 1999).

Similar to other phenomenological approaches, Gestalt practitioners must be extremely careful to not inadvertently force humanistic values and assumptions on clients, such as valuing emotional expression, preferring particular forms of "congruent" communication, or expecting different levels of emotional expression from women versus men (Gehart & Lyle, 2001).

Gestalt Case Study

Monica, a 27-year-old Mexican American female, has come to counseling because she began to have flashbacks and nightmares about her sexual abuse by her brother when she was 7 years old. She works as a grocery store clerk, and the nightmares started after one of her coworkers was raped in the parking lot one night. She reports that her parents minimized what happened by saying that he was just "exploring," but they agreed to not leave the two alone because of the issue. Her brother has never apologized. Over the years, Monica coped by being a "good girl" and playing by all of the rules and avoiding any type of risk. She had to work as soon as she turned 16 and started supporting herself as soon as she graduated from high school. She maintains her same friends from high school and has dated a few times but has not committed to anyone seriously after her high school sweetheart cheated on her with her best friend.

Gestalt Case Conceptualization

This case conceptualization was developed by selecting key concepts from "The Viewing: Case Conceptualization" section of this chapter. You can use any of the concepts in that section to develop a case conceptualization for this or other cases.

Assessing the Field

In assessing the field, AF (adult female) has a pattern of being and feeling victimized by others. It is likely that her unresolved issues related to being abused by her brother contributed to her choosing a boyfriend who eventually cheated on her and/or resulted in behaviors on her part that contributed to the problems in their relationship. Furthermore, her current pattern of avoiding risks, especially those related to relationships, is likely to continue to push others away from her.

Contact Boundaries and Encounters

AF has a long history of *deflection* and avoiding direct contact with others that can be traced back to her childhood sexual abuse. This pattern of deflection has become disabling in her social life.

Polarities and Disowned Parts

In order to cope with her abuse, AF has polarized, trying to become the "good girl" by avoiding risks, staying out of trouble, and always being responsible. Her avoidance of risk has truncated her development by choosing to work full-time rather than go to college and avoiding dating relationships in which she might get hurt.

"Shoulds"

AF has a long list of "shoulds": "I should not make a big deal of what happened," "I should always play itself and work at a safe job and avoid relationships where I might be hurt," "I should forgive and forget," and so on. These "shoulds" have kept her from living authentically in any area of her life.

Unfinished Business

AF has significant unfinished business with her brother and parents related to the abuse. The whole family has continued to go on like nothing ever happened by innocent child play, but AF feels otherwise. She has been too afraid to debunk this family myth but will likely need to speak her truth in order to live a more authentic life.

Gestalt Treatment Plan

Initial Phase of Treatment (First One to Three Sessions)
Initial Phase Therapeutic Tasks

1. *Develop working counseling relationship. Diversity note:* Adapt **emotional expression** to match AF's style as a Mexican American woman.
   Relationship building intervention:
   a. Confirmation of client's **unique self** and **validating her abuse experience** while counselor is also expressing authentic self.

2. *Assess individual, systemic, and broader cultural dynamics. Diversity note:* Adapt assessment of emotions, emotional expression, and authenticity to her family and cultural norms.
   Assessment strategies:
   a. Assess client's ability to make **authentic contact** with others and environment.
   b. Identify **polarities, disowned parts, "shoulds,"** and **unfinished business,** especially as they relate to abuse.

Initial Phase Client Goal

1. *Increase* tolerance of difficult emotions and **unwanted parts of self** that fuel crisis to reduce flashbacks and nightmares.
   Interventions:
   a. **Body awareness** and grounding exercises in session to help client identify and more effectively manage crisis emotions; developing grounding exercises in the present moment to help out of session.
   b. In structured in-session exercises, encourage client to **"stay with"** difficult **feelings** that fuel crisis and coach client through experiencing these emotions to defuse crisis out of session.

Working Phase of Treatment (Three or More Sessions)
Working Phase Counseling Task

1. *Monitor quality of the working alliance. Diversity note:* Adapt relationship to be responsive to AF's cultural forms of **emotional expression** as well as her need for safe **contact** due to abuse history.
   Assessment Intervention:
   a. Monitor frequency of **here-and-now experiencing,** willingness to tolerate differences between self and other, and **authentic expression of self**; use Session Rating Scale.

Working Phase Client Goals

1. *Increase* **integration of polarities** between "good girl" and "bad girl" to reduce shame related to the abuse and her fear of taking risks and being hurt or failing.
   Interventions:
   a. **Gestalt experiments** and **empty-chair** exercises to facilitate awareness and integration of polarities.
   b. **Modify language** both to allow for acceptance of polarities and to relax her fear of being "bad."

2. *Increase* ability to **self-regulate** in relationships to reduce avoidance of intimate relationships.

(continued)

Interventions:
a. Coach client on **staying with difficult feelings** related to rejection and being hurt to increase ability to self-regulate.
b. **Gestalt experiments** related to talking with men with alternative behaviors to increase self-regulation skills.

3. *Increase* ability to **accept "what is"** in relation to family's denial of abuse to reduce fear of risk and being hurt.
Interventions:
a. **Gestalt experiments** to practice raising the issue with her parents and/or brother; discuss pros and cons of doing these in real life and identify best strategies for resolving this old business.
b. **Language modification** to reduce "shoulds" in relation to "what is."

Closing Phase of Treatment (Last Four or More Sessions)
Closing Phase Counseling Task

1. *Develop aftercare plan and maintain gains. Diversity note:* Include strategies for early detection of trauma issues resurfacing.
Intervention:
a. Increase capacity for **organismic self-regulation** in relation to potential future stressors.

Closing Phase Client Goals

1. *Increase* capacity to **self-regulate** and expand **here-and-now experiencing** to be primary mode for daily living in all contexts to reduce potential for relapse of trauma symptoms, such as nightmares, relationship avoidance, and flashbacks.
Interventions:
a. Increasingly challenging **Gestalt experiments** to integrate spontaneity into all aspects of daily living.
b. **Dream work** to identify more subtle resistance and **polarities** that impeded full authenticity in daily living.

2. *Increase* **self-regulation** and **authentic expression of self** in intimate relationships while simultaneously allow for another's authenticity to reduce avoidance of intimate relationships.
Interventions:
a. **Empty-chair** experiments to develop awareness and skills for authentic relating to friends, family, and intimate partners.
b. **Gestalt experiments** in significant relationships that help to build capacity for authentic intimacy.

ONLINE RESOURCES

Associations and Training Institutes

Association for Humanistic Psychology
www.ahpweb.org

American Psychological Association, Division 32: Humanistic Psychology
www.apa.org/divisions/div32

Esalen Institute, Big Sur California
www.esalen.org

New York Institute for Gestalt Therapy
www.newyorkgestalt.org

Gestalt Institute of Cleveland
www.gestaltcleveland.org

Pacific Gestalt Institute
www.gestalttherapy.org

Gestalt Institute of San Francisco
www.gestaltinstitute.com/enter

Gestalt Institute of the Rockies
www.gestaltoftherockies.com

The Gestalt Therapy Institute of Philadelphia
www.gestaltphila.org

World Association for Person-Centered and Experiential Psychotherapy and Counseling
www.pce-world.org

Journals

British Gestalt Journal
www.britishgestaltjournal.com

Gestalt Review
www.gestaltreview.com

International Gestalt Journal
www.gestalt.org/igipromo

Journal of Humanistic Psychology
www.ahpweb.org/pub/journal/menu.html

Journal of the World Association for Person-Centered and Experiential Psychotherapy and Counseling
www.pce-world.org/pcep-journal.html

References

*Asterisk indicates recommended introductory readings.

Beisser, A. (1970). The paradoxical theory of change. In J. Fagan & I. Shepherd (Eds.), *Gestalt therapy now* (pp. 77–80). New York: Harper.

Clarke, K. M., & Greenberg, L. S. (1986). Differential effects of the Gestalt two-chair intervention and problem solving in resolving decisional conflict. *Journal of Counseling Psychology, 33*(1), 11–15.

Fernbacher, S., & Plummer, D. (2005). Cultural influences and considerations in Gestalt therapy. In A. L. Woldt & S. M. Toman (Eds.), *Gestalt therapy: History, theory, and practice* (pp. 117–132). Thousand Oaks, CA: Sage.

Gehart, D. R., & Lyle, R. R. (2001). Client experience of gender in therapeutic relationships: An interpretive ethnography. *Family Process, 40*, 443–458.

Greenberg, L. S., & Dompierre, L. M. (1981). Specific effects of Gestalt two-chair dialogue on intrapsychic conflict in counseling. *Journal of Counseling Psychology, 28*(4), 288–294. doi:10.1037/0022-0167.28.4.288

Greenberg, L., Elliott, R., & Lietaer, G. (1994). Research on experiential therapies. In A. Bergin & S. Garfield (Eds.), *Handbook of psychotherapy and behavior change* (pp. 509–539). New York: Wiley.

Greenberg, L. S., & Rice, L. N. (1981). The specific effects of a Gestalt intervention. *Psychotherapy: Theory, Research, and Practice, 18*, 31–37.

Hycner, R. (1995). The dialogic ground. In R. Hycner & L. Jacobs (Eds.), *The healing relationship in Gestalt therapy* (pp. 3–30). Highland, NY: Gestalt Journal Press.

Hycner, R., & Jacobs, L. (Eds.). (1995). *The healing relationship in Gestalt therapy*. Highland, NY: Gestalt Journal Press.

Lobb, M. S., & Lichtenberg, P. (2005). Classic Gestalt therapy theory: Field theory. In A. L. Woldt & S. M. Toman (Eds.), *Gestalt therapy: History, theory, and practice* (pp. 21–39). Thousand Oaks, CA: Sage.

Parlett, M., & Lee, R. G. (2005). Contemporary Gestalt therapy: Field theory. In A. L. Woldt & S. M. Toman (Eds.), *Gestalt therapy: History, theory, and practice* (pp. 41–63). Thousand Oaks, CA: Sage.

Perls, F. (1973). *The Gestalt approach and eyewitness to therapy*. Palo Alto, CA: Science and Behavior Books.

Perls, F., Hefferline, R. F., & Goodman, P. (1951). *Gestalt therapy: Excitement and growth in the human personality*. New York: Julian Press.

Polster, E., & Polster, M. (1973). *Gestalt therapy integrated*. New York: Brunner/Mazel.

Roberts, A. (1999). *From the radical center: The heart of Gestalt therapy: Selected writings of Erving and Miriam Polster*. Cleveland, OH: Gestalt Institute of Cleveland Press.

Smith, E. W. L. (1976). The roots of Gestalt therapy. In *The growing edge of Gestalt therapy* (pp. 3–36). Highland, NY: Gestalt Journal Press.

Wagner-Moore, L. E. (2004). Gestalt therapy: Past, present, theory, and research. *Psychotherapy: Theory, Research, Practice, Training, 41*(2), 180–189. doi:10.1037/0033-3204.41.2.180

Woldt, A. L., & Toman, S. M. (Eds.). (2005). *Gestalt therapy: History, theory, and practice*. Thousand Oaks, CA: Sage.

Yontef, G. (1993). *Awareness dialogue and process: Essays on Gestalt therapy*. Highland, NY: Gestalt Journal Press.

Yontef, G., & Jacobs, L. (2000). Gestalt therapy. In R. J. Corsini & D. Wedding (Eds.), *Current psychotherapies* (6th ed., pp. 303–339). Itasca, IL: Peacock Publishers.

CHAPTER

9

Cognitive-Behavioral Approaches

When people understand or have insight into how they needlessly disturb themselves and create unhealthy and dysfunctional feelings and behaviors, that insight often will help them change and make themselves less disturbed. But understanding and insight are not enough. In order to significantly change themselves, they almost always have to pinpoint their irrational philosophies and work at changing them to more functional and self-helping attitudes. They can do this in a number of cognitive, emotive-evocative, and behavioral ways.

—Ellis (2003, p. 220)

Lay of the Land

Behavioral, cognitive, and cognitive-behavioral approaches are a group of related counseling methods that emphasize using active techniques and psychoeducation to achieve changes in behaviors, cognition, and affect. They are favored by third-party payers, such as insurance, because they are brief, target medical symptoms rather than broader personality issues, and have a strong research tradition. These approaches can be divided into three streams of practice:

- *Behavioral approaches:* Using classical conditioning, operant conditioning, and social learning theory, behavioral approaches focus on analyzing and intervening on observable, measurable behaviors; in this approach, thought is conceptualized as a covert behavior that operates according to standard behavioral principles (Skinner, 1974). The evolution of behavioral approaches occurred in three waves (Hayes, 2004):
  - *The first wave of behaviorism:* The original "pure" behavioral approaches based on classical conditioning, operant conditioning, and social learning theory (see "The Viewing: Case Conceptualization").
  - *The second wave of behaviorism:* Integration of cognitive approaches with behavioral, which before the 1980s was a separate stream of research and practice.

- ○ *The third wave of behaviorism:* In the 21st century, mindfulness approaches are transforming behavioral practices to use compassionate acceptance of thoughts and feelings to paradoxically promote change.
- *Cognitive approaches:* Developed independently from behavioral approaches by Aaron Beck, cognitive approaches are based on the premise that (a) psychological disorders are characterized by dysfunctional thinking based on dysfunctional beliefs and that (b) improvement results from modifying dysfunctional thinking and beliefs (Beck, 1997). Cognitive theory can be used (a) separately from behaviorism, (b) as part of an integrated cognitive-behavioral practice, or (c) as *metatheory* for a general integrative approach (Alford & Beck, 1997).
- *Cognitive-behavioral approaches:* The mainstay of most contemporary practitioners, cognitive-behavioral approaches integrate both behavioral and cognitive techniques for changing problem thoughts, behaviors, and feelings. This chapter focuses on this commonly practiced combined approach. Several distinct forms of cognitive-behavioral approaches have been developed over the years:
  - ○ *Multimodal therapy:* An approach that uses an eclectic set of interventions, Arnold Lazarus's multimodal therapy is based on assessment of the BASIC-ID: behavior, affect, sensation, imagery, cognition, interpersonal relationships, and drug treatment.
  - ○ *Rational emotive behavior therapy:* Developed by Albert Ellis, counselors in rational emotive behavior therapy (REBT) use *A-B-C* analysis to help clients identify the *belief* (B) that results in symptomatic *consequences* (C) in response to *activating* (A) *events*. This approach uses a confrontational style to dispute irrational beliefs.
  - ○ *Reality therapy:* More philosophical than other cognitive-behavioral approaches, William Glasser's (1975, 1984) reality theory is based the premise that people are driven by five basic needs—survival, love, power, freedom, and fun—and emphasizes how people *choose everything* they do, including feeling miserable.
  - ○ *Mindfulness-based approaches:* The most recently developed, mindfulness-based approaches, such as mindfulness-based stress reduction and acceptance and commitment therapy, use observation of the mind and acceptance of thoughts and feelings to reduce anxiety, depression, addictive behaviors, and other symptoms. Because these put a paradoxical twist on traditional practices, they will be discussed in a separate section at the end of this chapter.

Cognitive-Behavioral Approaches

In a Nutshell: The Least You Need to Know

Cognitive-behavioral counselors have a no-nonsense, matter-of-fact approach to helping clients that is based on logic and education. Judith Beck (2005) wraps up cognitive approaches thusly: "In a nutshell, the *cognitive model* proposes that distorted or dysfunctional thinking (which influences the patient's mood and behavior) is common to all psychological disturbances. Realistic evaluation and modification of thinking procedures produces an improvement in mood and behavior" (p. 1; emphasis in the original; also, I did not pay her to mention nutshells). More simply stated, cognitive counselors believe unhelpful thoughts are the source of emotional and behavioral problems. Behaviorists add that maladaptive behavioral reinforcement also results in problem symptoms.

Cognitive-behavioral counselors use behavioral and cognitive techniques to directly treat symptoms either by creating new behavioral associations or by helping clients think and feel differently. More so than any other approach, they rely heavily on psychoeducation to help clients change their thinking and behavioral habits. The role of counselors is educational, using their expertise to help clients learn how to manage their thoughts, feelings, and emotions more effectively. Clients are actively engaged by performing homework tasks out of session. Unlike psychodynamic and humanistic approaches, the overarching goal is not personality change; instead, cognitive-behavioral counselors have the more modest goal of helping clients learn how to better manage troubling symptoms. Developed using the scientific method, cognitive behaviorists have a strong research tradition, generating a solid evidence base for its effectiveness with a wide range of clinical concerns.

The Juice: Significant Contributions to the Field

If you remember one thing from this chapter, it should be ...

A-B-C Theory

Originally developed by Albert Ellis (1962, 1996) using Beck's (1976) cognitive theory, the A-B-C theory is the centerpiece of rational emotive behavioral therapy. This model highlights the essence of all cognitive approaches: our *thoughts about a situation*—not the situation itself—are the source of emotional and behavioral problems. When you truly and deeply understand the wisdom in this statement, your life will never be the same—and you will be in a much better position to help others. So, to help lock this into your mind, I am going to put it in another one of those boxes:

> Our *thoughts about a situation*—not the situation itself—are the source of emotional and behavioral problems.

If you still need convincing, ponder how certain prisoners of war respond to torture. They experience forms of suffering far greater than most counselors and their clients face in the 21st century, making common presenting problems, such as having a critical parent or breaking up with a boyfriend, hard to label as a problem. For example, there are numerous Tibetan monks and nuns who were brutally tortured by the Chinese in the 1960s and 1970s and, when eventually released, did not report symptoms of trauma (Hayward & Varela, 1992). In fact, some described having compassion for those who tortured them *while being tortured*. Such responses defy Western psychological theories about trauma until the mediating beliefs are considered: these Buddhist practitioners have a different set of beliefs about "human rights" and maintain religious beliefs that emphasize learning to develop compassion for one's enemies as part of their spiritual development. Their beliefs informed their unusual response. Similarly, Viktor Frankl, who we learned about in Chapter 7, also noted that the attitude of prisoners in Nazi concentration camps dramatically affected their mental and physical survival, with those able to make meaning able to better survive the most horrifying of circumstances. These are extreme examples of how a person's thoughts shape emotional and behavioral responses to an event. The event itself is not the cause.

However, for most of us mere mortals, when we experience an adverse event, *it seems as though* it is clearly the cause of negative thoughts and feelings because the beliefs silently mediate the response in the background. Ultimately, cognitive behavioralists argue, it is the individual who is responsible for choosing thoughts and beliefs that result in healthy behaviors and positive emotions. Let's not kid ourselves: that is quite a challenge.

So, let's explore the other end of the spectrum and consider a mundane, nonclinical illustration. I feel hurt when you insult me, saying, "Your last example about the Tibetans and Nazis is moronic." Common sense (in Western cultures; after all, common sense is always culturally defined) would hold that feeling hurt after being insulted is "normal." However, that is not the cognitive-behavioral approach. Instead, the question would be, What belief do I hold that results in my feeling hurt? In this case, I would have to answer that on the basis of my culture, class, age, immigration status, and education, I believe that a person should not harshly criticize another even if there is disagreement; the person should find a more polite way to say it (i.e., "Your example did not convince me"), not say anything at all, or find an academic source to refute my claim. However, a cognitive behaviorist would be quick to point out that my feeling hurt is the result of *my beliefs*, not your comment. To further complicate matters, another person with slightly different but similar beliefs may feel angry, ashamed, or embarrassed. How one feels is a result of their belief, not the comment. The comment is only the trigger.

Cultural Considerations   At this point, you may be wondering when is a comment fairly labeled an "insult," "rude," or "appropriate." The general answer is that it depends on a complex matrix of age, social class, gender, education, ethnicity, ability, and sexual orientation as well as the level of intimacy of the persons involved. The cognitive behavioralist would add that a person should opt to not blindly follow a belief that doesn't work for them (Ellis, 1994). Thus, even if a person comes from a cultural context in which insults are considered rude and reason to be hurt or angry, that person should consider adopting new beliefs that do not result in negative emotions. From this perspective, although culture influences our every thought, action, and feeling, each person still has choice in terms of *how*. It should be noted that this highly individualistic belief is not shared in all cultures, and counselors must consider this when working with diverse clients (see "Snapshot: Working With Diverse Populations"). Perhaps now you have a better sense why cross-cultural communication becomes tricky quickly.

Clinical Applications   Finally, let's also consider the types of beliefs you are likely to work with in session, beliefs that fuel depression, anxiety, substance abuse, eating disorders, and so on. The basic rule still applies: beliefs are the missing link between a situation and the resulting feelings and behaviors. For example, many people experience the feelings and behaviors that characterize depression, such as feeling sad, avoiding once-pleasurable activities, and difficulty getting out of bed in the morning. Many beliefs can fuel these feelings, such as "I am worthless," "No one cares about me," or "I will never achieve my dreams" (note: You will read about Beck's and Ellis's specific cognitive theories on depression in "The Viewing: Case Conceptualization" section). The counselor's job is to help clients realize that it was not the specific event, such as losing a job or girlfriend, that caused these feelings; instead, it is the belief they have about these events that are causing the symptoms (e.g., "without that job or girlfriend, I am worthless").

Ellis developed the A-B-C model to illustrate how humans create their difficulties by the beliefs they hold. In this model, A is the "activating event" (the problem person, situation, etc.), B is the "belief" about the meaning of that event (that one is generally not aware of until a counselor points it out), and C is the emotional or behavioral "consequence" based on the belief (the symptoms).

A-B-C Model

A = Activating event → B = Belief about A → C = Emotional & behavioral consequences

(Trigger event or person)   (Symptoms)

Most clients come in able to see only the connection between A and C and thus report that A *causes* C: "I am depressed *because* my boyfriend broke up with me" or "I am angry *because* my boss favors my coworker." The counselor's job is to help the client identify the belief (B) that the client does not put into the equation, such as "I am worthless if a man decides not to be with me" or "I need to be the best in the office." These *irrational beliefs* are identified in assessment and targeted for change in the intervention phase by disputing these beliefs and adopting more realistic ones. If you are wondering, identifying the dysfunctional beliefs is far easier than changing them, but it is the requisite first step.

Rumor Has It: The People and Their Stories
Foundational Researchers
Ivan Pavlov A Russian physiologist and pioneer in behavior studies, Ivan Pavlov (1932) first described what is now referred to as *classical conditioning*: the ability to elicit a response (salivating) by pairing a natural stimulus (food) with a neutral stimulus (a bell).

B. F. Skinner Building on Pavlov's work, Skinner identified the principles of operant conditioning, which are used to shape new behaviors using consequences and schedules of reinforcement.

Albert Bandura A leading social learning theorist who built on Pavlov's and Skinner's work, Albert Bandura studied how people learn vicariously by observing others, their behaviors, and the consequences of those behaviors. His early experiments examined how children learn aggressiveness by watching adults act aggressively, a process now well known as *role modeling*. He advocated using behavioral methods not to control people but rather to help them develop their capacities for self-direction, sharing values similar to humanists (Bandura, 1974, 1986).

John B. Watson Considered the grandfather of behaviorism, Watson believed that behavior should be the sole focus of psychology, arguing that since cognitions were outside the realm of observation, they were inappropriate for empirical study. Most important, he established a culture of scientific research for the study of human behavior.

Joseph Wolpe Born in South Africa, trained as a Freudian, and conducting much of his research in the United States, Wolpe developed *systematic desensitization*, which is used to treat phobias and other anxiety disorders, after he found that traditional psychoanalytic approaches produced less-than-satisfactory results in treating posttraumatic stress in war veterans.

Leading Theorists and Practitioners
Aaron Beck One of the most disciplined researchers in the field of counseling and psychotherapy, Aaron Beck began his career attempting to scientifically validate Freud's theory of depression. When that failed, he began researching a cognitive model of depression (Beck, 1972, 1991) that resulted in his rejection and isolation from the psychiatric community for many years. Examining the underlying dysfunctional beliefs of psychopathology, Beck's (1988, 1991) research on depression, anxiety, substance abuse, eating disorders, relationship and personality disorders are considered some of the most significant in the field.

Albert Ellis A flamboyant, humorous, and often abrasive figure, Albert Ellis first articulated his highly influential REBT based on the A-B-C theory of change in 1955. He continued to developing his ideas, teaching, and writing until his death in 2007 at the age of 93. His theory used cognitive, behavioral, and affective techniques to help people make themselves less miserable.

Arnold Lazarus Grounding his work in cognitive and social learning theories, Lazarus developed *multimodal therapy*, which involves a multifaceted assessment and encourages technical eclecticism to effect change across all areas of functioning and experience.

Donald Meichenbaum Donald Meichenbaum's cognitive-behavioral modification approach focuses on changing clients' self-talk, intervening to help clients interrupt their negative internal scripts and replace these with more realistic thoughts. Meichenbaum (1997) is one of the few cognitive behavioralists who grounds his work in postmodern assumptions that people construct their realities through language, informing a greater "discovery orientation" than other cognitive behavioralists.

Big Picture: Overview of Counseling Process

The cognitive-behavioral approach involves four basic phases or steps:

- *Step 1: Assessment:* Counseling begins by obtaining a detailed behavioral and/or cognitive assessment of *baseline functioning*, including frequency, duration, and context of problem behaviors and thoughts.
- *Step 2: Target behaviors/thoughts for change:* Cognitive-behavioral counselors identify specific behaviors and thoughts for intervention (e.g., rather than the general goal of "improve mood," the counselor would target "increasing engagement in pleasurable activities," "initiating social contact," etc.).
- *Step 3: Educate:* Counselors educate clients on their irrational thoughts and dysfunctional patterns, helping to motivate them to make changes.
- *Step 4: Replace and retrain:* Finally, specific interventions are designed to replace dysfunctional behaviors and thoughts with more productive ones. Once the presenting symptoms have dissipated, treatment is ended.

Making Connection: Counseling Relationship

Educator and Expert

"REBT has always been very forceful, confrontative, and opposed to namby-pamby methods of therapy. It has particularly encouraged therapists to take the risks of quickly showing clients how they defeat themselves, rather than taking a long time to get to this point and rather than allowing clients to be evasive and defensive" (Ellis, 2003, p. 232).

Although the affective quality of connection exhibited by cognitive-behavioral counselors varies greatly—from cool and detached to warm and friendly to forceful and confrontative (but never namby-pamby)—the primary role of the counselor is the same: to serve as an expert who *directs* and *educates* the client and family on how to better manage their problems (Ellis, 2003). Especially in the working phase of counseling, the counselor's primary role is to educate clients on better ways to think and behave. Some cognitive-behavioral counselors, such as Ellis and Glasser, conceive of their role primarily as educators and adopt a highly directive approach. Others, such as Aaron Beck (1976), Judith Beck (2005), and Arnold Lazarus (1981), advocate a much warmer approach that "educates" using questions in Socratic style, requiring clients to critically and logically analyze their situation, offering a gentler means of guidance.

Empathy in Cognitive-Behavioral Counseling

True to their research foundations, cognitive-behavioral counselors increasingly use empathy, warmth, and a nonjudgmental stance to build a counseling alliance based on research results that indicate that these counselor qualities predict positive outcomes (Meichenbaum, 1997; see also the section "Common Factors Research" in Chapter 2). However, *the reason a cognitive-behavioral counselor uses empathy is quite different from the reason an humanistic counselor uses empathy.* This is frequently misunderstood, so I am going to say it again in case your mind was wandering: *cognitive-behavioral counselors use empathy for entirely different reasons than humanistic counselors.* Cognitive-behavioral counselors use empathy to create *rapport*, which then allows them to get to the "real" interventions that will change a client's behaviors, thoughts, and emotions. In dramatic contrast, for an experiential counselor, empathy *is* the intervention: they maintain that empathy is a curative process in and of itself (Rogers, 1961). The cognitive-behavioral counselor who uses empathy should not be seen as "manipulative" because in most cases the idea is to make the client feel more comfortable with the process, not to trick him or her. They should also not be seen as "integrating" experiential concepts because they are not using an experiential concept in the way an experiential counselor would use it. Instead, they are *adapting* it to work within their philosophical assumptions about counseling and the change process.

Contemporary Cognitive-Behavioral Alliance

Judith Beck (2005) describes five practices for fostering the counseling alliance that reflect more contemporary sensibilities:

1. *Actively collaborate with the patient:* Decisions about counseling should be jointly made with the client.
2. *Demonstrate empathy, caring, and understanding:* Expressing empathy helps clients trust the counselor.
3. *Adapt one's counseling style:* Interventions, self-disclosure, and directiveness should be adjusted for each client based on personality, presenting problem, and so on.
4. *Alleviate distress:* Demonstrating clinical effectiveness by helping clients solve problems and improving their moods enhances the counseling relationship.
5. *Elicit feedback at the end of the session:* By asking clients "how did it go?" at the end of each session, counselors can intervene early in cases of alliance rupture.

By building a collaborative and engaged alliance, counselors are more likely to be effective and work through possible dysfunctional beliefs the client may have about counseling or the counselor that interfere with the process, such as "My counselor doesn't understand me" or "This will never work."

Written Contracts

Cognitive-behavioral counselors are perhaps the most business-like when it comes to a counseling relationship (Holtzworth-Munroe & Jacobson, 1991), at least in terms of how they write about it on paper. And they are actually the most likely to write about it on paper. They frequently use *written contracts* spelling out the goals and expectations to help structure the relationship and to increase motivation and dedication with clients. Putting the goals and agreement in writing and having clients sign that they agree can be a very motivating experience for clients, creating a sense of commitment to the process.

The Viewing: Case Conceptualization

Baseline Functioning

At the beginning of treatment, sometimes even before the first session, cognitive-behavioral counselors conduct a baseline assessment of functioning that provides a starting point for measuring change. They ask clients to log the (a) frequency, (b) duration, and (c) severity of specific behavioral symptoms, such as depression, anxiety, panic, anger, social withdrawal, or conflict. Counselors may also include in the log identifying *antecedent* events that may have triggered the symptoms. Although it may seem that relying on clients' verbal recall of their symptoms is sufficient, most always a baseline assessment provides more detailed and accurate information than recall alone. In the case study at the end of this chapter, an assessment of baseline functioning is used to assess Maria's bipolar episodes.

A baseline log may look like this:

Problem Behavior	When?	How Long?	How Severe?	Events Before?	Events After?
Binging and purging	Monday evening: 7:00 p.m.; after a stressful day	1 hour	7 (on a 1–10 scale)	No breakfast; did not sleep well night before; tension with boss	Surfed Internet to distract self
Binging and purging	Friday night: 1:00 a.m.; after date	2 hours	9+	Fight with boyfriend during date; felt fat when saw other girls at club	Slept in next day; called boyfriend to make up

Cognitive-Behavioral Functional Analysis

Originally a purely behavioral assessment technique that was later adopted for cognitions also, *functional analysis* involves careful analysis of the antecedents and consequences of problem thoughts and behaviors in order to identify naturally occurring triggers, rewards, and punishments to clearly identify cause-and-effect patterns (Meichenbaum, 1977). Counselors use functional analysis to examine what a person was doing and thinking as well as what was going on in the environment *before, during*, and *after* an episode of the symptom. For example, if a person reports cutting to manage stress, the counselor would ask about what she was thinking and doing before the episode as well as ask about what was happening in her life at the time: the who, what, where, and when of her life. Similar questions are used to assess what she was feeling and thinking during and after cutting and what was going in her life. The counselor does this with several episodes early in treatment to identify patterns of what triggers and what reinforces the cutting. Functional analysis makes it easy to design successful interventions that are likely to quickly modify the problem behavior and thoughts.

Questions for Cognitive-Behavioral Functional Analysis

- What were you doing before (during and after) the episode? Where were you? Who was around? What time of day?

- What were you thinking before (during and after) the episode? Describe your inner conversation—thought by thought.

- What was going on in your life at the time (during and after)? What were the normal activities? What were atypical stressors?

- Repeat the above sequence of questions for "during" and "after" the episode.

Schemas and Core Beliefs

The cognitive approach of Aaron Beck (1976, 1997) focused on identifying and changing *schemas* and *core beliefs* that fuel problems in clients' lives, such as the belief that one must be perfect or that life should be fair. As the foundation for *dysfunctional thinking*, dysfunctional schemas are the root source of psychopathology; for the gains in counseling to be long term, the counseling process must modify core schemas, not just specific thoughts about a particular issue (Beck, 1997).

Schemas are the deepest of four levels in Beck's conceptualization of cognitions:

1. *Automatic thoughts:* These thoughts are "knee-jerk" reactions to distressing situations that run through a person's mind and that the person can generally identify, such as "If my friend does not return my call in 24 hours, she does not really like me."
2. *Intermediate beliefs:* Extreme or absolute rules that are more general and shape automatic thoughts, such as "Good friends always return calls quickly."
3. *Core beliefs:* Also global and absolute, core beliefs are about *ourselves*, such as "I am worthless." Beck identifies two general unifying principles or themes that underlie most core beliefs: (a) autonomy (beliefs about being effective and productive vs. helpless) and (b) sociotropic (beliefs about being lovable or unlovable).
4. *Schemas:* The deepest level of the cognitive structure, schemas are cognitive frameworks in the mind, organizing and shaping thoughts, feelings, and behaviors. Developed in childhood and informed by numerous other factors, including family, culture, gender, religion, and occupation, schemas may lie dormant until triggered by a specific event, such as "I am utterly worthless if even my best friend won't take the time to call me; no one really cares about me at all; what is the point of even trying to have friends if they only call when it's convenient for *them*?" Once triggered, information tends to be filtered to support the premise of the schema and valid evidence to the contrary is ignored; for example, even when the friend calls

apologizing that she didn't call back sooner because she felt ill, this is seen only as an excuse and further confirmation of being unlovable.

Assessing and correctly identifying schemas takes more time than assessing automatic thoughts and intermediate beliefs and adds greater depth to the counseling process. In the case study at the end of this chapter, the counselor identifies the core beliefs and schemas that fuel Maria's periods of depression and irritation.

Distorted Cognitions

Changing schemas is the ultimate goal in Beck's (1997) cognitive approach. To achieve this end, counselors often begin by identifying common *distortions* in automatic thoughts and intermediate beliefs that can then be changed using thought records (see "The Doing: Interventions"). These include:

1. *Arbitrary inference:* A belief based on little evidence (e.g., assuming your partner is cheating on you because she does not answer the phone immediately).
2. *Selective abstraction:* Focusing on one detail while ignoring the context and other obvious details (e.g., believing your boss/supervisor/instructor thinks you are incompetent because he or she identified areas for improvement in addition to strengths).
3. *Overgeneralization:* Just like it sounds, generalizing one or two incidents to make a broad sweeping judgment (e.g., believing that because your son listens to acid rock, he is not going to college and will end up on drugs).
4. *Magnification and minimization:* Going to either extreme of overemphasizing or underemphasizing based on the facts (e.g., ignoring two semesters of your child's poor grades is minimizing; hiring a tutor for one low test score is magnification).
5. *Personalization:* A particular form of arbitrary influence that is especially common in intimate relationships where external events are attributed to oneself (e.g., "My spouse has lost interest in me because she did not want to have sex tonight").
6. *Dichotomous thinking:* All-or-nothing thinking: always/never, success/failure, or good/bad (e.g., "If my husband isn't madly in love with me, then he really doesn't love me at all").
7. *Mislabeling:* Assigning a personality trait to someone based on a handful of incidents, often ignoring exceptions (e.g., saying one's husband is lazy because he does not help immediately on being asked).
8. *Mind reading:* A favorite in families and couple relationships, mind reading is believing you know what the other is thinking or will do without any supporting evidence and becomes a significant barrier to communication, especially when related to disagreements and hot topics, such as sex, religion, money, housework, and so on (e.g., before your spouse says a word, you are defending yourself).

In addition, Beck (1997) has identified dysfunctional schemas that are commonly associated with specific personality disorders:

- *Dependent:* "I am helpless."
- *Avoidant:* "I might get hurt."
- *Passive-aggressive:* "I might get stepped on."
- *Paranoid:* "People are out to get me."
- *Narcissistic:* "I am special."
- *Histrionic:* "I need to impress others."
- *Compulsive:* "Errors are bad."
- *Antisocial:* "People are there to be taken."
- *Schizoid:* "I need plenty of space."

Irrational Beliefs: The Three Basic Musts

Similar to assessing schemas in Beck's cognitive approach, Ellis (1994, 2003) assesses for *irrational beliefs*, which are typically flagged by words such as "should," "ought," and "must." These are preferences that get exaggerated into absolutist, extreme thinking, and unrealistic beliefs that lead to depression, anxiety, and a host of other unpleasant experiences. Over the years, Ellis (2003) has collapsed what were originally 11 categories into three basic categories of irrational beliefs:

1. *Perfection-based worth:* "'I must be thoroughly competent, adequate, achieving, and lovable at all times, or else I am an incompetent worthless person.' This belief usually leads to feelings of anxiety, panic, depression, despair, and worthlessness" (p. 236).
2. *Justice for me:* "'Other significant people in my life, must treat me kindly and fairly at all times, or else I can't stand it, and they are bad, rotten, and evil persons who should be severely blamed, damned, and vindictively punished for their horrible treatment of me.' This leads to feelings of anger, rage, fury, and vindictiveness and to actions like feuds, wars, fights, genocide, and ultimately, an atomic holocaust" (pp. 236–237).
3. *Effortless perfection:* "'Things and conditions absolutely must be the way I want them to be and must never be too difficult or frustrating. Otherwise, life is awful, terrible, horrible, catastrophic and unbearable.' This leads to low-frustration tolerance, self-pity, anger, depression, and to behaviors such as procrastination, avoidance, and inaction" (p. 237).

Negative Cognitive Triad

Beck's (1972, 1976) theory of depression describes a *negative cognitive triad* that characterizes depressed thinking. This triad consists of three sets of negative thoughts that characterize the thinking of person who is depressed:

1. Negative thoughts about the self (e.g., "I am worthless")
2. Negative thoughts about the world/environment (e.g., "life is unfair")
3. Negative thoughts about the future (e.g., "things will never get better")

Typically, people who are clinically depressed report having negative thoughts in all three areas rather than just one or two. For example, pessimism is defined by negative thoughts about the future but does not automatically lead to depression unless the person also has negative thoughts about self and the world.

BASIC-ID

Designed to be a brief, solution-oriented, yet comprehensive approach, Lazarus's (1981) *multimodal therapy* is "best described as *systematic eclecticism*" (p. 4) and is organized around the seven-pronged assessment of the BASIC-ID: behavior, affect, sensation, imagery, cognition, interpersonal relationships, and drugs/biology. The BASIC-ID questions can be used for a general global assessment or around a specific problem or symptom. (p. 17).

BASIC-ID Assessment for General Mental Health

- *Behavior:* What behaviors are getting in the way of your happiness? What behaviors do you want to stop or start doing and/or do more of?
- *Affect:* What makes you laugh? Cry? What makes you mad, sad, glad, scared? Are you troubled by any particular emotions?
- *Sensation:* What do you especially like/dislike to see, hear, taste, touch, and smell? Do you experience frequent unpleasant sensations (such as pain, dizziness, tremors, etc.)? What are some sensual and sexual turn-ons and turn-offs for you?
- *Imagery:* What do you picture yourself doing in the immediate future? How would you describe your self image? Body image? What do you like/dislike about these images? How do they influence your life?

(continued)

- *Cognition:* What are some of your most cherished beliefs and values? What are your main "shoulds," "oughts," and "musts"? What are your intellectual interests and pursuits? How do your thoughts affect your emotions?
- *Interpersonal relationships:* Who are the most important people in your life? What do they expect from you and you of them? How do they affect you and you affect them?
- *Drugs and biology:* Do you have any medical concerns? What are your diet and exercise habits? What type of medications do you use? Do you drink, smoke, or use recreational drugs? How much, how often?

BASIC-ID can also be used to assess a specific area or problem:

- *Behavior:* What are you doing in relation to the problems? (e.g., frequent crying, insomnia, bathing less often)
- *Affect:* What are your problematic emotional states? (e.g., depressed mood, no enthusiasm for or interest in favorite activities, worry)
- *Sensation:* What physiological sensations are you experiencing in relation to the problem? (tight back and jaw; abdominal discomforts, exhaustion, tightness in chest)
- *Imagery:* What images or metaphors do you associate with the problem? (e.g., nightmares of being chased, daydreams of quitting job)
- *Cognition:* What thoughts and beliefs are associated with the problem? (e.g., catastrophic thinking, self-blame, perfectionistic thinking)
- *Interpersonal relationships:* Which of your relationships impact and are affected by the problem? (e.g., shutting out boyfriend, drifting away from friends, avoiding family)
- *Drugs and biology:* What medications and physical conditions impact and are affected by the problem? (e.g., gaining weight, on antidepressants for 2 months, minimal progress)

A client-focused approach, multimodal assessment is used to fit the treatment to the client rather than requiring the client adapt to the treatment (Lazarus, 1981). Lazarus tailors treatment by *tracking* the clients' modality *firing order* or preferences and then sequences techniques accordingly. For example, if a client primarily describes the problem in behavioral terms, behavioral interventions will be the first line of intervention; then, if imagery were the second most salient, it would be targeted next and so forth. To keep treatment brief, Lazarus (1997) recommends using one of six modalities (B, S, I, C, I, D; basically, any modality *except* affect) to treat an issue "because affect cannot be directly modified but has to be accessed through one or more of the other six modalities" (p. 88). Lazarus contends that any shift in one area affects shifts in all the areas because they are interrelated.

DSM *Diagnosis*

Of all the mental health treatment approaches, cognitive-behavioral counseling is most closely aligned with the medical model, and thus they typically organize treatment using the diagnoses outlined in the *Diagnostic and Statistical Manual of Mental Disorders* (4th ed.; *DSM-IV*). Beck (1997) developed specific cognitive approaches for working with different diagnoses, such as depression, anxiety, eating disorders, substance abuse, and so on, having identified common dysfunctional cognitive patterns associate with each. Similarly, specific behavioral approaches have been developed for phobias, panic, depression, and various anxiety issues. Glasser (2003) is a notable exception, arguing that mental health symptoms are not "diseases" per se and that they can be changed when clients are supported in making new choices.

Targeting Change: Goal Setting

"When people accept the fact that they largely control their own emotional and behavioral destiny, and that they can make themselves undisturbed or less disturbed mainly by acquiring realistic and sensible attitudes about the undesirable things that occur or that they make occur in their lives, they then usually have the ability and power of changing their belief system, making it more functional, and helping themselves to feel and to behave in a significantly less disturbed fashion" (Ellis, 2003, p. 220).

Symptom and Problem Resolution

Unlike depth psychology and humanistic approaches, cognitive-behavioral counselors' primary goal is to reduce presenting symptoms and problems. Symptom resolution is considered a sufficient goal in and of itself, and broader, growth-oriented goals are not considered necessary. Furthermore, cognitive-behavioral counselors do not have a laundry list of "normal" thoughts and behaviors that all clients should exhibit to be considered healthy; instead, they work with clients to identify which beliefs and actions are resulting in problems and change *those and only those*, not adding other long-term goals based on a theory of personality or health.

Independent Problem Solvers

The long-term vision in cognitive-behavioral approaches is to enable clients to independently solve their own problems by recognizing dysfunctional thoughts and behaviors early enough to keep them from creating unnecessary emotional distress (Beck, 1997; Ellis, 2003). This goal is conceptually quite different from psychodynamic and humanistic goals that target personality change. Aspiring to be realistic, cognitive-behavioral counselors do not promise dramatic changes in the structure of the psyche but rather measure success by a client's ability to handle life stressors better, not perfectly. They also do not expect that life will be without future challenges and instead see the goal as preparing clients to better manage these on their own.

Behavioral and Measurable Goals

Specific treatment goals are identified through the above assessment procedures. Goals are stated in *behavioral* and *measurable* terms, such as "reduce arguments to no more than one per month." Once clear goals are agreed on, counselors also obtain a commitment from the client to follow instructions and complete out-of-session assignments in order to achieve the agreed-on goals. This agreement is often written down in the form of a written counseling contract. Getting client "buy-in" to complete assignments immediately on setting goals greatly increases the likelihood of client follow through.

Examples of middle phase cognitive-behavioral goals include the following:

- Reduce episodes of cutting and self-harm
- Replace perfectionist beliefs about work performance
- Reduce generalizations and mind reading with partner

Examples of late phase cognitive-behavioral goals include the following:

- Increase engagement in enjoyable activities, hobbies, and relationships
- End the use of substances to manage difficult moods; manage moods using healthy coping skills
- Redefine "I must be perfect to be loved" schema to increase capacity for intimacy

The Doing: Interventions
Psychoeducation

A hallmark of cognitive-behavioral counseling, psychoeducation involves teaching clients psychological principles and using them to handle problems (Ellis & Dryden, 1997;

Lazarus, 1981). Psychoeducation can be done in individual or groups sessions. The content typically falls into four categories:

- *Problem oriented:* Information about the patient's diagnosis and/or situation, such as attention-deficit/hyperactivity disorder, schizophrenia, alcohol dependence, depression, and so on. Counselors use this type of education to motivate clients toward taking new action.
- *Change oriented:* Information about how to reduce problem symptoms, such as improve communication, reduce anger, decrease depression, and so on. Counselors use this type of education to help clients actively solve their problems. For such education to be successful, clients must be highly motivated, and counselors need to introduce the new behavior in small, practical steps using everyday language.
- *Bibliotherapy:* "Bibliotherapy" is a fancy term for assigning clients readings that will be (a) motivating and/or (b) instructional for dealing with their presenting problem. Typically, counselors assign cognitive-behavioral self-help books, such as *Feeling Good* (Burns, 1988) or *The Worry Cure* (Leahy, 2005), to reinforce what is learned in session, but fiction or professional literature may also be assigned.
- *Cinema therapy:* Similar to bibliotherapy, cinema therapy involves assigning clients to watch a movie that will speak to the problem issues (Berg-Cross, Jennings, & Baruch, 1990).

Tips for Effectively Providing Psychoeducation and Task Setting (*Yes, these are similar to those used by Adlerians in Chapter 5*)

- *Practice!* Yes, I'm serious. There aren't too many counseling skills I recommend new counselors "practice" on family and friends, but psychoeducation is the major exception. Try explaining concepts and research outcome to people who haven't read books like this one. Notice the types of questions they ask after you explain a concept. That will help you learn what you might be leaving out, what type of jargon needs defining, and what people actually find useful.
- *Ask first:* Perhaps the single greatest secret to making psychoeducation work is *timing*: providing information when the client is in a receptive state. How do you know when they are ready? Ask them, "Would you be open to learning more about X?" If you fail to ask, you may not find a receptive audience. Alternatively, master the REBT style of confrontation and forget about timing.
- *Keep it very, very brief:* During a 50-minute sessions, I recommend keeping total psychoeducation time to 1 to 2 minutes—that's the max—and I am not exaggerating. Any other brilliant information you have to share should be saved for the following week because most clients cannot meaningfully integrate and act on more than a single principle at once.
- *Make one point—and one point only:* Try to teach only one concept, point, or skill in a session. Anything else is too much to be *practically* useful (see Judith Beck's recommendations in the section "Thought Records").
- *Ensuring understanding and acceptance:* After briefly providing information, *directly ask* if clients understand and if they believe it is useful and realistic for their life.
- *Apply it immediately:* After you provide information, immediately identify how it can be practically applied in the client's life to address a problem that occurred in the past week or upcoming week.
- *Step-by-step tasks:* After offering 2 minutes of psychoeducation, the following 48 minutes involve step-by-step instructions on how to apply the information to solve

(*continued*)

> a current problem. Get specific: who does what when and where and how often and any resistance or potential roadblocks.
>
> - *Follow up on tasks:* The next time you meet, ask the client if he or she used the information to any extent. If not, why? If so, what happened?

Socratic Method and Guided Discovery

Using the *Socratic method*, sometimes referred to as *guided discovery* or *inductive reasoning*, to gently encourage clients to question their own beliefs, cognitive counselors use open-ended questions that help clients to "discover" for themselves that their beliefs are either illogical (i.e., contrary to obvious evidence) or dysfunctional (i.e., not working for them; Beck, 2005). A less confrontational approach than other techniques, when questioning the validity of belief, counselors generally take a relatively neutral stance, allowing the client's own logic, evidence, and reason to do the majority of convincing. Although the term "change" is used to describe what happens, in actuality tightly held beliefs are slowly eroded over time by the client questioning and requestioning their validity in different situations.

Questions for Evaluating the Validity of Beliefs

- What evidence do you have to support your belief? What evidence is there to the contrary? So, what might be a realistic middle ground?
- What does respected person X (Y and Z) say about your situation? How could they all be wrong?
- If your child [or another significant person] were to say the same thing, how would you respond?
- What is the realistic likelihood that things will really go *that* badly? What is a more realistic outcome?
- You bring up one possible reason for X. Have you considered another explanation? Perhaps … ?
- How likely is it that person X's behavior was 100% directed at you? What else might have played a role in his or her behavior?

Thought Records

Cognitive counselors use thought records (Beck, 1995) to help clients learn how to better respond to automatic thoughts, the most readily accessible dysfunctional thoughts (see the section "Schemas and Core Beliefs"). Clients can use thought records to use Socratic questions to help them counter their own negative thinking and develop more adaptive responses. Thought records involve identifying (a) the triggering situation, (b) the automatic thought and strength of belief in terms of a percentage, (c) the resulting negative emotions and percentage of severity, (d) an alternative adaptive response, and (e) the alternative outcome in terms of percentage of belief, intensity of emotion, and new action.

One of the keys to the technique is to use *percentage* to measure *how much a person believes* an automatic thought and *how strong the emotions are.* By using percentage of emotion and belief, clients can begin to see how dysfunctional belief wax and wane and that not all negative emotions are as devastating as others. Simply noting the variability in symptom severity generates hope, greater sense of control, and motivation to change; "third-wave" behavioralists using mindfulness, and solution-focused counselors also focus on using these small indicators of control, change, and improvement to effect change. In the case study at the end of this chapter, the counselor uses thought records initially to help Maria counter her habitual pattern for interpreting others and later in the counseling to help her develop a relapse prevention plan related to her bipolar disorder.

Dysfunctional Thought Record (adapted from Beck, 1995, p. 126)

Date/ Time	Situation	Automatic Thought(s)	Emotion(s)	Adaptive Response	Outcome
	1. What event or stream of thoughts led to the unpleasant emotion? 2. What (if any) distressing physical sensations did you have?	1. What thoughts(s) and/or image went through your mind? 2. How much did you believe each one at the time (rate in terms of percentage)?	1. What emotion(s) did you feel at the time? 2. How intense (0–100%) were the emotions?	1. What cognitive distortions did you make (optional; use Beck's list)? 2. Use six questions below to develop a response to the automatic thought(s). 3. How much do you believe each of these new responses?	1. How much do you now believe the first automatic thought? 2. What emotion(s) do you feel now? How intense (0–100%) is the emotion? 3. What will/ did you do (or not do)?
Monday, 4/23 10:00 a.m.	In department meeting, boss praised Greg endlessly. I had cold, clammy hands.	My boss likes Greg better: 90%; I will never get any where in this company: 80%; I am a loser: 70%	Angry (at boss): 75%; Helpless: 100%; Hopeless: 80%	Magnification; personalization; Greg works harder and builds relationships better; I could do the same; I am a loser only if I don't try harder: 80%	20%; 30%; 20%; Angry (at self): 50%; Helpless: 20%; Hopeless: 10%; Motivated: 50%; Get to work earlier; goof off less; talk with boss

Questions to develop an alternative response; ask yourself these questions and see if you can develop a useful alternative to your automatic thought (note: Not all questions apply equally to all situations):

1. What is the evidence that the automatic thought is true? Not true?
2. Is there an alternative explanation for the situation?
3. What's the worst that could happen? Could I live through it? What's the best that could happen? What's the most realistic outcome?
4. What's the effect of my believing the automatic thought? What could be the effect of my changing my thinking?
5. What should I do about it?
6. If _____ was in the situation and had this thought, what would I tell him or her (or what would he or she do)?

The most important role is for counselors to *motivate* clients to use these outside of session instead of falling back into old patterns. Judith Beck (1995, p. 127) recommends the following to ensure success with this relatively involved homework task:

• Counselors need to develop competence using thought records *personally* before asking clients to do so.

- Before introducing the thought record, the counselors should determine if the client understands and responds well to the basic principles of the cognitive model.
- Before introducing the thought record, clients should (a) demonstrate an ability to readily identify automatic thoughts and (b) have had a positive experience with *successfully reducing negative emotions* using a *verbal* variation of this intervention or Socratic questioning.
- The counselor should introduce thought records in two stages: first describing how to identify the automatic thought in one session and then, in the second session, how to generate adaptive responses.
- Clients should successfully identify automatic thoughts in several situations before moving on to identifying adaptive responses.
- If the client fails to complete thought records once properly introduced, the counselor should explore automatic thoughts related to doing the homework, such as believing that "these will not make a difference" or that "I don't have time in my busy schedule."

Disputing Beliefs and the REBT Self-Help Form

Ellis's A-B-C theory has a second part: you guessed it, D-E-F, which describes the interventions for *disputing* (D) irrational beliefs and the new *effects* (E) and *feelings* (F) (see "The Juice" for A-B-C; Ellis, 1994, 2004; Ellis and Dryden, 1997). The D-E-F intervention is used both in and out of session to help clients dispute troubling beliefs and replace them with new ones. Not attacking any or all beliefs, cognitive-behavioral counselors specifically target "hot" beliefs, the ones that are the most emotionally charged, rather than "warm" or "cool" beliefs that tend to cause fewer problems (Ellis, 2003).

A-B-C Model

How Problems are Created A-B-C
A = Activating event → **B = Belief about A** → **C = Emotional & behavioral consequences**
(Trigger event or person)   ↑   (Symptoms)

How Problems are Resolved D-E-F ↑
↑   ↑
D = Disputing belief → **E = Effect** → **F = New feeling**
(Rational argument)

Counselors use the A-B-C-D-E-F model to provide clients a means to analyze their own cognitions and behaviors and develop more adaptive responses. Before assigning this as homework, counselors usually practice in session on a whiteboard to demonstrate the process. Clients are then asked to do the exercises on their own over the week as distressing events arise. Over the years, several REBT self-help forms have been available (Ellis, 1997), the most recent of which is an interactive online version available from the Rational Emotive Therapy Network website (Ross, 2006). The REBT self-help form walks clients through the A-E process. In the case study at the end of this chapter, the counselor uses the REBT self-help form to help Maria dispute irrational beliefs about how she interprets the comments and actions of others.

Step 1: Identify "A," the Activating or Trigger Event

What situation are you upset about?

Example: My girlfriend cheated on me.

Step 2: Identify "C," Unhealthy Negative Emotional and Behavioral Consequences

What negative feelings and behaviors are you experiencing in response to this event?

Unhealthy Emotions	*Unhealthy Behaviors*
Example: I feel hurt, angry, vengeful, depressed, jealous, and plain sad.	Example: I yelled at her; broke up with her; can't sleep or eat; don't want to see anyone.

Step 3: Identify "B," Irrational Beliefs

What beliefs do you have that lead you to interpret the event so that you feel and behave they way you do? Include unrealistic demands, awfulizing, low frustration tolerance, people rating, and overgeneralizing (one or more) beliefs as well as demanding (a) to be approved of and feel self-worth, (b) to be treated fairly, and (c) for life to be effortless.

Example: Demands: I must be with Yvonne; she should not have done this; I can't live without her.

Awfulizing: This is the worst thing in the world that has ever happened to me; my life is over.

Low frustration tolerance: I can't stand being treated like this.

People rating: Her actions prove I am worthless. She is a terrible person.

Overgeneralizing: I will never find anyone like her again.

Step 4: Identify "D," Irrational Beliefs Using Disputing Questions

Example: Demands: Why must I be with her? Why is she the only woman on the planet for me?

Awfulizing: Is this really the worst thing that could happen?

Low frustration tolerance: Where is it written that being cheated on should not happen to me?

People rating: How can something she did reflect on my self worth? She made a bad decision, but does that make her a bad person?

Overgeneralizing: Do I want to find someone like her if she cheated on me?

Step 5: Identify "E," Effective, Rational Beliefs

Example: Demands: I want to be with her—or at least I did want to be with her. I would have preferred having her in my life if she could have been faithful.

Awfulizing: Although this hurts, there are many things far worse that could happen to me. This only feels like the worst thing in the world. This type of thing has happened to millions of others for centuries; they survived, and I shall too.

Low frustration tolerance: I don't want to handle this, but I know that I can.

People rating: Her actions do not reflect on my self-worth; only my actions do that. I admire many of her qualities, but obviously she has flaws when it comes to faithfulness.

Overgeneralizing: When I am ready, I will look for someone whom I love as much and can be faithful to me.

(continued)

> ### Step 6: Identify New "F," Feelings and Behaviors, Such as "Healthy Negative Emotions" and Self-Helping Behaviors
>
> | *Healthy Negative Emotions* | *Healthy Self-Helping Behaviors* |
> | --- | --- |
> | Example: I am very disappointed and hurt, but I will be okay. | Example: I will start hanging out with my best friend to cheer me up; I will talk with people I trust about this; when I am ready, I promise myself I will meet someone new. |
> | *It may take a while, but I will find someone else.* | |

Labeling Cognitions

In addition to Socratic questioning and direct confrontation, some clients find it helpful to identify and label distorted thinking to reduce its sway on them. Counselors can help them practice labeling distorted thinking in session so that clients can transfer this skill to their everyday lives. Most frequently, counselors use Beck's (1976) categories of distorted thinking described earlier in "The Viewing: Case Conceptualization" section:

- *Arbitrary inference:* "jumping to conclusions"
- *Selective abstraction:* "filtering out the positive"
- *Overgeneralization:* "making sweeping conclusions without evidence"
- *Magnification and minimization:* "emphasizing the negative and ignoring the positive"
- *Personalization:* "exaggerating one's responsibility" and/or "misinterpreting neutral comments"
- *Dichotomous thinking:* "black-and-white thinking"
- *Mislabeling:* "attaching an extreme or overgeneralized label to a person or situation"
- *Mind reading:* "assuming negative thoughts and intentions on the part of other"
- *Catastrophizing:* "assuming the worst will happen"

Problem-Solving and Coping Skills Training

Meichenbaum (1977) noticed that while some times dysfunctional beliefs were the problem, at other times clients simply lacked problem-solving and coping skills. Thus, in addition to listening for the presence of erroneous beliefs, he listened for the "*absence* of specific, adaptive cognitive skills and responses" (p. 194). In the case of problem solving, the counselor engages in directly teaching clients how to (a) identify problems, (b) identify potential solutions, (c) select and act on a solution, and (d) evaluate the effectiveness of the solution. Similarly, with situations that are not easily solved, such as loss of a loved one or a chronic condition, the counselor helps clients learn coping skills using a similar format: (a) identifying the specific elements where the client could cope better, (b) identify potential coping strategies, (c) choosing and applying these strategies, and (d) evaluating their effectiveness.

Changing Self-Talk: Stress Inoculation Training

As an alternative to and/or in addition to confronting irrational beliefs, clients can use *stress inoculation training* to help them change their negative *self-talk* and unhelpful inner dialogues and increase coping skills (Meichenbaum, 1977, 1985). Stress inoculation involves three phases:

1. *Education:* Providing information on negative self-talk and how it creates stress
2. *Training:* Rehearsing and practicing skills that apply to the client's situation
3. *Practice:* Applying skills in real-world situations

The process of stress inoculation training helps clients change their self-talk in all phases of experiencing stress: (a) preparing for a stressor, (b) confronting and handling the stressor, (c) coping with the feeling of being overwhelmed, and (d) reinforcing self-statements after stress. In the case study at the end of this chapter, the counselor uses stress inoculation training to help Maria change her habitual patterns of interpreting stressful interactions with others in the worst possible way.

Positive Self-Talk in Stress Inoculation Training (adapted from Meichenbaum, 1977, p. 155)

Things clients can tell themselves in each phase of coping with a stressor:

Preparing for a stressor

"I can develop a plan to do deal with the stress."
"Just think about what I need to do rather than get anxious."
"Don't worry; worry won't help anything."

Confronting and handling the stressor

"One step at a time; I can handle this."
"Don't think about the fear: just think about what I have to do. Stay relevant. Just do it."
"This anxiety is what the counselor said I would feel; it's a reminder to use my coping skills."

Coping with the feeling of being overwhelmed

"Stay focused in the present. What is it that I have to do?"
"Don't try to eliminate the anxiety; just keep it manageable."
"When fear comes, just breathe."

Reinforcing self-statements

"You did it!"
"That wasn't as bad as I thought it would be."
"I am making good progress."

Cost-Benefit Analysis

Another common cognitive-behavioral technique, *cost-benefit analysis* helps confront dysfunctional thinking and create motivation by having clients identify the "costs" of a problematic behavior and the "benefit" (Ellis, 1991, 1994). Many problem behaviors develop by trying to avoid another problem, such as drinking to avoid feeling lonely. The counselor typically works with the client to make a written list of the costs and benefits or the pros and cons. The counselor has the client begin the list and prompts the client to rationally think through the list from both perspectives.

Classical Conditioning: Pavlov's Dogs and Relaxation

Frequently used to treat anxiety disorders, classical conditioning was developed by Ivan Pavlov (1932) in his famous experiments with salivating dogs. In these experiments, he was able to train dogs to salivate at the sound of a bell by *pairing* the dog's natural response to salivate at the sight of food with a bell. When the bell was rung each time food was presented, the dog learned that the bell signaled that food was coming and began salivating. After enough repetition, the dog began to salivate with just the sound of the bell. This procedure is technically described in terms of *conditioned/unconditioned stimuli and responses.*

Initially, these responses were believed to be purely behavioral and almost involuntary, but later behavioralists found that thought and conscious learning were required even in this most basic form of conditions: "Contrary to popular belief, the fabled reflexive conditioning in humans is largely a myth. *Conditioning* is simply a descriptive term for learning through paired experiences, not an explanation of how the changes come about. Originally, conditioning was assumed to occur automatically. On closer examination it turned out to be cognitively mediated" (Bandura, 1974, p. 859); or, more to the point, "Humans do not simply respond to stimuli: they interpret them" (Bandura, 1977, p. 59). Classical conditioning is used in clinical settings to address phobias, child behaviors, and anxieties.

> **How Classical Conditioning Works**
>
> *1. The Natural State of Affairs*
> Unconditioned Stimulus (UCS) $\longrightarrow$ Unconditioned Response (UCR)
>
> - Pavlov's Original Research: Dog Food $\longrightarrow$ Salivation
> - Treating Arachnophobia: Deep Breathing $\longrightarrow$ Relaxation Response
>   (slowed heart rate, decreased arousal)
>
> *2. Process of Pairing Conditional Stimulus With Response*
> UCS + Conditioned Stimulus (CS) $\longrightarrow$ Conditioned Response (CR)
>
> - Dog Food + Bell $\longrightarrow$ Salivation
> - Deep Breathing + Spider $\longrightarrow$ Relaxation
>
> *3. Resulting Pairing*
> Conditioned Stimulus (CS) $\longrightarrow$ Conditioned Response (CR)
>
> - Bell $\longrightarrow$ Salivation
> - Spider $\longrightarrow$ Relaxation

Operant Conditioning and Reinforcement Techniques: Skinner's Cats

Operant conditioning–based interventions use the principles identified by B. F. Skinner (1953, 1971) to modify human behavior, whether one's own or another's. The essential principle is to reward behavior *in the direction* of the desired behavior using small, incremental steps, a process called *shaping behavior*: "When a bit of behavior is followed by a certain kind of consequence, it is more likely to occur again, and a consequence having this effect is called a reinforcer" (Skinner, 1971, p. 27). Once a certain set of skills has been mastered, the bar is raised for which behavior will be reinforced, with ever closer approximations to the desired behavior. Thus, if parents are trying to teach a child how to complete homework independently, they may begin by overseeing when, where, and how the child completes homework and reinforcing success and failure under these conditions. Once the child regularly succeeds with full oversight, the child is given an area of responsibility to master—perhaps when the homework is done—and reinforced for success in this area. Next, the child may be rewarded for managing the list of homework assignments without oversight. This process continues until the child completes homework independently, much to the parents' delight. Individual clients can apply operant conditioning to themselves to change habits, such as developing a new exercise regimen, lose weight, reduce anxiety, increase social activity, or any number of behavioral changes.

Forms of Reinforcement and Punishment   In operant conditioning, desired behaviors can be positively or negatively reinforced or punished, depending on the desired behavior. The four options below are used alone or in combination to *shape* desired behavior.

> ## Types of Reinforcement and Punishment
>
> - *Positive reinforcement or reward:* Rewards desired behaviors by *giving* something desirable (e.g., a treat).
> - *Negative reinforcement:* Rewards desired behaviors by *removing* something undesirable (e.g., relaxing curfew; take a day off from a routine task).
> - *Positive punishment:* Reduced undesirable behavior by *adding* something undesirable (e.g., assigning extra chores; getting yourself to do a disliked task).
> - *Negative punishment:* Reduces undesirable behavior by *removing* something desirable (e.g., grounding; denying self something enjoyable).

To boil it down even more:

	Increase Desired Behavior	Decrease Undesirable Behavior
Add Something	Positive reinforcement; reward	Positive punishment
Remove Something	Negative reinforcement	Negative punishment

Frequency of Reinforcement and Punishment The frequency of reinforcement and punishment is key to increasing or decreasing behavior:

- *Immediacy:* The more immediate the reinforcement/punishment, the quicker the learning, especially with young children.
- *Consistency:* The more consistent the reinforcement/punishment, the quicker the learning. Consistency involves rewarding or punishing a behavior *every time* it occurs or on a consistent schedule (e.g., every other time), creating predictability.
- *Intermittent reinforcement:* Random and unpredictable reinforcement *increases* the likelihood of a behavior, for better or worse. Thus, if a parent inconsistently reinforces curfew (sometimes enforces it and other times not), the child is *more likely* to break it. Based on the same principle, random positive reinforcement of well-established desired behaviors helps sustain them (e.g., randomly reinforcing positive grades with an extra privilege or treat).

Point Charts and Token Economies Generally used with younger children but adaptable for adults, point charts (Patterson & Forgatch, 1995) or token economies (Falloon, 1991) are used to shape and reward positive behaviors by building up "points" that can be applied to privileges, treats, or purchases. The rewards must be motivating for the particular person involved; thus, what may work for one person may not work for another (Bandura, 1974). In addition, the rewards should follow the desired behavior closely in time and should be frequent enough for a person to feel motivated to do more. These principles can be used on children or adults to achieve behavioral change. For example, if parents want to increase a child's independence with homework, they can reward the child with a sticker that is placed on a chart; when the child accrues the target amount (perhaps five), the parents offer a motivating reward of some kind (e.g., a new book in a favorite series). Similarly, a typically shy adult wanting to increase his social connections could reward himself each time he contacts three friends in a week by buying a favorite CD or book.

Systematic Desensitization

A classic behavioral technique, *systematic desensitization* is a technique frequently used with anxieties and phobias in which a client begins with a low-intensity image and increasingly works toward direct contact with the stressful stimulus (Wolpe, 1997). Using classical conditioning, desensitization is achieved by pairing relaxation with the stressful stimulus, first in small amounts and then slowly increasing exposure, a process called *reciprocal inhibition*. The underlying assumption is that a person cannot be both anxious and stressed at the same time.

The process involves (a) teaching relaxation techniques, (b) creating a hierarchy of anxiety triggers, and (c) working up the hierarchy until the client no longer experiences anxiety related to the trigger. For practical reasons (such as having to bring spiders and snakes to the office), imagery is used for most of the desensitization process. Adding a cognitive component to this classic behavioral technique, Meichenbaum (1997) found that adding a *coping image*—imagining oneself coping rather than mastering the anxiety-provoking situation—resulted in better and more sustainable outcomes. For example, if a man feared public speaking, a counselor would first teach him how to get into a relaxed state using breathing and visualization techniques. He would also work with the client to create a hierarchy of anxiety-provoking speaking events. Next, the counselor would have him get into the relaxed state and then *imagine* himself coping well with making a point during a business meeting; the client would practice doing this until he could imagine it without feeling anxious. The next step would be to have him identify a slightly more anxious situation—such as making a presentation at a meeting—and repeat the procedure. As the client gains confidence, this learning is transferred to real-world situations until the client is able to cope well with speaking in public.

In Vivo Exposure and Flooding

A variation on systematic desensitization, *in vivo exposure* and *flooding* are used to treat anxiety and phobias. In vivo exposure refers to putting the client in real-life (in vivo), anxiety-provoking situations while supporting clients as they face their fears (Spiegler & Guevremont, 2003). Often a hierarchy similar to that used in systematic desensitization is used to expose the client in small doses to the feared situation or object, such as spiders or public speaking. In contrast, flooding refers to intense and prolonged exposure to the anxiety-provoking stimulus, either imagined or in vivo. In flooding, the client is not allowed to engage in the anxiety-reducing behaviors, and the fear generally resolves itself rapidly. Obviously, exposure treatments are appropriate for limited problems and are not appropriate for all clients, but when they are a good fit, they can be very effective in reducing phobias and anxiety.

Eye Movement Desensitization and Reprocessing

A highly specialized technique that requires additional training, eye movement desensitization and reprocessing (EMDR) is a form of exposure therapy used with trauma and stress. Although initially controversial, EMDR is recognized by the National Institute of Mental Health as a tier-1 intervention for trauma. The procedure involves having clients imagine the traumatic or anxiety-provoking event while using rapid eye movements to create bilateral stimulation of the brain (Shapiro, 2001). During the process, the counselor asks questions about the associated memories that surface. The eye movements are used to help reconnect memory networks with more adaptive semantic memory networks. The EMDR specialist identifies negative and positive cognitions to structure the treatment, using the eye movements to defuse the negative cognition and associated bodily sensations. As this wanes, the client is then asked to "install" new positive cognitions, again using eye movements to affect memory networks. The effectiveness of EMDR has been the subject of ongoing debate, with research and meta-analyses having mixed results (Nowill, 2010).

Putting It All Together: Cognitive-Behavioral Treatment Plan Template

Use this treatment plan template for developing a plan for clients with depressive, anxious, or compulsive types of presenting problems. Depending on the specific client, presenting problem, and clinical context, the goals and interventions in this template may need to be modified only slightly or significantly; you are encouraged to significantly revise the plan as needed. For the plan to be useful, goals and techniques should be written to target specific beliefs, behaviors, and emotions that the client is experiencing. The more specific, the more useful it will be to you.

Cognitive-Behavioral Treatment Plan

Initial Phase of Treatment (First One to Three Sessions)
Initial Phase Therapeutic Tasks

1. *Develop working counseling relationship. Diversity note:* Adapt use of warmth, "expertise," and emotional versus rational focus based on ethnicity, gender, age, and so on.
   Relationship building intervention:
   a. Use warmth and **empathy** to build rapport; establish **credibility**.

(continued)

2. *Assess individual, systemic, and broader cultural dynamics. Diversity note:* Determine whether traditional **individualistic goals** are appropriate for client's personal and cultural background
   Assessment Strategies:
   a. Obtain **baseline** of problem behavior; **functional analysis** of problem behaviors and thoughts; *DSM-IV* diagnosis.
   b. Identify specific **schemas** and **irrational beliefs** related to presenting problem.

Initial Phase Client Goals *(One to Two Goals):* Manage crisis issues and/or reduce most distressing symptoms

1. *Decrease* [name specific crisis-related behavior] to reduce [crisis] symptoms.
   Interventions:
   a. Use **functional analysis** to identify one behavior the client is willing to do to reduce severity of symptoms.
   b. Use **control theory** to motivate client to *choose* functional behaviors that move towards desired life goals.

Working Phase of Treatment (Three or More Sessions)
Working Phase Counseling Tasks

1. *Monitor quality of the working alliance. Diversity note:* Ensure that goals and premises are a good fit for diverse clients.
   Assessment Intervention:
   a. Use Session Rating Scale; verbally ask clients if sessions are beneficial and if they feel understood by counselor.

Working Phase Client Goals *(Two to Three Goals).* Target individual and relational dynamics using theoretical language (e.g., decrease avoidance of intimacy, increase awareness of emotion, increase agency)

1. *Decrease* [specify: **distorted cognitions**; e.g., overgeneralizing] and [specify: **irrational beliefs**; e.g., "I must be loved at all times"] to reduce depression/anxiety and so on.
   Interventions:
   a. **Disputing** irrational beliefs in session and using **REBT self-help form.**
   b. **Socratic questioning** related to depressive (anxious) beliefs.
   c. **Label dysfunctional cognitions** to counter automatic thoughts.

2. *Increase* [specify: **functional behaviors**] and choices to reduce depression and anxiety.
   Interventions:
   a. Use **operant conditioning** and **in vivo exposure** to develop positive behavioral choices.
   b. Use **choice theory** and **cost-benefit analysis** to motivate clients to make positive behavioral choices.

3. *Increase* positive **self-talk** related to [specify: presenting problem] to reduce feelings of hopelessness, anxiety, fear, and so on.
   Interventions:
   a. **Stress inoculation training** and **problem-solving training** related to presenting problem.
   b. Use **thought records** to develop alternative thoughts related to presenting problem.

Closing Phase of Treatment (Last Two or More Sessions)
Closing Phase Counseling Task

1. *Develop aftercare plan and maintain gains. Diversity note:* Include individual, family, and community resources as supports.

(continued)

Intervention:
   a.   Use thought records and REBT self-help form for potential future problems.

Closing Phase Client Goals *(One to Two Goals):* Determined by theory's definition of health and normalcy

1.   *Increase* **positive self talk** about self worth and expectations from life to reduce feelings of hopelessness, anxiety, fear, and so on.
     Interventions:
     a.   **Socratic dialogue** to help client develop positive views of self and life.
     b.   Use **thought records** to develop realistic self-talk about personal worth.

2.   *Decrease* **dysfunctional schemas and core beliefs** about self, others, and life to reduce depressive, anxious, and compulsive symptoms.
     Interventions:
     a.   Dispute three basic "musts," negative cognitive triad, and related core schemas.
     b.   **Thought records** to develop alternative, realistic schema, and core beliefs above worth as person and relationships.

Reality Theory

In a Nutshell: The Least You Need to Know

Arguably the original "get-real" counseling approach, reality theory counseling is an active approach that incorporates many elements of behavioral and cognitive approaches but is based on a different model of human motivation. Developed by William Glasser, who was dissatisfied with the outcomes of psychoanalytic therapy when working in a girls' prison, reality theory is based on *choice theory*, which posits that the choices people make determine the quality of their lives and are the means for both creating and resolving problems. In a matter-of-fact manner, reality counselors simply allow reality to confront clients and help them identify what needs to change: "Is what you doing getting you what you want?" The counselor then helps clients identify alternative choices and behaviors that are more likely to get them what they really need.

Choice Theory

Developed from his early *control theory*, which that conceptualized people as driven by inner control systems, Glasser's (1975, 1997, 1998, 2000) *choice theory* posits that the choices people make determine the quality of their lives. Glasser believed that five basic needs motivated the choices people make:

*   Belonging/relationships
*   Power/achievement
*   Fun
*   Freedom/independence
*   Survival

The choices people make inform their behaviors, which Glasser conceptualized as *total behavior*, which incorporates acting, thinking, feeling, and physiology. Using the metaphor of four car wheels, any one behavior is inherently connected to all other elements. For example, a person cannot decide to get drunk (or stay sober) without the choice impacting thoughts, feelings, and physiology.

Similar to behaviorists and solution-focused counselors (see Chapter 11), Glasser believed that when a person wants to change, *action* is generally the easiest and most effective place to start. Thus, when assessing clients, counselors use choice theory to identify the actions clients choose that drive the negative thoughts, feelings, and physical symptoms (e.g., nagging a partner or not giving one's best at the office) and target these for later intervention. In the case study at the end of this chapter, the counselor uses choice theory to help Maria make better choices about how she uses her time and interacts with others.

Reality Theory Behavioral Analysis

In reality therapy, counselors analyze behavior to help motivate clients to take responsibility for the quality of their lives and make choices to improve their situations using the WDEP (Wants-Doing-Evaluation-Planning) system (Glasser, 2000; Wubbolding, 2008).

W = Exploring Wants, Needs, and Motivations

Counselors explore clients' wants using a series of questions to assess what clients really want and need in all areas of their lives: family, friends, job, self, health, and so on (Wubbolding, 2008):

- What do you want that you *are* getting? What do you want that you *are not* getting? What are you getting that you don't want?
- What are you willing to settle for?
- How much effort are you willing to exert to get what you want? How committed are you?
- What do you have to give up to get what you want? Are you willing to do this?

Doing = Discussing What Clients Are Doing and the Resulting Direction

Compared to thoughts, feelings, and physiology, Glasser believed that behaviors were the easiest thing for people to control. Thus, he asked clients to examine their actions and if they were helping them move toward their wants and needs:

- What actions are you taking right now that are helping you fulfill your wants?
- What actions are taking *away from* your wants?
- When you are feeling bad [name the symptom], what actions do you take? What thoughts inform your choice to take this action?

E = Evaluating the Effectiveness of Actions and Choices

Next, counselors encourage clients to *self-evaluate* the effectiveness of their actions and choices. Some ways counselors encourage this is to ask evaluative questions:

- Are these actions helpful or hurtful to you in the short run? Long run?
- Are these actions improving your relationships or destroying them?
- Are these actions your best effort or least effort?

P = Planning a Course of Action

Based on clients' evaluations of their actions, counselors help them develop a doable, realistic plan for getting more of what they want. They strive to keep plans simple and attainable with measurable goals that are within the client's control.

Mindfulness-Based Approaches

In a Nutshell: The Least You Need to Know

Described as the third wave of behavioral therapy (with "pure" behavioral therapy the first wave and cognitive-behavioral therapy the second), mindfulness-based approaches add a paradoxical twist to cognitive-behavioral approaches: *accepting* difficult thoughts and emotions in order to transform them (Hayes, 2004). Counselors using mindfulness-based approaches encourage clients to curiously and compassionately observe difficult thoughts and feelings *without the intention to change them*. By changing *how* clients relate to their problems—with curiosity and acceptance rather than avoidance—they experience new thoughts, emotions, and behaviors in relation to the problem and thus have many new options for coping and resolving issues. These practices require counselors to have their own mindfulness practice and training before trying to teach clients to do the same.

A Brief History of Mindfulness in Mental Health

Mindfulness has an unusual history as a cognitive-behavioral technique: it was not developed in a researcher's lab or from a Western philosophical tradition. Instead, mindfulness comes from religious and spiritual traditions, making it a surprising favorite for cognitive-behavioral counselors who ground themselves almost exclusively in Western scientific traditions. Most commonly associated with Buddhist forms of meditation, mindfulness is found in virtually all cultures and religious traditions, including Christian contemplative prayer (Keating, 2006), Jewish mysticism, and the Islamic-based Sufi tradition. Although it has religious roots, mindfulness entered mental health as a nonreligious "stress reduction" technique and was intentionally separated from religion and spiritual elements and adapted for use in behavioral health settings (Kabat-Zinn, 1990).

Over 30 years ago, Jon Kabat-Zinn (1990) began researching the mindfulness-based stress reduction (MBSR) program at the University of Massachusetts, which has been highly influential in making mindfulness a mainstream practice in behavioral medicine. The MBSR program is an 8-week group curriculum that teaches participants how to practice mindful breathing, mindful yoga postures, and mindful daily activities. Participants are encouraged to practice daily at home for 20 to 45 minutes per day. MBSR shows great promise as an effective treatment for a wide range of physical and mental health disorders, including chronic pain, fibromyalgia, psoriasis, depression, anxiety, attention-deficit/hyperactivity disorder, eating disorders, substance abuse, compulsive behaviors, and personality disorders (Baer, 2003). Closely related, Teasdale, Segal, and Williams (1995) have adapted the MBSR curriculum for depression relapse in their program, mindfulness-based cognitive therapy (MBCT). With 50% of "successfully" treated cases of depression ending in relapse within a year, MBCT counselors are using mindfulness to reduce the high relapse rate with promising findings.

In addition to including MBSR (Kabat-Zinn, 1990) and MBCT (Teasdale et al., 1995), mindfulness has been integrated into two counseling approaches that have also shown great promise in treating a wide range of clinical conditions: dialectic behavioral therapy (Linehan, 1993) and acceptance and commitment therapy (Hayes, Strosahl, & Wilson, 1999).

Mindfulness Basics

The most common form of mindfulness involves observing the breath (or focusing on a repeated word, a *mantra*) while quieting the mind of inner chatter and thoughts (Kabat-Zinn, 1990). Focus is maintained on the breath, grounding the practitioner in the present moment *without judging* the experience as good or bad, preferred or not preferred. Usually within seconds, the mind loses focus and wanders off—thinking about the exercise, a fight that morning, to-do lists, past memories, or future plans; feeling an emotion or itch; or hearing a noise in the room. At some point, the practitioner realizes that the mind has wandered off and then returns to the object of focus without berating the self for "failing" to focus but rather with compassion understanding that the loss of focus is part of the process—refraining from beating oneself up is usually the most difficult part. This process of focusing, losing focus, regaining focus, losing focus, and regaining focus continues for an established period of time, usually 10 to 20 minutes.

Gehart and McCollum (2007, 2008; McCollum & Gehart, 2010) have used mindfulness to help first-year counselors and therapists learn how to develop therapeutic presence with encouraging reports from trainees who say that they notice significant changes both in and out of the therapy session. Trainees report being better able to be emotionally present with clients, less anxious in session, and better able to respond in difficult moments. Most report that their overall level of stress noticeably decreases within 2 weeks of practicing 5 days per week for 2 to 10 minutes; they also report better relationships and a greater sense of inner peace—not bad for a 10- to 50-minute-per-week investment. So you might want to give it a try.

Starting Your Personal Mindfulness Practice

1. *Find a regular time*: The most difficult part of doing mindfulness is finding time—2 to 10 minutes several days a week. My colleague Eric and I have our students do 5 days per week. It is best to "attach" mindfulness practice to some part of your regular routine, such as before or after breakfast, working out, brushing your teeth, seeing clients, coming home, or going to bed (if you are not too tired).

2. *Find a partner or group (optional)*: If possible, find a partner or meditation group with whom you can practice on a regular basis. The camaraderie will help keep you motivated.

3. *Find a timer (highly advisable)*: Using a timer helps structure the mindfulness session, and many find that it helps them focus better because they don't wonder if time is up. Most mobile phones have alarms and timers that work well; you can also purchase meditation apps with Tibetan chimes for iPhones and other smart phones. Digital egg timers work well too—avoid the ones that tick.

4. *Sit comfortably*: When you are ready, find a comfortable chair to sit in. Ideally, you should not rest your back against the chair; rather, sit toward the front so that your spine is erect. If this is too uncomfortable, sit normally with your spine straight—but not rigid.

5. *Breathe*: Set your timer for 2 minutes initially and watch yourself breathe while quieting the thoughts and any other discourse in your mind:

   - Don't try to change your breathing; just notice its qualities, not judging it as good or bad.

   - Know that your mind will wander off numerous times to both inner and outer distractions. Each time it does, gently notice it without judging. Perhaps imagine it disappearing like a cloud drifting off or soap bubbles popping or say "ah, that too" and then gently return your focus to watching your breath.

   - Accept your mind how it is each time you practice; some days it is easier to focus than others. The key is to practice acceptance of "what is" rather than fall into the common pattern of being frustrated with what is not happening.

   - The goal is *not* to have extended periods without thinking but rather to practice nonjudgmental acceptance and cultivate a better sense of how the mind works.

6. *Notice*: When the bell rings, notice how you feel. The same, more relaxed, more stressed? Try only to notice without judging. You may or may not feel much difference; the most helpful effects are cumulative rather than immediate. If you happen to notice that you wish to go on, go ahead and add a minute or two the next time you practice. Slowly, you will add minutes until you find a length of time that works well for you. Don't extend the time until you feel a desire to do so.

7. *Repeat*: Our students report the best outcomes with shorter regular practices rather than longer but infrequent practices. Thus, doing five 2-minute practices is likely to produce better outcomes than one 10-minute session each week.

Resources to Support Your Practice

- *Free meditation podcasts:* You can download free guided mindfulness meditations and other free resources to support your practice from my website (www.dianegehart.com) and from UCLA's Mindfulness Awareness Research Center (www.marc.ucla.edu).

- *Workbooks: The Mindfulness-Based Stress Reduction Workbook* (Stahl & Goldstein, 2010) and *Get Out of Your Mind and Into Your Life: The New Acceptance and Commitment Therapy* (Hayes & Smith, 2005) are excellent workbooks to teach your practical techniques.

Specific Mindfulness Approaches
MBSR and MBCT

Not primarily about becoming a good meditation practitioner, these mindfulness-based group treatments are designed to help clients change *how they relate to their thoughts and internal dialogue.* Using a highly structure group process, clients are introduced to mindfulness breathing (similar to the instructions discussed earlier) as well as mindful yoga (stretching) positions and mindful daily activities (e.g., washing dishes mindfully, walking; Kabat-Zinn, 1990). Depending on the group's focus, clients may be taught to apply mindfulness to physical conditions, difficult emotions, depressive thinking, and so on. The group format is ideal for motivating clients to practice regularly at home and report back to the group on progress.

The eight groups in MBSR cover the following:

Session 1: Introduction to mindfulness: Foundations of mindfulness and body scan meditation

Session 2: Patience: Working with perceptions and dealing with the "wandering mind"

Session 3: Nonstriving: Introduction to breathing meditation; mindful lying yoga; qualities of attention

Session 4: Nonjudging: Responding versus reacting; awareness in breath meditation; standing yoga; research on stress

Session 5: Acknowledgment: Group check in on progress; sitting meditation

Session 6: Let it be: Skillful communication; loving-kindness meditation; walking meditation; daylong retreat

Session 7: Everyday mindfulness: Mindful movement and everyday applications; practicing on one's own life

Session 8: Practice never ends: Integrating with everyday life

The eight groups of MBCT cover the following (Segal, William, & Teasdale, 2002):

Session 1: Automatic pilot: Introduce mindfulness; eating mindfulness exercise; mindfulness body scan

Session 2: Dealing with barriers: Explore mental chatter using the body scan exercise

Session 3: Mindfulness of the breath: Introduce mindfulness breath focus and 3-minute breathing space exercise

Session 4: Staying present: Link mindfulness to automatic thoughts and depression

Session 5: Allowing and letting be: Introduce acceptance and allowing things to just be

Session 6: Thoughts are not facts: Reframe thoughts as just thoughts and not facts

Session 7: How can I best take care of myself?: Introduce specific techniques for depressive thoughts

Session 8: Using what has been learned to deal with future moods: Motivate to continue practice.

Through these mindfulness exercises, clients learn to do the following:

- Deliberately direct their attention and thereby better control their thoughts
- Become curious, open, and accepting of their thoughts and feelings, even those that are unpleasant
- Develop greater acceptance of self, other, and things as they are
- Live in and experience themselves in the present moment

Dialectical Behavior Therapy

Originally developed for treating suicidal borderline clients, *dialectical behavior therapy* (DBT; Linehan, 1993) is named for the fundamental dialectical tension between change and acceptance: "The paradoxical notion here is that therapeutic change can only occur in the context of acceptance of what is; however, 'acceptance of what is' is itself change" (p. 99). In contrast to other cognitive-behavioral approaches, this approach is based on the premise that emotion *precedes* the development of thought and that strong emotions, traumatic experiences, and attachment wounds are the source of psychopathology. In a nutshell, the process of DBT helps clients be present with, tolerate, and accept strong emotions in order to transform them. In a sense, it is a client's desperate attempts to avoid painful emotions that are the root of the problem.

DBT counselors help clients "be with" difficult emotions by encouraging clients to manage dialectic tension, that is, the tension between two polar opposites, such as both loving and hating someone. Rather than retreating to either pole, the counselor encourages clients to experience how they can both simultaneously feel love and dislike by acknowledging the multiple levels of truth and reality in a given situation. These contradictory feelings and thoughts are first tolerated and then explored and eventually synthesized so that the reality of both extremes can be recognized. For example, an adult might come to acknowledge both ultimately loving a critical parent but at the same time hating how that parent speaks to her. As the client becomes able to accept having both loving and hateful feelings toward the parent, she will find herself less reactive and emotional about the situation. The process of DBT involves helping clients learn to increase balance in their lives by better managing the inherent dialect tensions in life:

- Being able to both seek to improve oneself as well as accept oneself
- Being able to accept life as it is and also seek to solve problems
- Taking care of one's own needs as well as those of others
- Balancing independence and interdependence

Acceptance and Commitment Therapy

A behavioral approach that shares philosophical assumptions with postmodern, narrative, and feminist approaches (see Chapter 13), acceptance and commitment therapy (ACT, pronounced "act," not "A-C-T") is based on the postmodern premise that we construct our realities through language, which shapes our thoughts, feelings, and behaviors. ACT practitioners believe that human suffering is in large measure created and sustained through language: "It is not that people are thinking the wrong thing—the problem is thought itself and how the verbal community (contemporary culture) supports its excessive use as a mode of behavioral regulation" (Hayes et al., 1999, p. 49). Unlike traditional cognitive behavioralists, ACT practitioners assert that attempts to control thoughts and feelings and avoid direct experience are the *problem*, not the solution. Instead, they advocate mindfulness-based *experiencing* to promote acceptance of the full range of human emotions: "In the ACT approach, a goal of healthy living is not so much to feel *good*, but rather to *feel* good. It is psychologically healthy to feel bad feelings as well as good feelings" (Hayes et al., 1999, p. 77).

The same acronym, ACT, is used to outline the process of counseling:

A = Accept and embrace difficult thoughts and feelings
C = Chose and commit to a life direction that reflects who the client truly is
T = Take action steps towards this life direction.

The first phase in ACT is to accept and embrace the very thoughts and feelings clients have been trying to avoid via their symptoms: accepting loss, feeling fear, and acknowledging anger. They caution clients to not "buy into" their thoughts and challenge them to see the flimsy link between reasons (i.e., excuses) and causes of their behavior. At the same time, they help clients develop a *willingness* to experience difficult thoughts and feelings with their *observing self*. Through this process of observation, clients are better able to identify their true values and selves, which helps them not only readily identify a life direction but commit to pursuing it. As you might imagine, this is not as simple as it sounds. In the action phase, most clients reexperience the resistance to experience and negative thoughts that brought them to counseling in the first place. However, with increased ability to accept these and a renewed commitment to pursue a meaningful life direction, the counselor can work with the client when obstacles arise in pursuing new action.

Snapshot: Research and the Evidence Base

Quick Summary: Arguably the best-researched approach, cognitive-behavioral approaches have strong empirical support for their effectiveness in treating several specific disorders.

Because of their conceptual home in experimental psychology, research is part of the culture of cognitive-behavioral counseling (Beck, 1976); therefore, they are some of the best-researched approaches in counseling. More so than any other approach, cognitive-behavioral counselors integrate research into their conceptualization of theory development and intervention, carefully researching specific interventions for specific populations (Beck, 1997). Additionally, true to their belief in using research to guide practice, cognitive-behavioral counselors have become increasingly attentive to a nonjudgmental counseling alliance because of research indicating the importance of this aspect of therapy. Although cognitive-behavioral counseling has an extensive research history, counselors need to be careful to assume that it is therefore superior to other approaches. As discussed in Chapter 2, when confounding factors such as researcher allegiance are controlled for, no therapy is consistently found to be superior to any other (Sprenkle & Blow, 2004).

The meticulous and extensive research efforts of cognitive behavioralists enable counselors to better know when and how their methods work. In a recent meta-analysis (analysis of the findings from several studies) of well-controlled studies on cognitive-behavioral approaches, Lynch, Laws, and McKenna (2010) found that cognitive-behavioral therapy was not effective in treating or preventing relapse with schizophrenia; it was effective in treating and reducing relapse in depression, although the effect size was small; and it was not effective in preventing relapse in bipolar disorder. To the untrained eye, these may seem like less-than-flattering findings, but the specificity is unparalleled, with no other approach able to provide similar information or superior findings.

With an impressive range of applications, cognitive-behavioral therapies dominate the National Institute of Mental Health's list of evidence-based treatments (empirically supported treatments; Chambless et al., 1996) and include but is not limited to the following:

- Cognitive-behavioral therapy for panic disorder
- Cognitive-behavioral therapy for generalized anxiety disorder
- Exposure treatment for agoraphobia
- Exposure/guided imagery for specific phobias
- Exposure and response prevention for obsessive compulsive disorder
- Stress inoculation for coping with stressors
- Behavior therapy for depression
- Cognitive therapy for depression
- Cognitive-behavior therapy for bulimia
- Behavior modification for enuresis
- Applied relaxation for panic disorder and generalized anxiety disorder
- Cognitive-behavioral therapy for social phobia
- Cognitive therapy for obsessive compulsive disorder
- Exposure treatment for posttraumatic stress disorder
- Stress inoculation training for posttraumatic stress disorder
- Relapse prevention program for obsessive-compulsive disorder
- Behavior therapy for cocaine dependence
- Cognitive therapy for opiate dependence
- Cognitive-behavioral therapy for benzodiazepine withdrawal in panic disorder patients
- Trauma-focused cognitive-behavioral therapy

Detailed descriptions of these and other evidence-based programs can be found on the National Registry of Evidence-Based Practices and Programs website at **http://nrepp .samhsa.gov.**

Snapshot: Working With Diverse Populations

Quick Summary: Widely used with diverse range of clients, counselors must thoughtfully adapt the level of directiveness and the relative emphasis on behavior versus thought versus emotion when working with diverse populations.

At a purely theoretical and less-than-romantic level, cognitive behavioralists define culture as a set of socially reinforced contingences of reinforcement: each culture has a defined set of "good behaviors" and socially reward and punish around these definitions (Skinner, 1971). Thus, on the basis of their theory, cognitive behavioralists are cultural relativists, meaning that what is good or normal is culturally defined. However, in the world of everyday practice, the directive and expert stance of cognitive behavioralists make it easy for counselor bias to creep in and subtly shape the direction of counseling according to the counselor's beliefs and values more than the client's. Additionally, these approaches are predicated on distinct Western values of individual independence, rationality, and autonomy, which cross-cultural research has demonstrated is not shared by all and, in fact, disagreed with by some diverse clients (Scorzelli & Reinke-Scorzelli, 1994). Thus, cognitive-behavioral counselors must reflect on the use of their influence and the valuing of individuality and rationality when working with diverse clients.

Another area of potential quagmire, cognitive-behavioral assessment and conceptualization techniques locate problems *in the individual* clients' thoughts and behaviors, not in the social environment, thus potentially putting undue blame on diverse individuals for their situation. Furthermore, disputing irrational beliefs, such as "life should be fair," can minimize the challenges and pain of being in a marginalized group, such as ethnic or sexual minority. Counselors have to then consciously modify assessment methods to account for the social and political forces of being different. On the other hand, the directive counseling relationship and education-based techniques of cognitive-behavioral approaches may be an excellent fit for many diverse clients. Men and certain culture groups, such as Latino, Asian, and Native Americans, often prefer active, directive counseling and interventions (Gehart & Lyle, 2001; Pedersen, Draguns, Lonner, & Trimble, 2002). Wong, Kim, Zane, Kim, and Huang (2003) found that the level of acculturation affected Asian American's perceptions of cognitive therapy, with those having less Western identities preferring cognitive to psychodynamic premises and those with more westernized identities receptive to both.

Cognitive-Behavioral Case Study and Treatment Plan

A 34-year-old woman of Puerto Rican descent, Maria was recently diagnosed with bipolar disorder, for which she is taking medication and is seeking counseling because she wants to manage her life better. She reports numerous and long bouts of depression, the most recent after her second child was born 2 years ago. During these periods, she can barely drag herself out of bed to go to her job in retail; avoids her friends, who she says don't really care; and watches television all night when she comes home. Her husband tries to cheer her up, but she finds his attempts mostly irritating because "he doesn't really understand me." Her manic episodes take the form of being highly irritated with her husband and children, who she says do nothing to help around the house and expect her to be their maid and cook more than anything. Similarly, she feels that customers at work see her as a doormat. She tries not to lose her temper when she feels "super irritable" and instead becomes snappy and icy cold; she also reports having lots of headaches during these periods. Also during these periods, she stays up and paints nature scenes at night, which is the one thing that she reports enjoying.

Cognitive-Behavioral Case Conceptualization

This case conceptualization was developed by selecting key concepts from "The Viewing: Case Conceptualization" section of this chapter. You can use any of the concepts in that section to develop a case conceptualization for this or other cases.

Schemas and Core Beliefs

One of AF's (adult female) core beliefs is that if she is respectful and helpful to others, she is entitled to be treated similarly. Although this is an excellent ideal to aspire to, AF has rigidified this ideal to a mandate; when someone fails to treat her as well as she believes she is entitled to, she is harsh and shuts them out of her life. This is contributing to her problems with friends and family.

Distorted Cognitions

- *Selective abstraction:* AF focuses on the one or handful of times she is treated poorly by others and ignores the overall pattern.
- *Overgeneralization:* AF quickly feels that *all* customers treat her poorly or that her whole family *always* takes her for granted.
- *Magnification and minimization:* AF is quick to magnify disrespectful behavior from others and minimizes acts of generosity and kindness.
- *Personalization:* AF takes the behaviors of customers quite personally when most of their moods and attitudes have little to do with her personally.

Irrational Beliefs: The Three Basic "Musts"

Of the three basic "musts," AF struggles most with "justice for me" and wants others to always treat her fairly.

BASIC-ID

- *Behavior:* AF has difficulty getting up alternating with staying up late at night.
- *Affect:* AF has periods of feeling very depressed and worthless as well as feeling irritable and taken advantage of by others.
- *Sensation:* AF reports frequent headaches.
- *Imagery:* AF reports that nature scenes help her feel better about her life and problems.
- *Cognition:* AF believes most all of the people in her life do not really care for or respect her or what she does for them.
- *Interpersonal relationships:* AF often feels as though others are not appreciating her, both at home and at work. She often isolates herself from her friends for similar reasons.
- *Drugs and biology:* AF is taking mood stabilizing medication for her bipolar disorder.

Cognitive-Behavioral Treatment Plan

Initial Phase of Treatment (First One to Three Sessions)
Initial Phase Therapeutic Tasks

1. *Develop working counseling relationship. Diversity note:* Ensure a respectful, accountable, and engaged relationship that is attentive to Puerto Rican norms.
   Relationship building intervention:
   a. Use warmth and **empathy** to build rapport; establish **credibility**; demonstrate respect and ensure that AF feels sense of dignity.

(continued)

2. *Assess individual, systemic, and broader cultural dynamics. Diversity note:* Ensure that goals are responsive to communal as well as individualist values that are appropriate for acculturation.
   Assessment strategies:
   a. Obtain **baseline** of problem AF's behavior; **functional analysis** of problem behaviors and thoughts; *DSM-IV* diagnosis.
   b. Assess BASIC-ID to identify effects of bipolar disorder.
   c. Identify specific **schemas** and **irrational beliefs** that relate to her relational issues and bipolar concerns.

Initial Phase Client Goals

1. *Decrease* hopeless and fatalistic thinking related to bipolar and relationships to reduce depressed mood and social isolation.
   Interventions:
   a. **Psychoeducation** on bipolar disorder and depressed thinking to create sense of hope that change is possible.
   b. Use **control theory** to motivate AF to *choose* one behavior to engage in over the week that will reduce her social isolation at home or with friends and/or reengage her in normal activity.
   c. Use **functional analysis** to identify one behavior the AF is willing to do to reduce severity of depression and manic symptoms.

Working Phase of Treatment (Three or More Sessions)
Working Phase Counseling Task

1. *Monitor quality of the working alliance. Diversity note:* Monitor to ensure that AF is related to in a way that respects cultural and gender values and forms of emotional expression.
   Assessment Intervention:
   a. Use Session Rating Scale; verbally ask AF if sessions are beneficial and if she feels understood by counselor.

Working Phase Client Goals

1. *Decrease* selective **abstraction** and **overgeneralization** that magnify sense of victimization and ill treatment by others to reduce depressive and manic symptoms.
   Interventions:
   a. **Disputing** irrational beliefs in session and using **REBT self-help form**.
   b. **Label dysfunctional cognitions** to counter automatic thoughts.

2. *Decrease* rigidity of **core belief/basic "must"** that she must be treated fairly at all times to reduce depressive mood.
   Interventions:
   a. **Socratic questioning**, such as, "What evidence do you have to support your belief? What evidence is there to the contrary? What might be a realistic middle ground?"
   b. Use **choice theory** to motivate AF to make positive choices: What do you want that you *are* getting? What do you want that you *are not* getting? What are you willing to differently to get more of what you want.

3. *Increase* positive **self-talk** related to how people are viewing and seeing her to reduce feelings of irritation, depression, and so on.
   Interventions:
   a. **Stress inoculation training** and **problem-solving training** to help AF learn to interpret others' actions and words in more realistic way.
   b. Use **thought records** to develop alternative thoughts when she encounters a situation in which she feels that others are not appreciating her.

(continued)

Closing Phase of Treatment (Last Two or More Sessions)
Closing Phase Counseling Tasks

1. *Develop aftercare plan and maintain gains. Diversity note:* Include individual, family, and community resources to support AF in maintaining gains; consult with prescribing physician about her progress.
   Intervention:
   a. Use **thought records** and **REBT self-help form** for potential future problems.

Closing Phase Client Goals

1. *Increase* **positive self-talk** about self-worth and relationships to reduce feelings of depression, irritation, and so on.
   Interventions:
   a. **Socratic dialogue** to help AF develop positive views of self and others' behaviors.
   b. Use **thought records** to reinforce realistic self-talk about personal worth and how others see her.

2. *Increase* **proactive and responsible** approach to managing bipolar symptoms to reduce risk of relapse.
   Interventions:
   a. **Socratic dialogue** to increase AF's sense of empowerment and responsibility related to bipolar diagnosis and symptoms; include husband in plan to prevent relapse.
   b. **Thought records** to teach AF how to self-monitor symptoms and identify early warning signs of relapse.
   c. Teaching **mindfulness** to reduce risk of depression relapse.

ONLINE RESOURCES

Associations and Training Institutes

Academy of Cognitive Therapy
www.academyofct.org

American Institute for Cognitive Therapy
www.cognitivetherapynyc.com

Association for the Behavioral and Cognitive Therapies
www.abct.org

Beck Institute
www.beckinstitute.org

Mindfulness Awareness Research Center: UCLA
http://marc.ucla.edu

Mindfulness Based Stress Reduction Clinic: Jon Kabit-Zinn
www.umassmed.edu/cfm/mbsr

National Association of Cognitive-Behavioral Therapists
www.nacbt.org

Rational Emotive Behavioral Therapy Network
www.rebtnetwork.org

REBT self-help form (thought record exercise)
www.rebtnetwork.org/library/shf.html

William Glasser Institute
www.wglasser.com

Journals

Behavior Therapy
www.elsevier.com/wps/find/journaldescription.cws_home/707105/description#description

Cognitive Therapy and Research
www.springer.com/medicine/journal/10608

International Journal of Cognitive Therapy
www.guilford.com

International Journal of Reality Therapy
www.journalofrealitytherapy.com

Journal of Behavior Therapy and Experimental Psychiatry
www.sciencedirect.com/science/journal/00057916

Journal of Cognitive Psychotherapy
www.springerpub.com/product/08898391

Journal of Rational Emotive Behavioral Therapy
www.springerlink.com/content/104937

References

*Asterisk indicates recommended introductory readings.

Alford, B. A., & Beck, A. T. (1997). *The integrative power of cognitive therapy*. New York: Guilford.

*Baer, R. A. (2003). Mindfulness training as a clinical intervention: A conceptual and empirical review. *Clinical Psychology: Science and Practice*, 10(2), 125–143. doi:10.1093/clipsy.bpg015

Bandura, A. (1974). Behavior theories and the models of man. *American Psychologist*, 29, 859–869. doi:10.1037/h0037514

*Bandura, A. (1977). *Social learning theory*. Englewood Cliffs, NJ: Prentice Hall.

Bandura, A. (1986). *Social foundations of thought and action: A social cognitive theory*. Englewood Cliffs, NJ: Prentice Hall.

Beck, A. T. (1972). *Depression: Causes and treatment*. Philadelphia: University of Pennsylvania Press.

*Beck, A. T. (1976). *Cognitive therapy and the emotional disorders*. New York: International Universities Press.

Beck, A. T. (1988). *Love is never enough*. New York: Harper and Row.

Beck, A. T. (1991). Cognitive therapy: Reflections. In J. K. Zeig (Ed.), *The evolution of psychotherapy: Third conference* (pp. 55–64). New York: Brunner/Mazel.

*Beck, J. (1995). *Cognitive therapy: Basics and beyond*. New York: Guilford.

Beck, A. T. (1997). The past and future of cognitive therapy. *Journal of Psychotherapy Practice and Research*, 6(4), 276–284.

*Beck, J. (2005). *Cognitive therapy for challenging problems: What to do when the basic don't work*. New York: Guilford.

Berg-Cross, L., Jennings, P., & Baruch, R. (1990). Cinematherapy: Theory and application. *Psychotherapy in Private Practice*, 8, 135–157.

Burns, D. (1988). *Feeling good: The new mood therapy*. New York: Signet.

Chambless, D. L., Sanderson, W. C., Shoham, V., Johnson, S. B., Pope, K. S., Crits-Christoph, P., et al. (1996). An update on empirically validated treatments. *The Clinical Psychologist*, 49(2), 5–18. Available: http://www.apa.org/divisions/div12/journals.html

Ellis, A. (1962). *Reason and emotion in psychotherapy*. New York: Lyle Stuart.

Ellis, A. (1991). Using RET effectively: Reflections and interview. In M. E. Bernard (Ed.), *Using rational emotive therapy effectively* (pp. 1–33). New York: Plenum.

Ellis, A. (1994). *Reason and emotion in psychotherapy* (2nd rev. ed.) New York: Kensington.

*Ellis, A. (1996). *Better, deeper, and more enduring brief therapy: the rational emotive behavior therapy approach*. New York: Brunner/Mazel.

Ellis, A. (2003). Early theories and practices of rational emotive behavior therapy and how they have been augmented and revised during the last three decades. *Journal of Rational-Emotive and Cognitive Behavior Therapy*, 21(3–4), 219–243. doi:10.1023/A:1025890112319

Ellis, A. (2004). *The road to tolerance: The philosophy of rational emotive behavior therapy*. Amherst, NY: Prometheus Books.

Ellis, A., & Dryden, W. (1997). *The practice of rational emotive behavior therapy* (2nd ed.). New York: Springer.

Falloon, I. R. H. (1991). Behavioral family therapy. In A. S. Gurman and D. P. Kniskern (Eds.), *Handbook of family therapy*, volume 2 (pp. 65–95). Philadelphia, PA: Brunner/Mazel.

Gehart, D. R., & Lyle, R. R. (2001). Client experience of gender in therapeutic relationships: An interpretive ethnography. *Family Process*, 40, 443–458. doi:10.1111/j.1545-5300.2001.4040100443.x

*Gehart, D., & McCollum, E. (2007). Engaging suffering: Towards a mindful re-visioning of marriage and family therapy practice. *Journal of Marital and Family Therapy*, 33, 214–226. doi:10.1111/j.1752-0606.2007.00017.x

Gehart, D., & McCollum, E. (2008). Teaching therapeutic presence: A mindfulness-based approach. In S. Hicks (Ed.), *Mindfulness and the healing relationship* (pp. 176–194). New York: Guilford.

Glasser, W. (1975). *Reality therapy.* New York: Harper and Row.

Glasser, W. (1997). Teaching and learning reality therapy. In J. K. Zeig (Ed.), *The evolution of psychotherapy: Third conference* (pp. 123–130). New York: Brunner/Mazel.

Glasser, W. (1984). *Control theory in the classroom.* New York: Harper and Row.

Glasser, W. (1998). *Choice theory: A new psychology of personal freedom.* New York: HarperCollins.

Glasser, W. (2000). *Counseling with choice theory: the new reality therapy.* New York: HarperCollins.

Glasser, W. (2003). *Warning: Psychiatry can be hazardous to your mental health.* New York: HarperCollins.

Hayes, S. C. (2004). Acceptance and commitment therapy, relational frame theory, and the third wave of behavior therapy. *Behavior Therapeutic, 35,* 639–666.

*Hayes, S. C., & Smith, S. (2005). *Get out of your mind and into your life: The new acceptance and commitment therapy* Oakland, CA: New Harbinger.

*Hayes, S. C., Strosahl, K. D., & Wilson, K. G. (1999). *Acceptance and commitment therapy: An experiential approach to behavior change.* New York: Guilford.

Hayward, J. W., & Varela, F. J. (1992). *Gentle bridges: Conversations with the Dali Lama on the sciences of the mind.* Boston: Shambhala.

Holtzworth-Munroe, A., & Jacobson, N. S. (1991). Behavioral marital therapy. In A. S. Gunman & D. P Kniskern (Eds.), *Handbook of family therapy* (Vol. 2, pp. 96–132). New York: Brunner/Mazel.

Kabat-Zinn, J. (1990). *Full catastrophe living: Using the wisdom of your body and mind to face stress, pain, and illness.* New York: Delta.

Keating, T. (2006). *Open mind open heart: The contemplative dimension of the gospel.* New York: Continuum International Publishing Group.

Lazarus, A. A. (1981). *The practice of multimodal therapy: systematic, comprehensive and effective psychotherapy.* New York: McGraw-Hill.

Lazarus, A. A. (1997). Can psychotherapy be brief, focused, solution-oriented, and yet comprehensive? A personal evolutionary perspective. In J. K. Zeig (Ed.), *The evolution of psychotherapy: Third conference* (pp. 83–89). New York: Brunner/Mazel.

Leahy, R. L. (2005). *The worry cure: Seven steps to stop worry from stopping you.* New York: Harmony Books.

*Linehan, M. M. (1993). *Cognitive-behavioral treatment of borderline personality disorder.* New York: Guilford.

Lynch, D., Laws, K., & McKenna, P. (2010). Cognitive behavioural therapy for major psychiatric disorder: Does it really work? A meta-analytical review of well-controlled trials. *Psychological Medicine: A Journal of Research in Psychiatry and the Allied Sciences, 40*(1), 9–24. doi: 10.1017/S003329170900590X

McCollum, E., & Gehart, D. (2010). Using mindfulness to teach therapeutic presence: A qualitative outcome study of a mindfulness-based curriculum for teaching therapeutic presence to master's level marriage and family therapy trainees. *Journal of Marital and Family Therapy, 36,* 347–360. doi:10.1111/j.1752-0606.2010.00214.x

Meichenbaum, D. (1977). *Cognitive behavioral modification: An integrative approach.* New York: Plenum.

Meichenbaum, D. (1985). *Stress inoculation training.* New York: Pergamon Press.

Meichenbaum, D. (1997). The evolution of a cognitive-behavior therapist. In J. K. Zeig (Ed.), *The evolution of psychotherapy: Third conference* (pp. 95–106). New York: Brunner/Mazel.

Nowill, J. (2010). A critical review of the controversy surrounding eye movement desensitization and reprocessing. *Counselling Psychology Review, 25*(1), 63–70.

Patterson, G. R., & Forgatch, M. S. (1995). Predicting future clinical adjustment from treatment outcome and process variables. *Psychological Assessment, 7*(3), 275–285. doi: 10.1037/1040-3590.7.3.275

Pavlov, I. P. (1932). Neuroses in man and animals. *Journal of the American Medical Association, 99,* 1012–1013.

Pedersen, P. B., Draguns, J. G., Lonner, W. J., & Trimble, J. E. (Eds.). (2002). *Counseling across cultures* (5th ed.) Thousand Oaks, CA: Sage.

Rogers, C. (1961). *On becoming a person: A therapist's view of psychotherapy.* Boston: Houghton Mifflin.

Ross, W. (2006). REBT self-help form. Available: http://www .rebtnetwork.org/library/shf.html

Scorzelli, J. F., & Reinke-Scorzelli, M. (1994). Cultural sensitivity and cognitive therapy in India. *The Counseling Psychologist, 22,* 603–610.

Segal, Z. V., William, J. M. G., & Teasdale, J. D. (2002). *Mindfulness-based cognitive therapy for depression: A new approach to preventing relapse.* New York: Guilford.

Skinner, B. F. (1953). *Science and human behavior.* New York: Macmillan.

Skinner, B. F. (1974). *About behaviorism.* New York: Knopf.

Skinner, B. F. (1971). *Beyond freedom and dignity.* New York: Knopf.

Shapiro, F. (2001). *EMDR as an integrative psychotherapy approach: Experts of diverse orientations explore the paradigm prism.* Washington, DC: American Psychological Association.

Spiegler, M. D., & Guevremont, D. C. (2003). *Contemporary behavior therapy* (4th ed.). Pacific Grove, CA: Wadsworth.

Sprenkle, D. H., & Blow, A. J. (2004). Common factors and our sacred models. *Journal of Marital and Family Therapy, 30,* 113–129.

Stahl, B., & Goldstein, E. (2010). *The mindfulness-based stress reduction workbook.* Oakland, CA: New Harbinger.

Teasdale, J. D., Segal, Z. V., & Williams, J. M. C. (1995). How does cognitive therapy prevent depressive relapse and why should attentional control (mindfulness) help? *Behaviour Research and Therapy, 33,* 25–39.

Wolpe, J. W. (1997). From psychoanalytic to behavioral methods in anxiety disorders: A continuing evolution. In J. K. Zeig (Ed.), *The evolution of psychotherapy: Third conference* (pp. 107–119). New York: Brunner/Mazel.

Wong, E., Kim, B., Zane, N., Kim, I., & Huang, J. (2003). Examining culturally based variables associated with ethnicity: Influences on credibility perceptions of empirically supported interventions. *Cultural Diversity and Ethnic Minority Psychology, 9,* 88–96. doi:10.1037/1099-9809. 9.1.88

Wubbolding, R. (2008). Reality therapy. In J. Frew & M. D. Spiegler (Eds.), *Contemporary psychotherapies for a diverse world* (pp. 360–396). Boston: Lakhasa.

CHAPTER
10

Systemic Family Counseling and Therapy

The family is not a static entity. It is in the process of continuous change, as are its social contexts. To look at human beings apart from change and time is solely a construct of language. Therapists, in effect, stop time when they look at families, like stopping a motion picture to focus on one frame.

—Minuchin and Fishman (1981, p. 20)

Lay of the Land

Got to love 'em even though they drive us batty: our parents, partners, children, in-laws, extended family—thank goodness we can add a dog, good book, headphones, and a few hundred miles of space into the mix to preserve our sanity. What is it about our families and partners that can push our buttons: that can make us act—dare I say—crazy? Hmmm. We might be on to something here.

The vast majority of clients present with some form of relational issue: I'm depressed because I broke up with my boyfriend, or my anxiety started in childhood when my mother would correct everything I said and did. For this reason, all counselors should consider the larger relational system and how it relates to the concerns that clients bring. Systemic counselors make this their primary means of understanding and intervening.

Systemic approaches were originally developed for work with couples and families. They represent a unique set of theories that conceptualize an individual's symptoms as arising within and helping to balance family and relational dynamics. Developed in the 1960s, systemic approaches represented such a radically new way of working that they inspired a separate discipline and license to support this distinctive approach. In fact, the field of family therapy, which is the focus of those who study to become marriage and family therapists, has enough theories to fill its own textbook, and many textbooks have been written on this topic, including one by myself (Gehart, 2010).

Thus, I will not endeavor in this text to scantily cover the same material that fills another book—that would guarantee my failure and a funky treatment plan and would most likely leave even the brightest readers more confused than when they began. Furthermore, I have had several students report hurling confusing texts across the room, so my most modest goal here is to not go splat! Instead, this chapter will present a *general, integrated systemic counseling approach* that counselors, psychologists, social workers, and family counselors can use as their primary theoretical approach for working with individuals, couples, and families. At the very least, systemic ideas are useful to counselors of any theoretical stripe during the initial case conceptualization process to identify systemic dynamics that may be affecting an individual (see Chapter 15) or when working with couples or families. In short, I hope to provide a meaningful, coherent, integrated systemic counseling approach rather than briefly review each of the over 15 family therapy approaches that rightly deserve their own book.

In this chapter, I distinguish *systemic family counseling* from generic *family counseling*, which can refer to wide range of counseling models, including Adlerian, solution-focused, or psychodynamic family counseling. I use the term "systemic" as it is generally used in counseling, psychology, and social work, which is quite different than the use of the term "systemic" within the field of family therapy, where virtually all of the theories are systemic, and thus they must make far finer distinctions. Translated into the more delicately delineated language in the field of family therapy, this chapter will specifically cover a primarily structural-strategic family therapy approach, which is the most commonly used, especially in newer evidence-based approaches. This systemic approach also covers many key principles that are shared with other major family therapy schools, such as Bowen's intergenerational and Satir's human growth model; however, to fully understand the unique methods of conceptualization and intervention in these theories, I encourage curious readers to read Gehart (2010) or a similar text for further details (note that single chapters on these theories can be purchased separately for a minimal fee).

The systemic counseling approach in this chapter is based on several of the seminal models of family counseling:

- *Mental Research Institute (MRI):* Located in Palo Alto, California, next to Stanford University, MRI was established after Gregory Bateson (see "Rumor Has It: People and Places") and his research team concluded their groundbreaking research on communication in families that have a member diagnosed with schizophrenia. Richard Fisch and Don Jackson worked together to found MRI, which has since served as the most influential training center in family therapy, inspiring Jay Haley's strategic therapy, the Milan team's systemic approach, Virginia Satir's human growth model (see Satir's Human Growth Model), and solution-focused brief therapy (see Chapter 11). A gifted clinician, Don Jackson developed many of the foundational theories of the field at MRI before his early passing. Later, using action-based interventions, Paul Watzlawick, John Weakland, and Richard Fisch began the ambitious Brief Therapy Project to find the quickest possible resolution to client complaints, developing the original brief therapy model (Watzlawick & Weakland, 1977; Watzlawick, Weakland, & Fisch, 1974; Weakland & Ray, 1995).
- *Milan systemic (long-term brief counseling):* Originally working with anorectic and schizophrenic children, Mara Selvini Palazzoli, Gianfranco Cecchin, Giuliana Prata, and Luigi Boscolo constituted the Milan team, who studied at MRI and returned to Italy with the goal of designing a counseling model that embodied a pure cybernetic (see the section "Systems 101: Philosophical Foundations") systems theory as articulated by Gregory Bateson (1972, 1979). Less action oriented than their California peers, Milan counselors closely attend to how client language shapes the family dynamics and then use this language to alter family interaction patterns (Selvini Palazzoli, Cecchin, Prata, & Boscolo, 1978).
- *Strategic:* One of the original associates at MRI, Jay Haley developed his own form of systemic therapy with his wife at the time, Cloe Madanes. Their approach focuses on the use of power and, in their later work, love in family systems (Haley, 1976).
- *Structural:* The most down-to-earth and practical, the structural approach developed by Salvador Minuchin involves mapping family structure—boundaries, hierarchy, and subsystems—and then actively engaging the family to help them develop a relational structure that eliminates the needs for symptoms and enables all members to thrive.

Systems 101: Philosophical Foundations

Before we get to what happens in the counseling room, we should first explore the philosophical foundations of the often counterintuitive practice of systemic counseling. These ideas, which are also presented in full detail in chapter 8 of *Mastering Competencies in Family Therapy* (Gehart, 2010), are known for making heads spin, ache, and fog over—or so my students report. So, read slowly and on a steady surface.

General Systems and Cybernetic Systems Theories

Systems theory has its origin in the cross-disciplinary study that began at the Macy Conferences, which were attended by rocket scientists building self-guided missiles, anthropologists studying intertribal interactions, and ecologists studying the interactions between species, among others. These researchers discovered that whether studying mechanical parts, social groups, or animals, they were noticing that systems operated using the same basic principles. From these conferences, von Bertalanffy (1968) developed *general systems theory*. Closely related but more focused on social systems was *cybernetic systems theory*, articulated by Gregory Bateson (1972), which has had the most influence on mental health counseling approaches.

Cybernetics, Homeostasis, and Self-Correction

The term "cybernetic" refers to "steersman" in Greek, which hints at the functional principles of cybernetic systems: they are *self-correcting* and therefore able to "steer" their own course, unlike a computer, for example, which needs an outside entity to steer it (Bateson, 1972). What does a cybernetic system steer toward? *Homeostasis.* Homeostasis, in the case of families, refers to the unique set of behavioral, emotional, and interactional norms that create stability for the family (or other social group). Despite what the name might imply, homeostasis is not static but *dynamic.* Much like a gymnast constantly moves to maintain her balance on a beam, systems must be constantly in flux in order to maintain a sense of stability. In all living systems, it takes work to maintain balance, whether it be mood, habits, weight, or overall health. The key to maintaining stability is the ability to self-correct, which requires feedback.

Negative and Positive Feedback

You can pretty much guarantee that negative and positive feedback will be on any multiple-choice test about family counseling. Why? Because the disciplinary use of the terms are *opposite* of the colloquial use of the terms. So, remember, the negative and positive feedback questions are always *trick questions*—that is, if you haven't studied. Here's how to remember it:

> **Negative Feedback** = *No* new information to steersman = waters are the *same* = Homeostasis
>
> **Positive Feedback** = *Yes*, new information is coming in to the steersman = waters are choppy, moving faster, colder, etc. = Something is *changing*

Negative feedback is "more of the same" feedback, meaning there is no new news or change (Bateson, 1972; Watzlawick, Bavelas, & Jackson, 1967). Much like "positive test results" in medical parlance, positive feedback is news that things are not within expected parameters, which is or may be experienced as a problem or crisis, depending on the situation. The problem or change could be due to what is generally considered "bad news" (death of a loved one, a fight with a spouse, a problem at work, etc.) or "good news" (graduation from college and needing to find a job, getting married and starting a new household, moving to a new city for a job, etc.). Both good and bad news can create positive feedback loops, which result in one of two options: (a) return to former homeostasis or (b) create a new homeostasis.

In most cases, a system's response to positive feedback is to try to get back to its former homeostasis as quickly as possible. After a fight, most couples quickly want to make up and "get back to normal." After a death, most talk about how "getting back to normal" will take a while; depending on how significant that person was, this may or may not be possible, as sometimes it is not possible to get back to the "old normal," and a new normal needs to be created. The need for a new norm or homeostasis is also referred to as "second-order change."

First- and Second-Order Change

Second-order change refers to when a system restructures its homeostasis in response to positive feedback and rules that govern the system fundamentally shift (Watzlawick et al., 1974). *First-order change*, of course, then refers to when the system returns to its previous homeostasis after positive feedback. In first-order change, the roles can reverse (e.g., a former distancer in a relationship could start pursuing—which seems like a radical change if you are in the relationship), but the underlying family structure and rules for relating stay essentially the same. This type of first-order shift is frequent in the early stages of counseling with couples when they shift roles being the pursuer and distancer. For example, if in the beginning the woman was asking for more closeness from her husband and he was asking for more space, as counseling progresses they may shift roles, and so the problem may appear solved on the surface. However, functionally there has been no shift in the rules that regulate intimacy in the relationship; they just have switched roles so that it looks and feels different.

A second-order shift with this couple would involve reducing the overall pursuer–distancer pattern and increasing each person's ability to tolerate more togetherness and more distance. It is also important to remember that second-order change is not always necessary in counseling, depending on the client's situation. In terms of how clients experience them, first-order solutions make logical sense; second-order solutions seem odd and illogical because they introduce new rules into the system.

"One Cannot Not Communicate"

The early work of the Bateson team resulted in Watzlawick et al.'s (1967) classic text *Pragmatics of Human Communication*, in which they proposed the following axiom: "One cannot not communicate." In addition to blatantly ignoring high school English teachers' rules about double negatives, this axiom seems to contradict the most common presenting problem by couples and families: "We can't (or don't) communicate." So, where did this axiom come from? What the Bateson team learned from their research of families with members diagnosed with schizophrenia was that even schizophrenic attempts to not communicate (e.g., nonsense, immobile states, etc.) still sent a message, often communicating a desire to not communicate. Since all behavior is a form of communication and it is impossible to not be engaged in some form of behavior (at least while we are alive), it follows that we are always communicating. As we all know, silence speaks volumes, as does nonsense, withdrawal, or a frozen pose; thus, even the most creative attempts to not communicate inherently send a message. More commonly, the claim that "we just can't communicate" means that the interlocutors reject what the other has to say, at which point it is helpful to examine the anatomy of the communicated messages, namely, the report and command aspects of communication.

Double Binds

Double-bind theory goes back to the Bateson group's earliest research on families with a member diagnosed with schizophrenia (Bateson, 1972). Watzlawick et al. (1967) identify the ingredients of a double-bind communication:

1. Two people are in an *intense relationship* that has a high degree of survival value, such as familial relations, friendship, religious affiliation, doctor–patient, counselor–client, social norms, and so on.

2. Within this relationship, a message is given that is structured with (a) *primary injunction* (e.g., a request or order) and (b) a simultaneous *secondary injunction* that *contradicts* the first, usually at the metacommunication level.

3. Finally, the receiver of the contradictory injunctions has the sense that he or she *cannot escape* or step outside the cognitive frame of the contradictions either by metacommunicating (e.g., commenting on the contradiction) or by withdrawing without threatening the relationship. The receiver is made to feel "bad" or "mad" for even suggesting there is a discrepancy.

Common examples are the commands "love me" or "be genuine," in which one person orders another to have spontaneous and authentic feelings. In their research, the MRI team noticed that this type of communication characterized families who had a member diagnosed with schizophrenia. A common type of exchange they noticed in these families was a mother who gives her child a cold, distant hug (command aspect communicates distance) and then says, "Why are you never happy to see me?" (report aspect suggests closeness). No matter how the child responds, the mother can prove him or her wrong. Thus, the "logical" response is a *nonresponse* or *nonsense response*, which characterizes schizophrenic behavior, such as word salad (spoken words that have no real meaning), loose associations (tangentially relating words or topics), or catatonic behavior (rigid, repetitive behavior that has no interactive meaning). Although the double-bind theory does not account entirely for how schizophrenia develops or who develops it, it is often useful for clinicians working with families that get stuck—whether or not there is a member diagnosed with schizophrenia.

Family as a System

The defining feature of systemic approaches to family counseling is viewing the family as a system: an entity in itself, the whole greater than the sum of its parts (Watzlawick et al., 1967). What does this really mean? Systemic counselors view the interactional patterns of the family as a sort of "mind" or organism that is not controlled by any single member, nor can it be controlled by an outside entity, such as a counselor. This view results in several startling propositions:

- *No single person orchestrates the interactional patterns:* The rules that govern family interactions are not consciously constructed like the U.S. Constitution; instead, they emerge through an organic process of interaction—feedback (reaction)—correction until a norm or homeostasis is formed. In fact, many of the arguments early in a relationship serve as feedback to shape the emerging relationship's homeostatic norms. In most cases, this whole process occurs with minimal metacommunication about how the relational rules are being formed.
- *All behavior makes sense in context:* Read that again—and then sit and think about it. Because if you really believe this and lead your life accordingly, everything changes (generally for the better), especially if applied to every other person you meet or hear about. Because all behavior is a form of communication, each behavior makes sense in the context in which it is expressed, within the rules of that particular system. Thus, even the most outrageous, inappropriate, or unexpected communication of those you meet on the street, at work, or at home make sense in the appropriate context.
- *No single person can be blamed for family distress:* Because no one consciously creates the rules but instead the patterns emerge naturally through ongoing interactions, it follows that no single person can be fully to blame for family problems; this means not that individuals do not simultaneously have moral and ethical obligations in cases of abuse but rather that the interactions "made sense" or at least are made possible by the dynamics of the system.
- *Personal characteristics are system dependent:* Although a member may display certain characteristics or tendencies, these are not inherent personality characteristics that exist independent of the system but rather emerge from the interactional patterns in the system. Thus, even when a family reports that "Suzie has always been like this" (e.g., angry, helpful, forgetful, etc.), the counselor takes this to be a statement more about the rules and likely rigidity of the system than an inherent truth about Suzie.

In a Nutshell: The Least You Need to Know

Systemic counselors always view a person as inherently part of larger *relational systems*, which include the *family of origin* (mother, father, siblings, extended family), *family of procreation* (spouse, partner, children, step children, etc.), social communities (e.g., church, neighborhoods, and even online communities), as well as broader societal groups (e.g., gay/lesbian communities, ethnic communities, state, nation, etc.). Systemic counselors radically propose that a person's problems or symptoms are inherently related to the dynamics of these systems; thus, an individual's depression (or fill in the blank with any other symptom) plays a role in maintaining a sense of "normalcy" in the system. At the same time, systemic counselors maintain a *nonpathologizing* position, not blaming persons within the system or the system itself for the symptoms. Instead, symptoms are viewed more *neutrally* and with curious enthusiasm—much like an anthropologist trying to understand a long lost culture—as a set of behaviors, feelings, and beliefs that help the system maintain a sense of balance or *homeostasis*. In the tiniest of nutshells, systemic counselors see their jobs as helping individuals and families find new relational patterns that do not require the symptom for the system or its members to feel balanced and connected.

Systemic counselors are the martial artists and Zen masters of the counseling world in that their interventions are rarely logical on the surface and often involve unusual Zen-like koans that serve to get people thinking in new ways. Much like a martial artist, they work *with* the symptoms, taking their energy and redirecting it in more productive ways rather than trying to forcefully stop a problem behavior, thought, or feeling. Thus, they *do not* reeducate individuals and families on how to better relate as do Adlerians and cognitive counselors. Instead, they use a wide variety of techniques to interrupt and redirect problem behavior sequences, often allowing the family to develop its own new ways of responding. They conceptualize families using two basic paradigms: (a) family structure: boundaries, hierarchy, and subsystems and (b) systemic interaction patterns: repetitive interaction cycles related to the problem. Systemic counselors are *strength focused*, never seeing individuals or families as dysfunctional but rather seeing people who need assistance in expanding their repertoire of interaction patterns to adjust to the ever-changing developmental and contextual demands.

The Juice: Significant Contributions to the Field

If there is one thing you remember from this chapter, it should be ...

Enactments

Perhaps the most practical and researched systemic intervention, counselors use *enactments* to redirect symptom-laden interactions to interaction patterns that are more effective and satisfying (Colapinto, 1991; Minuchin, 1974; Minuchin & Fishman, 1981). Regardless of whichever counseling model you prefer to use in the end, you will need to master enactments. Why? Because most couples and families are going to start arguing in your office whether you ask them to or not, and even individual clients may need to be coached in how to appropriately communicate, so you better be prepared. Enactments are one of the best ways to handle dicey, difficult moments in session (or even the waiting room).

Systemic counselors prefer enactments to talking about interactions because often people describe themselves as being one way but behave quite differently (clearly, this does not apply to you or me; we are speaking hypothetically, of course). This incongruity is not because people are malicious or hypocritical but because it often is difficult to clearly see how our behavior looks from the outside (Minuchin & Fishman, 1981). Enactments are used to both assess and alter the problematic interactional sequences, allowing the counselor to *map*, *track*, and *modify* the family structure or an individual's interaction patterns.

As a counselor becomes more experienced, it requires only a couple of minutes of listening to an individual recount a problem situation or watching a family interact to quickly know where and how to *restructure* boundaries and other relational structures.

Restructuring may take the form of creating a clearer boundary in enmeshed relationships (e.g., stopping people from interrupting and speaking for one another), increasing engagement by encouraging the expression of empathy or direct eye contact, or improving parental effectiveness by helping the parent successfully manage a child's in-session behavior.

An enactment occurs in three phases (Minuchin & Fishman, 1981):

Phase 1: Tracking and mapping: Observation of spontaneous interactions: When talking with an individual or family, the counselor closely follows both content and metacommunication, listening for the assumptions that coordinate the interactions, such as demands for intimacy, independence, or control, as well as strengths and abilities. When talking with clients, the counselor more closely *tracks actual transactions* (what is done in session) than verbal accounts (Colapinto, 1991). Gathering information from what is observed, the content of what is said, and the metacommunication, the counselor develops a working hypothesis that *maps* the family's boundaries and hierarchy (Minuchin & Fishman, 1981). Once counselors identify an area for change, they are ready to invite the individual or family into the active phase of enactment.

Phase 2: Eliciting interaction: The invitation: Counselors issue an "invitation" for an enactment in one of two ways: either by the counselor directly requesting the individual or family to enact a real-world interaction or by the clients spontaneously engaging in the problematic behavior, usually in the form of an argument or stone-cold silence (Colapinto, 1991). Obviously, the counselor does not need to do much when the client spontaneously begins; otherwise, the counselor must issue an explicit invitation for the client to "show" the problem:

- "Can you reenact what happened last night?" or
- "Please show me what happens at home when he is 'defiant'; can you act out an incident of defiance that happened last week so I have a good idea of what the problem really is?"

Enactments can also be used with individuals by having them enact their half of the encounter and summarizing—or even using a puppet to say—what the other person said. Using enactments is important when working with individuals because it is easy to collude with them in blaming others. Although it solves nothing and typically makes the situation far worse (see the discussion of triangulation below), blaming others without holding oneself responsible for one's half of the dynamic is a favorite recreational sport for many. Counselors can avoid this common helper's pitfall when working with individual clients by using enactments to keep both counselor and client focused on the only element in the system that they can affect: the client.

Phase 3: Redirecting alternative transactions: Up to this point, the enactment process has just been the more-of-the-same interaction pattern and does not count as an intervention (and actually isn't helpful) until counselors actually help clients *do something different*. Thus, in this phase, the counselor redirects interaction patterns to clarify boundaries, hierarchy, subsystems, and other structural issues. How exactly counselors redirect the interaction depends on the particular dynamics assessed in the first phase. Some of the more common ways that systemic counselors redirect interactions include the following:

- *Reduce enmeshment:* Allow each person to finish speaking and stop interruptions
- *Reduce disengagement:* Encourage couples to share thoughts and feelings on difficult topics
- *Reduce triangulation:* Ask two people to talk directly to each other while asking a third (typically intrusive person) to remain quiet

- *Clarify boundaries:* Rearrange chairs physically to increase or decrease emotional closeness
- *Alter pattern with individual:* Direct him or her to rephrase or "redeliver" a request or response as if the other person were present
- *Increase parental hierarchy:* Direct a parent to set limits for a child in session (rather than the counselor doing it)

Minuchin and Fishman (1981) identify several benefits of enactments, including providing real-life practice in new behaviors, shattering the illusion that the problem belongs to "the other" person, and increasing a person's sense of competence and confidence in handling the problem situation better.

Rumor Has It: People and Places

Gregory Bateson

Participating in the Macy Conferences with his then wife Margaret Mead, Bateson was a British anthropologist who explored cybernetic theory studying intertribal interactions in New Guinea and Bali (Bateson, 1972, 1979; MRI, 2002). Bateson's elegant and thoughtful articulations of cybernetic theory influenced numerous disciplines, including communications, anthropology, and family therapy. As part of his research of human communications, he assembled what was later known as the Bateson group: Don Jackson, Jay Haley, William Fry, and John Weakland. For 10 years, he worked with the team studying communication in families with members diagnosed with schizophrenia, providing consultation on cybernetic theory, and introducing them to the trance work of Milton Erickson. Together with the team, they developed the *double-bind theory of schizophrenia* (Bateson, 1972), in which they reconceptualized psychotic behavior as an attempt to meaningfully respond in a family system characterized by double-bind communications. Bateson's prior anthropological research provided the team with a theoretical framework through which to view problematic human behavior as a function of the larger social systems rather than being purely intrapsychic.

Don Jackson

A student of the founder of interpersonal psychoanalysis, Harry Stack Sullivan (who, I am sure you remember from Chapter 3, was criticized for relying on observable data more than interpretation of the unconscious), Don Jackson was a key figure in the development of systemic family theories, taking a leading role in the development of foundational concepts such as family homeostasis, family rules, relational quid pro quo, conjoint therapy, interactional theory, and, along with others at MRI, the double-bind theory (MRI, 2002; Watzlawick et al., 1967). Jackson also was one of the first psychiatrists to question the myth of normality (Jackson, 1967), which 50 years later has finally been adopted as part of the international *recovery movement*.

John Weakland

Originally trained as a chemical engineer, Weakland joined the Bateson group helping to articulate the application of communication theory, emphasizing the importance of developing theory based on concrete and observable behaviors rather than inferences or constructs, which are not observable (MRI, 2002). Along with Haley, Weakland was key in integrating Milton Erickson's (see Chapter 11) work at MRI as part of the Brief Therapy Project.

Richard Fisch

After initially proposing the creation of MRI, Richard Fisch was appointed by Jackson to be the director of the new Brief Therapy Project at MRI, a project inspired by Erickson's brief hypnotic work; the goal was to develop a highly teachable form of brief psychotherapy (Watzlawick et al., 1974). In addition to spearheading the development of the therapy model for which MRI is most famous, Fisch's research and contributions centered on how to influence others with words and indirect influence (Fisch & Schlanger, 1999; Fisch, Weakland, & Segal, 1982; MRI, 2002).

Paul Watzlawick

Born in Austria, Paul Watzlawick (Vats-la-vik—rhymes with "not Slavic") was a communications theorist who cofounded the Brief Therapy Center at MRI with Weakland and Fisch, the center's goal to develop an ultrabrief approach to therapy (Watzlawick, 1977, 1984, 1990, 1993a). In his later writings, Watzlawick explored the implications of radical constructivism for therapy and human communication in cleverly titled books such as *How Real Is Real?* (1977), *The Invented Reality* (1984), *Ultra Solutions: How to Fail Most Successfully* (1988), and *The Situation Is Hopeless but Not Serious: The Pursuit of Unhappiness* (1993b).

Salvador Minuchin

Trained as a pediatrician and child psychiatrist, Salvador Minuchin developed the structural family counseling approach (Colapinto, 1991; Minuchin, 1974). Leading a life that taught him about diversity on numerous fronts, Minuchin was born and raised in Argentina, lived in Israel during two periods of his life, and settled in the United States, where he spent most of his professional life. Like Don Jackson, Minuchin studied with Harry Stack Sullivan (see Chapter 4), whose psychoanalytic work emphasized interpersonal relationships rather than unconscious processes. After his psychoanalytic training, Minuchin accepted a position at the Wiltwyck School for delinquent boys and suggested to his colleagues—Dick Auerswald, Charlie King, Braulio Montalvo, and Clara Rabinowitz—that they see the entire family of these problem children. With no formal models to follow, they used a one-way mirror to observe each other and developed a working model as they went along. In 1962, Minuchin visited MRI, where Haley, Watzlawick, Fisch, and others were at the forefront of developing family approaches. There he befriended Jay Haley, and the two formed an influential relationship in developing both structural and systemic forms of counseling; in fact, this cross-fertilizing friendship is the foundation for the integrated systemic approach presented in this chapter.

From 1965 to 1976, Minuchin severed as the director of the Philadelphia Child Guidance Clinic, and in 1975 he founded the Family Therapy Training Center (later renamed the Philadelphia Child and Family Therapy Training Center, which still operates today). In 1967, Minuchin, Montalvo, Guerney, Rosman, and Schumer published *Families of the Slums*, considered the first book to describe structural therapy, a book that also reveals an inherent sensitivity to viewing families with attention to poverty and diversity issues at a time when the term "multiculturalism" was not yet coined. This book is still a seminal piece for mental health providers working with poor families. Minuchin is still an active leader in the field, continuing to teach new generations of family practitioners (Minuchin, Nichols, & Lee, 2007). His influential students and colleagues include Harry Aponte, Jorge Colapinto, Charles Fishman, Jay Lappin, and Michael Nichols.

Jay Haley and Cloe Madanes

Jay Haley, one of the original members of the Bateson team, student of Milton Erickson, and cofounder of the Brief Therapy Project at MRI, developed his own systemic approach: strategic therapy (Haley, 1963, 1973, 1976, 1980, 1981, 1984, 1987, 1996; Haley & Richeport-Haley, 2007; MRI, 2002). He and his then wife Cloe Madanes (1981, 1990, 1991, 1993), founded the *Family Therapy Institute* in Washington, D.C. Their approach distinguishes itself by conceptualizing families using hierarchy, power, and love and their use of *directives* for interventions. As he and Minuchin carpooled for many years while developing their ideas, each man's work influenced the other's.

The Milan Team

Founded in 1967 to study families with children diagnosed with anorexia in Italy, the *Milan team* included Mara Selvini Palazzoli, Gianfranco Cecchin, Luigi Boscolo, and Guiliana Prata (Campbell, Draper, & Crutchley, 1991). They traveled to MRI in California to study the work of Bateson and continued an ongoing relationship with Watzlawick as they developed their unique theory that focused more on language than MRI's brief approach or Haley's strategic approach. In 1979, the team separated along interest and gender lines: Selvini and Prata, primarily researchers, wanted to continue their investigation treating families diagnosed with psychosis or anorexia, while Cecchin and Boscolo worked together, their attention focused on clinical and training applications. The later work of Selvini and Prata centered on the *invariant prescription* (see "Invariant Prescription to Sever Coalitions"), while Cecchin and Boscolo explored *second-order cybernetics* (see "First- and Second-Order Change"), attending to language and the construction of meaning through multiple descriptors, eventually moving toward a more postmodern, social constructionist stance (see Chapter 12).

The Big Picture: Overview of Treatment

Systemic counseling focuses on resolving the presenting problem with the counselor imposing no other goals or agendas based on theories of normalcy. Systemic counselors view the presenting problem not as an individual problem but as a relational one, specifically an *interactional* one, even if the counselor is working with an individual (Cecchin, 1987; Haley, 1987). Systemic counselors conceptualize interaction using two lenses: (a) identifying problematic interaction sequences and (b) mapping family structure, including boundaries, hierarchy, and coalitions. In this approach, neither an individual nor a relationship is considered "dysfunctional"; instead, the problem is viewed as part of the interactional sequence of behaviors that have emerged through repeated exchanges with no one person to blame (the sure sign that a counselor does not understand systems theory is when he or she uses the word "dysfunctional" or implies that if only person X changed, everyone else in the system would be fine).

In the early phase, the counselor observes and maps the problem behavior by obtaining a detailed description of the behavioral sequence surrounding the problem and by observing how clients interact. Often counselors achieve this by having them *enact* the problem situation (see "The Juice"). Once the counselor has identified the interactional behavioral patterns and meanings associated with the problem, the counselor uses one of many potential interventions to *interrupt* and *alter* this sequence—not necessarily correct it. By simply interrupting highly repetitive and rigid interaction patterns that constitute a problem (a problem wouldn't be a problem if it weren't highly repetitive and resistant to change), the system—which is inherently self-correcting and seeking balance—will effortlessly reconfigure itself around the new information that has been introduced. For example, if a man complains of frequent arguments with his partner, the counselor does not try to educate him in better communication skills. Instead, the counselor strives to simply *interrupt* the sequence by having him do *one thing different*, often a small, personally symbolic, easily achieved behavioral change, such as scheduling arguments at random times during the week or passing a symbolic object during the argument. Alternatively, the counselor may offer a reframe to give new meaning to the arguments that radically alter how they are viewed, such as a way to build connection and in some special way show love. Another option would be an enactment to help the client find new ways to interact more effectively. Any of these tactics of change will interrupt the problem sequence and allow for self-correction, resulting in new actions, thoughts, and behaviors.

Counselors frequently give clients some form of homework, sometimes a specific behavioral task or a cognitive reframing that highlights the systemic nature of the problem. Each week, the counselor follows up on the prior week's homework and then designs another task or reframe based on their response. This continues just as long as is necessary to resolve the presenting problem, and then counseling is terminated. To recap, the general flow of systemic or strategic therapies is as follows:

> ### The Process of Systemic Counseling
>
> *Step 1: Assess the interactional sequence, family structure, and associated meanings:* Identify interactional behavior sequences that constitute the problem, including the actions and reactions of everyone in the system and the associated meanings; assess boundaries, hierarchy, subsystems, and coalitions (see "The Viewing: Case Conceptualization and Assessment" section).

(continued)

Step 2: Intervene by interrupting and redirecting the interactional sequence: Using a reframing technique or a task, the counselor interrupts the sequence, allowing the family to reorganize itself in response to the intervention. *The differences between the specific schools of MRI, strategic, Milan, and structural are seen primarily in the preferred method of interrupting the interactional sequence.* Contemporary practitioners generally borrow freely from all of these systemic approaches (hence, they are presented together in this chapter).

Step 3: Evaluate outcome and client response: After the intervention, the counselor assesses the client's response and uses this information to design the next intervention.

Step 4: Interrupt the new pattern: Then the counselor interrupts the new pattern with another intervention. This continues—interrupting behavioral sequence, allowing family to reorganize and respond, and intervening again—until the problem is resolved.

Who's Involved

When possible, systemic counselors prefer to begin counseling with the persons most significant to the identified client in attendance, often family or partner, to assess the relational system (Colapinto, 1991). Once the relational system has been assessed, the counselor may meet with specific subsystems and individuals to achieve particular goals. For example, often sessions with the couple alone are necessary to strengthen the boundaries between the couple and the parental subsystems and to sever cross-generational coalitions with children or in-laws. If seeing only an individual, the counselor still assesses the *entire relational system* as much as possible, often using *circular questions* (see "The Doing: Interventions") that trace how each person in the system responds to the other in situations involving the problem.

Making Connection: The Counseling Relationship
Joining

Rather than thinking in terms of empathy, transference, or rapport, systemic counselors build relationships with clients by recognizing that they are *joining* with system that has its own distinct set of rules for communicating, showing respect, and making meaning (Minuchin, 1974; Minuchin & Fishman, 1981; Minuchin & Nichols, 1993). Rather than demonstrating understanding by verbally expressing empathy, systemic counselors "join" a system by accommodating to its style: how people talk, forms of emotional expression, pacing, and so on. In the historical context of mental health, this is a radical concept in that the counseling relationship accommodates to the client rather than the inverse, making it more adaptable to various cultural groups.

Much like an anthropologist observing and studying a new culture, systemic counselors approach clients with abundant curiosity about how they make meaning, organize their relationships, handle power, solve problems, express love, hang tough, entertain themselves, and otherwise move through life (Minuchin, 1974). The process of joining can also be likened to learning a new dance. Do they talk fast or slow? Do they talk over one another, or do they wait for clear pauses to speak? Do they use teasing and humor, or are their words gentle and soft? A successful systemic counselor needs to have a wide repertoire of social skills to successfully join with families, especially when working with diverse populations.

Respecting and Trusting the System

Systemic counselors respect the *system* of which the client is a part and view it as an entity that has its unique *epistemology* or way of knowing and understanding the world. Fully and humbly aware that they do not have direct control over a system, systemic counselors have an abiding trust that the system will reorganize itself in new and better ways without the counselor forcing the change. Instead, the counselor provides opportunities—sometimes many opportunities—for the system to reorganize itself using various interventions that are designed not to be the "solution" for the client but rather to shake the system up and allow it to naturally resettle into its own solution. Symptoms are seen not as indicators of individual pathology but rather as the by-product of interactional sequences in relational systems that have served a purpose (if you are paying attention, you will notice I repeat this point because it is hard to grasp, taking years to fully appreciate the implications).

Neutrality and Multipartiality

As you can imagine, when you start working with more than one person in the room, counselors are invited many, many times both verbally and nonverbally to take sides: "Counselor [wink, wink] is it healthy, natural, or normal for a person to do or feel X?" Breathlessly, everyone in the room awaits your response to see whose side you will join. Answering this or other innocent-sounding questions typically leads down a painful, slippery slope and the erosion of a good counseling relationship. All new counselors slip and slide several times before they finally learn, but at least you have been forewarned.

Knowing this, systemic counselors advocate a *neutral* stance when working with clients (Selvini Palazzoli, Boscolo, Cecchin, & Prata, 1980; Selvini Palazzoli et al., 1978). Neutrality is practiced in two ways: *nonpartiality*, not taking sides on particular issues, and also *multipartiality*, the willingness to honor all perspectives. Cecchin (1987) of the Milan team emphasizes that neutrality applies to how the counselor relates to clients as well as problems.

Neutrality in Relation to Clients Cecchin described neutrality the *pragmatic effect* the counselor has on the client: if at the end of the session the client cannot say which "side" the counselor was on, then the counselor has had the pragmatic effect of being neutral. A counselor may appear to take sides with each person's view simply by discussing it, understanding it, and empathizing with it; thus, the key is for clients to leave without feeling the counselor is on anyone's side—or if the client's epistemology includes the view that the counselor *must* be on someone's side, the client is at least quite confused about whose that may be. This type of neutrality is even more important when working with individual clients because if a counselor gives the impression of literally being on the client's side, especially in terms of a relational dispute, the client will not be motivated to change and instead will more likely go home, tell the other that "my counselor says you are wrong" (reality check: even if you try very, very hard to be neutral, it is very likely that clients will do this anyway, but at the very least you should not encourage it; this is a form of triangulation discussed).

Neutrality in Relation to the Problem More abstractly, counselor neutrality also implies not getting overly invested in particular meanings, descriptions, or outcomes (Boscolo, Cecchin, Hoffman, & Penn, 1987). The Milan team carefully avoided "falling in love with" (they were Italian and actually described it this way) any one description of the problem, *including their own*. Thus, neutrality also requires that the counselor not rigidly hold onto his or her own hypotheses and case conceptualization ideas: the case conceptualization should be constantly evolving and changing rather than rigidly remaining the same. Using a fluid problem description, the counselor has more maneuverability and can see more possibilities for intervention rather than focusing on the single solution.

Maneuverability

Perhaps the most adaptable and flexible in terms of forming a working alliance, systemic counselors do not use a one-size-fits-all approach to developing the counseling relationship. Systemic counselors highly value *maneuverability*, the freedom to use personal judgment in defining the counseling relationship so that it is most likely to quickly effect change (Nardone & Watzlawick, 1993; Segal, 1991; Watzlawick et al., 1974). Depending on (a) the relational rules of the particular system and (b) the presenting problem, the counselor may play the role of an expert or take a one-down helpless stance (see One-Down Stance), depending on which stance seems to help clients reach their goals quicker, not what the client simply prefers. Furthermore, the counselor may choose to be disliked by the client or be the "bad guy" in order to achieve the desired change in the system. Thus, in the working phase, the counselor may use different relational roles with different clients to promote change.

One-Down Stance

The one-down stance operates at two different levels: a general one-down stance in relation to the system and a strategic use of the one-down stance to promote change with certain clients (Segal, 1991). At one level, the one-down stance is sincere and genuine for systemically trained counselors because they respect each system as an entity that has its owns rules and integrity that must be respected, much in the sense that a mountain climber must respect the awesome forces of nature or the sailor an ocean: there is way to forcibly control or predict it; one can only defer to it and learn to gracefully and skillfully dance with its natural rhythms.

The second and more common use of the one-down stance refers to the counselor paradoxically claiming, "I'm not sure if I am able to handle such a problem" in order to motivate clients to change. Frequently used with clients who relentlessly complain that their situation is utterly hopeless yet do not take action, when the counselor *instead* takes the hopeless stance, the logic of the system impels the client to take up the role of being the hopeful one. Systemically, this works because in most systems there is a counterbalance where if one person is hopeless, the other feels compelled to be hopeful to maintain a balance. This same dynamic is also observed between couples in crisis: generally, one person will manage the crisis, allowing the other one to more fully feel the panic and trauma in that moment.

Social Courtesy

A rare and refreshing use of social norms in counseling relationships, Haley (1987) describes the initial stage of counseling as the *social stage*, a time during which the counselor engages in casual social conversation (e.g., about the weather or traffic) as a way of making clients comfortable and reducing their sense of shame: "the model for this stage is the courtesy behavior one would use with guests in the home" (p. 15). Before moving onto discussing the problem, the counselor ensures that all members have been properly greeted. During the social stage, the counselor is assessing interactions and mood in order to know how to begin moving into discussing the problem (Haley & Richeport-Haley, 2007). Even a few moments of "normal" social conversation can help clients feel more empowered, connected, and engaged because the counseling relationship involves something familiar.

Spontaneity

Counseling spontaneity refers to the ability to flow naturally and authentically in a variety of contexts and situations, but it does not imply a throw-caution-to-the-wind and say-what-you-please approach. Instead, systemic spontaneity is a relationally and contextually responsive expression of self that is constrained by the relational rules of the system (Minuchin & Fishman, 1981, p. 3). Much the way driving a car becomes "natural" after years of practice, systemic spontaneity is cultivated and shaped through the training process, increasing counselors' repertoire for "being natural" in a wide range of clinical situations.

Observation Team

A trademark practice of systemic approaches, counselors work with an *observation team* to better observe systemic patterns (Watzlawick et al., 1974). This practice evolved from the Bateson team's early research methods where they would sit behind a one-way mirror to observe the "conductor of the session" working with the family. The team could "see" the systemic dance more rapidly and completely because the person in the room very quickly falls in sync with the family system and has a more difficult time seeing the entirety of the interaction. Anyone who has spent time behind a mirror and in front of it knows that you are always "smarter" behind it. The distance created by not being part of the interactional dance of the family increases one's ability to see the steps more clearly and quickly. Arguably the main reason that family counselors still train with a mirror is to develop the ability to "see" the systemic dynamics. This is never to say that a counselor in the room *can't* see the systemic dynamics; it is just harder and takes more practice.

The Viewing: Case Conceptualization and Assessment

Systemic counselors conceptualize work with individuals, couples, and families using the following concepts:

Areas of Systemic Case Conceptualization

1. **Strengths and Development**
   - Strengths
   - Family life cycle stage of development
2. **Systemic Dynamics**
   - Interactional patterns and behavioral sequences
   - Role of symptom in the relational system
3. **Structure of the Relational System**
   - Subsystems
   - Triangles and cross-generational coalitions
   - Boundaries
   - Hierarchy
   - Complementarity

Strengths

Systemic counselors are fundamentally *strengths based*, keeping their focus on clients' strengths and advocating strongly against labeling families or individuals as "dysfunctional." In particular, systemic counselors focus on unique cultural and idiosyncratic strengths, such as religious beliefs or unusual hobbies, using these to design interventions (Minuchin & Fishman, 1981; Minuchin & Nichols, 1993; Watzlawick et al., 1974). Minuchin and Fishman (1981) powerfully argue against seeing the family as an enemy of its individual members, as is frequent in psychological literature, encouraging counselors to recognize how the family provides support, protection, and a foundation for its individual members. Family strengths are used to design interventions and promote the goals of individual and family growth as well as symptom reduction (see Chapter 15 for a full description of assessing strengths).

Family Life Cycle Stage of Development

Rather than a static entity, the family is viewed as continually growing and changing in response to predictable stages of development as well as unexpected life events, such as a death, moving, or divorce (Carter & McGoldrick, 2005; Minuchin & Fishman, 1981). Successfully navigating each stage requires changes in how the family balances *interdependence* and *independence* to meet each person's changing developmental needs. Whether working with individuals or families, systemic counselors identify their stage in the life cycle to better understand their developmental needs and challenges. Although this cycle can look vastly different based on cultural norms and family structure, the typical cycle involves the following developmental tasks:

1. *Leaving home: Single adult:* Accepting emotional and financial responsibility for self.
2. *Marriage/committed partnership:* Commit to new system; realigning boundaries with family and friends.

3. *Families with young children:* Adjust marriage to make space for children; join in child-rearing tasks; realign boundaries with parents/grandparents.
4. *Families with adolescent children:* Adjusting parental boundaries to increase freedom and responsibility for adolescents; refocus on marriage and career life.
5. *Launching children:* Renegotiating marital subsystem; developing adult-to-adult relationships with children; coping with aging parents.
6. *Family in later life:* Accepting the shift of generational roles; coping with loss of abilities; middle generation takes more central role; creating space for wisdom of the elderly.

Carter and McGoldrick (2005) also discuss alternative family life cycle models for gays/lesbians, single adults, divorce families, single-parent families, and remarried families, all of which center around the fundamental tension of balancing a sense of connection with significant others while maintaining a sense of individuality. At each stage of the process, family members need to renegotiate boundaries to define levels of closeness and independence that support the growth needs of individual members. Families often get stuck transitioning from one stage to another if they fail to renegotiate boundaries and hierarchy as the family develops. For example, after the birth of a child, couples need to radically reorganize how they manage independence and interdependence as they add the high-maintenance needs of a newborn into their juggling act. On the other end of the spectrum, as in the case study at the end of this chapter, Navid's family is adjusting to his leaving for college and establishing himself as a responsible adult, which he is not doing as well as the parents expected. His parents step in using authoritarian rules to try and force Navid to stop smoking pot, thus delaying the need to reorganize the system and adapt to his launching.

Interaction Patterns and Behavioral Sequences

Of critical importance when working with individuals who do not have others to share the "other side of the story," systemic counselors always assess the *interaction patterns* and *behavioral sequences* surrounding a symptom. Assessing interaction patterns involves tracing the behavioral sequences in the homeostatic dance in which the symptom is embedded. The interactional sequence is traced through four general phases: (a) things being normal (homeostasis), (b) tensions escalating (early positive feedback), (c) the symptomatic feelings and behaviors (positive feedback), and, finally, (d) self-correction with the ultimate return to normal (homeostasis). Depending on the symptom, this sequence can take several minutes or several months. Clients typically only describe the symptom, but by tracing the symptom from homeostasis to homeostasis, systemic counselors have a much better sense of how to intervene.

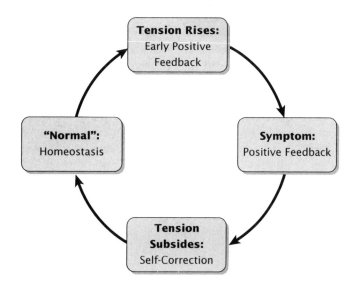

For example, if a client complains that she is anxious in public situations, a systemic counselor would explore the behaviors and interactions when the client feels "okay" or normal and then identify the behaviors, contexts, and relational and interactions when the anxiety starts to rise, what she does when she feels the anxiety at its height and how others respond, and then trace the behaviors and interactions until she feels "okay" or back to normal again. Similarly, when working with a couple who argues, the counselor first asks about what types of things they are doing when things are good between the two of them, what each starts to do as tensions rise, what each says and does in response to the other during the argument, and how they get back to a sense of "normal" again.

In addition to observing actual interactions, systemic counselors *ask* a series of questions to assess the interaction sequence. For example, with the couple who is having trouble with the defiant child, in addition to observing, the counselor would ask, What is happening just before the problem incident? What is each person saying and doing? How does the child respond? How does each parent and anyone else involved respond to the defiance? How does the child respond to this?

Questions for Assessing Interactional Sequence

- *Counselor asks about "life as normal" related to the presenting issue.*

  Example: "What is going on when you feel normal (okay, good, etc.)?"

- *Counselor asks client to describe how the problem begins, inquiring about contexts and persons that seem to trigger the symptom if these are not obvious.*

  Example: "Describes what typically happens prior to feeling anxiety. Then how does the anxiety ultimately begin? Does it seem to happen in particular contexts or with certain people?"

- *Counselor inquires about the behavioral sequence that comprises the symptom.*

  Example: "So what do you do at the height of the anxiety? What type of dialogue is going on in your head? How do others respond to you? How do you respond to them? What happens next?"

- *Counselor continues to trace these* back-and-forth interactional patterns *until things return to "normal" or homeostasis.*

  Example: How do things get back to normal? Do you have to do something? Does someone say or do something that helps? Does it generally happen the same way every time?

- *Counselor also inquires about how significant others in the system respond to the problems situation.*

  Example: Are others affected by this anxiety? How do they respond during or afterward? How do you respond to them?

- *Counselor continues assessing the interaction pattern until it is clear that the entire system has returned to its sense of "normalcy."*

Role of the Symptom

Systemic counselors view symptoms as playing a role in maintaining relational homeostasis and sense of normalcy (Colapinto, 1991). Symptoms can help maintain a sense of normalcy in a number of ways: limiting emotional intimacy, creating physical distance, forcing connection, creating distraction, or delaying developmental changes, just to name a few. Even though the symptoms are unwanted, they are often preventing or minimizing an even more distressing situation. For example, fear of going to public places (agoraphobia) often serves to force connection with a select few while creating great distance from others and avoiding numerous other responsibilities. Systemic counselors never view the *symptom bearer* or *identified patient* as the sole source of intervention, and instead the family interaction patterns are targeted for intervention. In the case study at the end of this chapter, Navid's substance use is considered as part of the family's homeostasis, helping to maintain his dependent status and his parents' caretaking roles.

Subsystems

Using Minuchin's (1974) structural theory, systemic counselors conceptualize a family as a single system that consists of multiple *subsystems*. Certain subsystems exist in all families: couple, parental, sibling, and each individual as a separate subsystem. In addition, in some families other influential subsystems develop along gender lines, hobbies, and interests (e.g., sports, music, etc.), and even personality style (e.g., serious vs. fun loving). When assessing a client's family (also see Chapter 15), the most important subsystem issues to consider are the following:

- Is there a clear distinction between the *parental* and *couple* subsystems?
- Is there a clear boundary between the *parental* and *child* subsystems? Alternatively stated, is there an effective *parental hierarchy*?
- Is the family divided along subsystem lines?

Many couples need help distinguishing the marital from parental subsystem when all their energy goes into caring for the children with nothing left for the relationship. Frequently parents need help distinguishing the parental and child subsystems by establishing a hierarchy (see "Hierarchy"). Additionally, many subsystems create unhelpful dynamics that need correcting, such as coalitions across generations.

Triangles and Cross-Generational Coalitions

One type of subsystem is particularly damaging: *triangles* (Bowen, 1985), which often take the form of *cross-generational coalitions* (Minuchin & Fishman, 1991; Minuchin & Nichols, 1993). Triangles can form in any relationship in which a third person is pulled in to reduce tension in a dyad, often taking the form of "confiding" in a friend or family member who takes the side of person in the dyad against the other. Cross-generational coalitions are a *triangle* that forms between a parent and child *against* the other parent or other key caretaker. This is a common family dynamic, often involving a parent who "teams up" with one or more children against the other parent, undermining the other parent, taking the child's side in an argument, using the child as a confidant, or simply being more invested in the parent–child relationship. In a divorce, this pattern is almost universal as parents vie to create coalitions against the other. Triangles can be *overt*, readily identifiable, or *covert*, not directly addressed or spoken about in the family but evident by secrets between the parent and child ("Don't tell your mom/dad about this") or comments that compliment the child and disparage the other spouse ("I am so glad you didn't inherit your father's/mother's gene for X").

Boundaries

"*Boundaries*" refer to the relational patterns and rules for relating in a system. Each individual family has a unique set of boundaries that closely tied to their family, cultural, socioeconomic, gender, educational, and other background variables. When initially assessing boundaries, they seem two-dimensional: too weak or too strong. But the more you work with them, the more you learn that they are far more complex than they appear at first glance. Nonetheless, let's start with the simple two-dimensional definition.

Boundaries are rules for managing physical and psychological distance between family members, defining the regulation of closeness, distance, hierarchy, and family roles (Minuchin & Fishman, 1981). Although they may sound static, they are an organic, living process. Systemic counselors identify three basic types of boundaries:

- *Clear boundaries:* Clear boundaries refer to a range of "normal" boundaries that allow for close emotional contact with others while also allowing each person to maintain a sense of clear identity (Colapinto, 1991). Each culture defines a range of "normal" boundaries that define appropriate expressions and levels of independence versus interdependence. For example, in some cultures, more physical space is typical of clear boundaries than others, and within a given culture, families can have a wide variety of expressions of this that are considered normal. Import those same rules to another culture (e.g., from anywhere to the United States), and the once-normal boundaries may not be "normal" in the new context. Thus, immigrant and multiracial families have much more complex boundary dynamics to navigate the multiple worlds in which they live.

- *Enmeshment and diffuse boundaries:* If boundaries are blurry, diffuse, or weak, this leads to relational *enmeshment*, which is evidenced by a lack of clear distinction between members and a strong sense of mutuality and connection at the expense of individual autonomy (Colapinto, 1991). When talking with an enmeshed family, counselors typically see family members do the following:
    - Interrupting one another and/or speaking for one another
    - Mind reading and making assumptions
    - Insisting on high levels of protectiveness and over-concern
    - Demanding loyalty at the expense of individual needs
    - Feeling threatened when there is disagreement or difference

How do you sort through family and cultural differences and determine whether a particular relationship has clear or enmeshed boundaries? Simple. If there are symptoms and problems in one or more individuals and/or complaints about family interactions, then the boundaries are too diffuse for the current developmental stage and context. Thus, behaviors that constitute problematic boundaries in one cultural context may be clear in another cultural context, making it difficult for families and counselors alike to sort out relational rules in immigrant and other bicultural families because there is more than one cultural context at play (Minuchin & Fishman, 1981). Counselors must proceed slowly and mindfully to accurately assess where and how boundaries are a problem to avoid inadvertently imposing dominant cultural norms or psychological theory on clients. That said, rarely in the early stages of counseling are boundaries clear because generally some boundary patterns need to be renegotiated to resolve the presenting complaint.

- *Disengagement and rigid boundaries:* Boundaries can also become highly rigid, resulting in relational *disengagement*. Families with rigid boundaries value autonomy and independence over emotional connection, creating isolation that may be more emotional than physical (Colapinto, 1991). These families have excessive tolerance for deviation, often failing to mobilize support and protection for one another. Counselors working with disengaged families notice the following:
    - A lack of reaction and repercussions even to problems
    - Significant freedom for most members to do as they please
    - Few demands for or expressions of loyalty, affection, or commitment
    - Parallel interactions (e.g., doing different activities in the same room) consistently substituting for reciprocal interactions and engagement

Like enmeshed boundaries, rigid boundaries cannot be accurately assessed without taking cultural and developmental variables into consideration. High levels of independence are not considered problematic unless one or more persons are experiencing symptoms.

Hierarchy

A painful, shocking reality that I was very slow to believe as a new counselor is that most child behavior issues boil down to an ineffective *parental hierarchy*—or at least greatly improve when hierarchical issues are address. The parental hierarchy refers to the power differential between the parent and child and the parent's ability to manage the child's behavior (Colapinto, 1991; Minuchin, 1974; Minuchin & Fishman, 1981). There are three basic forms of parental hierarchy:

- *Effective:* An effective parental hierarchy is evidenced by two things: (a) parents can effectively set boundaries and limits while (b) still maintaining emotional connection with their children. For better or worse, children keep changing, and thus the behaviors that constitute an effective parental hierarchy at one point in time do not work at another—thus, it is hard for parents to continually shift and balance these two roles as children grow.

- *Insufficient:* A common parenting pattern, an insufficient parental hierarchy means that the parent is not able to effectively manage the child's behavior, commonly referred to as a permissive parenting style. In these families, parents cannot sufficiently influence their children's behavior to avoid problems from erupting. Often these parents hope that the counselor will "teach" their children to obey rules, be polite, and take responsibility. Alas, such a hope is in vain. Each adult must establish an effective hierarchy with a child on a one-to-one basis: this includes parents, teachers, stepparents, and, yes, counselors too. In fact, it is commonly the case that one parent has an effective hierarchy and the other does not, thus providing evidence that the burden is on the adult rather than the child to effectively establish a hierarchy. Similar to boundaries, the outward expression of an effective versus an insufficient hierarchy can be determined only by examining the cultural context, family life stage of development, and symptomatic behavior.
- *Excessive:* The other extreme is an excessive hierarchy in which the parent maintains rules that are developmentally too strict and unrealistic and consequences that are too severe to be effective. The children typically behave well (until they decide to rebel) but at the expense of emotional closeness. These parents need assistance in developing age-appropriate rules and expectations and in developing a stronger emotional bond with their children.

Complementarity

One of the most elegant and subtle areas assessed by systemic counselors, "complementarity" refers to rigidly adopted patterns of opposite roles in a relational system (Colapinto, 1991). Like jigsaw puzzles, individuals develop complementary roles in their couple, family, and organizational relationships: the over/underfunctioner, good/bad child, understanding/strict parent, logical/emotional, role model/rebel, and so on. Over time, these systemically generated roles become viewed as inherent personality characteristics that seem unchangeable within that particular relationship, even if the same dynamic is not manifested in other contexts. The more exaggerated and rigid these roles become, the more of a problem they create. After years, the individuals involved do not believe they could behave any differently, although they have ample evidence that they did in fact possess these qualities prior to being in the relationship. One of the most distinguishing features of systemic counselors is that they are able to recognize rigid complementary patterns as part of the system dynamics rather than individual personalities and can help clients move beyond them.

Targeting Change: Goal Setting
Four Steps for Setting Systemic Goals

In the MRI brief approach, counselors use a four-step process for setting goals based on the axiom that "the problem is the attempted solution," meaning that the problem is that the client has been using the wrong class or type of solution (Watzlawick et al., 1974). The counselor's task then is to identify the type of solution that *hasn't been working* and then identify what solutions would represent a solution that uses an alternative logic or premise. For example, if a person is trying to reduce worry by trying to control or manage it—and all those attempts have failed—the counselor would identify solutions with an alternative logic to control, such as indulging the worry by instructing the client to worry at specific times (see the section "Paradoxical Intervention and Symptom Prescription").

Setting systemic goals involves four distinct steps:

Step 1: Clearly define the problem: Define the problem in concrete, behavioral terms, including the actions and reactions of all involved: When a systemic counselor hears from a client, "I worry too much," the counselor has not really heard a meaningful problem statement. The counselor's job at this point is to help the client turn this into a clear problem statement that is behavioral and concrete: "When I am assigned an important project at work, I end up thinking about it before I go to bed, during my commute, and when working on other projects; I ask my boss a thousand questions and she gets annoyed with me; I second-guess myself when talking with my partner at dinner, and she keeps trying to reassure me that I am doing great, but I don't believe her because she is just saying that to make me feel better." Now *that* is a clear problem.

Step 2: Identify prior attempted solutions: Identify the attempted solutions thus far: The counselor may ask, "How have you attempted to deal with this problem?" and listens for patterns in the various attempted solutions (e.g., I tell myself to stop worrying but can't stop; I look to others to reassure me but don't believe them either; etc.). Although a seemingly obvious thing to assess, attempted but failed solutions often are not spontaneously mentioned because they are typically not remembered or flagged as important because they didn't work.

Step 3: Develop clear description of preferred change: Develop a behavioral description of the things to be changed: Systemic counselors take goal writing very seriously. *How* the goal is languaged is a critical part of the intervention. If systemic goals are not crafted carefully using clear descriptions of *behavioral change*, failure is more likely. Watzlawick et al. (1974) identify three characteristics of helpful goals: realistic, specific, and time limited:

- *Realistic:* Systemic counselors avoid pie-in-the-sky, utopian goals that clients hope they can achieve by seeking professional help, such as *always* be happy, *never* fight with a partner, or have a child who *always* obeys. If humans are involved, "always" and "never" are not a part of realistic goals. Instead, he counselor helps the client develop more human goals that "increase the frequency" of desired behaviors and decrease that of undesirable ones. For many clients, accepting realistic goals is a significant form of change in and of itself, often resulting in improvements just from setting a realistic goal.
- *Specific:* Goals should target clearly defined behaviors and interactions rather than vague intentions, such as "communicate better," "feel happier," or "relax more." Vague goals can set up false hopes and reduce the counselor's effectiveness. Instead, goals should be written so it is easy to determine when they have been attained: "increase frequency of asserting needs at work" or "increase time spent with friends."
- *Time limited:* Systemic counselors set clear time limits (e.g., achieve goal in 4 weeks or 4 months) to help motivate and focus both client and counselor. A written time limit helps set realistic expectations. When time limits are not met, systemic counselors view this as feedback indicating that something may be amiss and needs to be addressed, such as an unassessed dynamic, an inadequately joined counseling system, poorly designed interventions, or unrealistic initial goals.

Step 4: Develop a systemic treatment plan: Develop a plan that is based on systemic principles to achieve change: When developing a plan, systemic counselors use two basic principles:

- The *target of change* is the *attempted solution*, meaning that a new logical premise is used (e.g., rather than forcefully trying to control a behavior, the new logic is to allow it in some form).
- The *tactic of change* is to use the *client's own language* to speak directly to the client's view of reality (e.g., if the client is athletically inclined, a sports metaphor may be used).

When designing a treatment plan, systemic counselors *never* use commonsense logic or basic psychoeducation on how to solve problems: that is the type of approach used in cognitive-behavioral or Adlerian counseling. Instead, systemic counselors alter the interaction pattern, trusting that the system will reorganize itself using its innate ability to self-correct—the counselor's role is simply to give the system a gentle nudge in the right direction, which is in the *opposite* direction of the prior attempted solution.

Systemic and Structural Goals

Systemic counselors target similar basic goals for clients that can generally be categorized as goals for (a) systemic dynamics and (b) family structure (Colapinto, 1991; Madanes, 1991; Minuchin, 1974; Watzlawick et al., 1974).

General Goals for Systemic Dynamics

- Develop relational patterns that maintain *flexible interaction and behavior patterns* without the presenting symptom(s)
  Example: Reduce pursuer–distancer pattern and increase ability to tolerate higher levels of intimacy

General Goals for Family Structure

- *Clear boundaries* between all subsystems that allow for *intimacy* and *individuation* appropriate within client's cultural contexts
  Example: Reduce enmeshment between client and mother to increase client's ability to make independent decisions
- Clear distinction between the *marital/couple subsystem* and *parental subsystem* (if children are involved)
  Example: Increase separation of parental and marital subsystems to increase emotional intimacy and solidarity in the partnership
- *Effective parental hierarchy* and the severing of cross-generational coalitions (if children are involved)
  Example: Increase the effectiveness of the parental hierarchy and the ability of the parents to consistently set and reinforce limits
- Relational structures that promote the *development and growth of individuals and relationships*
  Example: Increase sense of emotional connection with father

The Doing: Interventions

Enactments and Modifying Interactions (see "The Juice")

Systemic Reframing

One of the most frequently used interventions, systemic counselors use *systemic reframing* to alter interaction and behavior patterns related to the problem by offering new frameworks for viewing the problem (Colapinto, 1991; Minuchin, 1974; Minuchin & Fishman, 1981; Watzlawick et al., 1974). Systemic counselors reframe problems in a very specific way, which distinguishes their work from other forms of counseling. Specifically, *systemic reframes illuminate how a client's symptom is part of a larger interactional pattern.* For example, if a person's worrying elicits sympathy from others creating a sense of connection, a systemic reframe would highlight this dynamic in the reframe.

Systemic reframing focuses on reciprocal interactions, meaning that person A affects person B's response, which then affects person A's response, which affects B's response, ad infinitum ($A \rightleftarrows B$). This process requires piecing together the interaction patterns that involve the client and others involved in the problem interaction sequence and reframing it so that the broader systemic dynamic is revealed.

How to Generate Systemic Reframes

1. *Assess broader interactional patterns:* Complementary relationships, hierarchy, boundaries, and so on.
   Example: The counselor assesses a hero/damsel-in-distress pattern in which a woman's husband responds to her fear of a manic episode relapse by taking over many of her household tasks and chores; the more he does, the less capable she seemingly becomes.

(continued)

> 2. *Redescribe the problem in a systemic frame:* Use interactional pattern to describe problem in larger context.
> *Example:* The counselor can reframe the situation thusly: "Your fear and your husband's fear of relapse has resulted in him taking over many of the household tasks you dislike: cooking, cleaning, doing homework with the children, paying bills, and so on. Now you are in a situation where you have to stay worried about relapse in order to avoid those tasks. It's a tough situation you are in. If you allow yourself to feel better, you have new problems to deal with."

Circular Questions

In my humble estimation, circular questions are some of the best questions in the field of mental health because they have a consistent one-two punch: assessment and intervention. They are invaluable when working with clients who complain about or compare themselves to others (okay, I guess that covers virtually all of us). Developed by the Milan team, circular questioning is an elegant and highly efficient technique that simultaneously assesses interactional patterns while reframing them: thus, this is a winning two-for-one assessment/intervention combination. Circular questions make overt the systemic dynamics and interactive patterns in the system and by doing so inherently *reframe* the problem for all participants without the counselor directly proposing a reframe (Selvini Palazzoli et al., 1978, 1980). They are perhaps the most effective way means of "confronting" clients on patterns that they don't want to acknowledge without the counselor having to directly confront: instead, *the clients* are the ones who reveal the pattern by responding to questions. It's always harder to not believe oneself than another.

Specific forms of circular questions (Cecchin, 1987) include the following:

- *Behavioral sequences questions:* These questions trace the entire sequence of behaviors that constitute the problem, such as "When you start to get depressed, what is your first sign? What do you do next? What do others see and how do they respond? How do you respond in turn to them? What happens next?" The counselor follows the sequence of interactions until homeostasis is restored again.
- *Behavioral difference questions:* Behavioral difference questions shatter the illusion a particular behavior is part of a person's inherent personality. For example, if a client claims, "I am a worrier," the counselor would ask, "What do you do that makes you a worrier?" The *behavioral definition* of the problem behavior, "plan for how to handle potential problems," is then used to compare with others: "How does your partner plan for potential problems? How did your parents plan for potential problems? Others that you know? What is similar and what is different about these approaches?"
- *Comparison and ranking questions:* Comparison and ranking questions reduce labeling and other rigid descriptions of self and others; they also help illuminate problem interaction patterns: "Who is the most anxious person you know (or in your family, office, etc.)? The least anxious? Who does each deal with anxiety? Who is the most upset by your anxiety? The least upset by it?"
- *Before-and-after questions:* When a particularly notable positive or negative event has occurred, counselors use "before" and "after" questions to assess nuances in the relational dynamics: "Before your depressive episode, did you and your partner fight more or less? Who was happier at that time? Who did more of the chores then?"
- *Hypothetical circular questions:* Hypothetical questions can be helpful in assessing how a person responds to stress and to better understand the subtle relational dynamics. For example, "If you were to suddenly lose your job, what would you do? Who would you turn to first? Who would be the first to offer help? Who would you not want to tell?"

In the case study at the end of this chapter, the counselor uses circular questions to enable Navid to better see how his substance use is related to the family dynamics and rather than a form of "rebellion" is actually serving to keep the family functioning the same, namely, his parents treating him like a child.

Directives

Frequently misunderstood because they do not follow commonsense logic, directives are a signature systemic technique (Madanes, 1991). As the name implies, directives are directions for the client to complete a specific task, usually between sessions but sometimes within the session. The key element is that the tasks are rarely "logical" or linear solutions to the problem; instead, they interrupt the system's interaction patterns in minor but meaningful ways to create new interactions (Haley, 1987). More simply stated, they are designed to "trip up" the problem and get the pattern slightly off-kilter so that clients have to rebalance. Systemic counselors trip up the problem with the *smallest change possible*. For example, if part of a client's "depression ritual" (or pattern) involves eating a pint of his favorite ice cream, a directive might involve tripping this pattern up with the least amount of change (client more likely to do it) that is still meaningful (shakes things up): such a directive might be to read a favorite poem aloud or eat a pint of less desirable flavor, such as strawberry. Although this may sound quite ridiculous at first, for the person involved, just shifting that one element often results in "waking up" and seeing the pattern more clearly and also feeling more motivated to do something different. Because they are based in action, directives inspire a visceral form of insight because the person is in the middle of the action that needs changing, which is quite different from the more distant, cognitive insight in traditional psychodynamic theory.

Designing Directives

Step 1: Assess the problem sequence of behaviors: Identify the sequence of behaviors that constitute the presenting problem (e.g., client encounters problems with a project at work, becomes intensely focused on project, or is snippy with coworkers and ignores family; when work problem is solved, client is happy but has alienated people in his life).

Step 2: Target a small change in behavioral sequence: Identify one small behavioral change in the sequence that the client can reasonably make that would alter the problem sequence (e.g., put on a object of clothing, hang a sign, or otherwise send a signal to others that symbolizes he is unavailable for normal human interaction until the problem is resolved).

Step 3: Motivate the client to follow through: Haley (1987) emphasizes the importance of motivating the client *before* the task is issued. This is usually done by appealing to the ultimate goal: that the client and significant others wants the problem behavior to stop.

Step 3: Give precise, doable instructions for the directive: The key to directives is to be very specific: when, where, how, who, and on which day of the week. The counselor should consider variations in schedules, such as vacations, illness, weekends, and so on. Furthermore, the directives should be *given* rather than casually suggested. For example, "It sounds like you would really like to do something different the next time you get pulled into a work project. So here is what I want you to do. The next time you start to feel the 'pull,' I want you to email your coworkers and family that you will unfortunately be absent in their lives until this problem is resolved. Feel free to add playful references to your metaphoric death, by perhaps signing it, 'Temporarily departed.'" The counselor avoids theoretical or logical explanations about "why" and "what for" and simply says, "I think this might be helpful" if the client asks.

Step 4: Review the task in painful detail: Have the client describe precisely what he is to do and how he is going to do it (e.g., "Just to review and make sure we understand, can you review what you are going to do this week when you feel the pull of a project?").

Step 5: Request a task report: The following week, the counselor asks the client "how it went?" Generally, one of three things happens: the client (a) does it, (b) does not do it, or (c) partially does it (Haley, 1987). Obviously, if clients complete their tasks, they are congratulated, and the counselor discusses how it went. If they have partially done the task, the counselor does not excuse them too quickly because that would send the message that undermines the counselor's authority. If they fail to attempt the task, Haley uses two responses, one nice and one not so nice. In the nice way, the counselor says, "I must have misunderstood you or your situation to ask that of you—otherwise you would have done it" (Haley, 1987, p. 71). In the not-so-nice approach, the counselor emphasizes that the client has missed an opportunity to make changes for their own good and that this is a loss for him or her (*not* that the counselor is disappointed); the counselor does not ask them to redo the task even if they say they want to. Instead, the counselor uses this experience to increase motivation for the next task.

Paradoxical Intervention and Symptom Prescription

Perhaps the most misunderstood of systemic interventions, *paradoxical intervention* and *symptom prescription* involve instructing clients to engage in the problem behavior in some fashion, such as assigning a client to worry each morning from 8:00 to 8:15 a.m. Symptom prescription and other paradoxical interventions are "paradoxical" because they seem as though they will make the problem worse rather than better—or at least at first glance. I guess I should mention that, yes, indeed they can make things worse if they are used at the wrong time or for the wrong problem, so these should be used only under careful supervision until you understand how they work.

You will know when it is time to use one of these interventions because *when it is appropriate to use paradox, it will not seem paradoxical—at least in the mind of the counselor—it will be the only logical, obvious action to take.* Generally, it takes many years of practice (and good supervision) until paradox seems like a good idea. Not a garden-variety technique that works for everybody, paradoxical interventions are appropriate for two types of problems: (a) when making any other change disrupts the client's current level of stability or (b) when the problem seems "uncontrollable" from the client's perspective: "I can't keep myself from worrying, nagging, eating, fighting, dancing a jig, and so on."

Paradox With Clients Resisting Change Some clients seem to resist any and all attempts at change even though they say they really, really want to change (the "really, really" part should be your first clue that things may not go as planned). No matter how great the idea and how much these clients agree to it, they never seem to follow through on anything that actually would promote change. As maddening as they can be for the counselor, these clients are not bad, hypocritical, or actively resisting. They simply need an intervention that honors the fact that this symptom is very important in maintaining homeostasis for the them. Thus, they—often realistically—fear that giving it up may create *more* discomfort and chaos than they are currently experiencing; in these situations, paradox can be useful (Haley, 1987). In such a situation, the counselor may restrain or caution against certain changes, such as "perhaps the couple needs to argue to keep their passion strong; if they stopped, things may get worse." Paradoxical tasks are difficult to effectively deliver because the counselor must communicate several messages at once:

- I want to help you resolve your problem.
- I am sincerely concerned about you.
- I think you can be normal but perhaps you cannot.

When paradox is successful, change is usually spontaneous. Systemic counselor also often use paradoxical intervention in the later stages of counseling to prevent relapse by paradoxically encouraging it (Haley, 1976): "I know that you are saying that you aren't worrying any more, but now I am a bit worried about that. You might just want to let yourself worry for 5 to 10 minutes a day a few times a week, just in case you find that it really did solve problems for you."

Paradox With "Uncontrollable" Symptoms When clients report symptoms they claim to have no control over, systemic counselors use *symptom prescription* as an intervention. Symptom prescription changes the *context* (where, when, who, and what) of the problem behavior without requiring clients to stop having the symptom. If the context changes, the *meaning* of the behavior must also change. When the meaning changes, thoughts, feelings, and subsequent behaviors automatically change too. A common example of using paradox is worrying, which is particularly difficult to intervene on because it is a thought and emotional process often with limited associated behaviors. When a client is given the directive to set an egg timer to worry for 10 minutes at a particular time in the day, it radically changes worrying from a vague, free-floating experience to a consciously chosen activity that they can voluntarily start and that most often they quickly discover can also stop at will. By changing the context, the meaning and experience of worrying changes, often creating significant movement on a symptom that seemed totally out of the client's control.

Shifting Epistemologies: Expanding and Challenging the Client's Worldview

Systemic counselors carefully examine the rules, logic, and premises that clients construct their worldviews on: what is "necessary," what is prohibited, how does one show love, and what does one owe to others. Most people cannot list the majority of these epistemological assumptions that inform their every action, interaction, thought, priority, and emotion. By identifying and commenting on them, systemic counselors affect the operating premises that fuel the problem (Colapinto, 1991; Minuchin, 1974; Minuchin & Fishman, 1981).

As you might have guessed this far into the chapter, systemic counselors generally don't directly confront these premises but instead use existing beliefs and *expand* and *reinterpret* them in more helpful directions. Again, this intervention involves using the symptom—not asking clients to relinquish it—and recontextualizing, stretching, and/or reordering it to resolve issues. For example, if a client tends to be a perfectionist who never stops to enjoy life, you might help them become perfect at relaxing. Alternatively, if parents were great at structuring and setting limits with young children and start to struggle with teens, they can be challenged to learn how to get the teen to structure himself or herself and set his or her own behavioral standards. Like a martial artist, the systemic counselor takes a fundamental premise that has been supporting the problem and redirects its logic to support an alternative set of behaviors and interactions, allowing clients to maintain their core beliefs but use them in new ways.

Complimenting Strengths and Shaping Competence

Compliment strengths and *shaping competence* are used to augment and reinforce the clients' natural positive interaction patterns and strengths. When systemic counselors identify client strengths, they are quick to compliment and encourage. A similar process, *shaping competence* involves noticing and complimenting small successes along the way to reaching goals. For example, if a client was able to stop a panic attack once during the week or keep it from getting out of control, systemic counselors compliment and encourage the client for these small successes.

Shaping competence also refers to not overfunctioning for the client, meaning doing things that the client is capable of doing and/or needs to be learning to resolve an issue. This can include setting limits with a child, jotting down an idea from session, following up on a phone call, or making a decision about how to proceed. Depending on a client's presenting problem, all of these common in-session occurrences are opportunities for clients to shape their competence rather than have counselor do it for them, depriving them of an opportunity to learn in a safe and supported environment. In the case study at the end of this chapter, the counselor helps shape Navid's competence by complimenting his behaviors and decisions that include taking responsibility and avoiding trouble, such as choosing not to use and focus on his studies.

Interventions for Specific Problems
Invariant Prescription to Sever Coalitions

As the name implies, the *invariant prescription* is a directive that is not varied across families because this one task quickly severs inappropriate parent–child coalitions (Selvini

Palazzoli, 1988). The prescription is essentially this: the parents are instructed to arrange to go on a date (or other outing), and they are not to tell the children where they were going or why. The desired effect is to create a *secret* between the parents, ending inappropriate coalitions by creating a clear boundary between the parents as a unified team and the symptomatic child. The child loses the status of being a special confidant of the one parent, which also lessens the emotional burden on the child, resulting in fewer problem symptoms. Although originally designed for severe pathology such as anorexia or psychosis in the child, this intervention is also effective with parents who overemphasize transparent and open communication with their children to the extent that one parent creates a coalition with the child and/or the parental hierarchy is ineffective.

Ordeals for Compulsive Behaviors

Inspired by the work of Milton Erickson (see Chapter 11), *ordeals* are often used in situations where the client feels helpless in controlling a symptom, such as overeating, smoking, nail biting, drinking, and so on, and is based on a simple premise: "If one makes it more difficult for a person to have a symptom than to give it up, the person will give up the symptom" (Haley, 1984, p. 5). Rather than try to develop linear, logical means for stopping the behavior (that would be a cognitive-behavioral approach), the strategic counselor *allows* the symptom with a twist (by now, you should recognize this theme): the client must complete another task, an "ordeal" first or afterward.

The ordeal need not be directly related to the undesired activity but often carries a metaphoric relation to it. For example, if a person were trying to reduce his or her "emotional eating" to sooth difficult emotions, the ordeal would target the behavior and internal tension by logical means (e.g., write for 10 minutes in a journal, jog for 10 minutes, do a calorie log before the binge, etc.) or metaphorically (e.g., "clean out" the refrigerator, pantry, etc.; set an elaborate table for a feast) or with a seemingly unrelated task (e.g., perform a random act of kindness for a stranger or loved one, answer three emails, etc.). In most cases, ordeals are less about creating a horrific, unappealing ordeal to stop undesired behavior and more about shaking up or perturbing the systemic pattern so that new behavioral sequences can evolve. The ordeal isn't a behavioral deterrent or punishment as much as it is adding a new—often neutral—behavior that forces clients to interrupt their patterns. As the individual or family adjusts to this rather small and innocuous twist, it *must* change to create new steps and is able to do so with less fear and resistance than if it were told to stop.

Boundary Making to Increase or Decrease Engagement

Boundary making is a special form of enactment that targets over- or under-involvement to help families soften rigid boundaries or strengthen diffuse boundaries (Colapinto, 1991; Minuchin, 1974). Systemic counselors use this technique to direct who participates and how. By actively setting boundaries, counselors interrupt the habitual interaction patterns, allowing members to experience underutilized skills and abilities. Boundary making may involve several different directives:

* Asking family members to change seats
* Asking family members to move seats farther or closer together or turn toward one another
* Having separate sessions with individuals or subsystems to strengthen subsystem boundaries.
* Asking one or more members to remain silent during an interaction
* Asking questions that highlight a problem boundary area (e.g., "Do you always answer for your son when he is asked a question?")
* Blocking interruptions or encouraging pauses for less dominant persons to speak

Putting It All Together: Systemic Treatment Plan Template

Use this treatment plan template for developing a plan for clients with depressive, anxious, or compulsive types of presenting problems. Depending on the specific client, presenting problem, and clinical context, the goals and interventions in this template may need to be modified only slightly or significantly; you are encouraged to significantly revise the plan as needed. For the plan to be useful, goals and techniques should be written to target specific beliefs, behaviors, and emotions that the client is experiencing. The more specific, the more useful it will be to you.

Treatment Plan

Initial Phase of Treatment (First One to Three Sessions)
Initial Phase Counseling Tasks

1. *Develop working counseling relationship. Diversity note:* Adapt style for ethnicity, gender, family dynamics, and so on.
   Relationship building intervention:
   a. **Join** with client using **social courtesy** and by respecting larger systemic culture and maintaining neutral position between clients and others.

2. *Assess individual, systemic, and broader cultural dynamics. Diversity note:* Include larger cultural systemic dynamics.
   Assessment Strategies:
   a. Obtain detailed description of **problem behavioral sequences.**
   b. Identify **boundary, subsystems, triangles, hierarchy,** and **complementary patterns** that contribute to the problem.

Initial Phase Client Goals (One to Two Goals): Manage crisis issues and/or reduce most distressing symptoms

1. *Decrease* [name specific crisis behavior] to reduce [crisis] symptoms.
   Interventions:
   a. Directives to **interrupt crisis escalation** and enable alternative means to manage crisis.
   b. **Reframing** crisis situation to reduce sense of urgency and crisis.

Working Phase of Treatment (Three or More Sessions)
Working Phase Counseling Task

1. *Monitor quality of the working alliance. Diversity note:* Ensure positive alliance with clients and significant others not in session.
   Assessment Intervention:
   a. Use Session Rating Scale; verbally ask client about alliance.

Working Phase Client Goals (Two to Three Goals). Target individual and relational dynamics using theoretical language (e.g., decrease avoidance of intimacy, increase awareness of emotion, increase agency, etc.)

1. *Increase* **interruptions to problem interaction cycle** to reduce depression/anxiety and so on.
   Interventions:
   a. **Directives** to do one small thing different to interrupt problem interaction pattern.
   b. **Systemic reframing** to alter response to problem pattern.
   c. **Paradoxical injunctions** to engage in symptomatic behavior in new context or with restraints.

2. *Increase* **clear boundaries, relational structure,** and **communication** to reduce depression and anxiety.
   Interventions:
   a. **Enactments** to clarify boundaries, triangles, and hierarchy.
   b. **Circular questions** to make problem dynamics overt.

(continued)

3. *Increase* developmental, relational, and cultural appropriateness of **worldview** and **rules for relating** to reduce feelings of hopelessness, anxiety, fear, and so on.
    Interventions:
    a. **Circular questions** to increase awareness of relational assumptions.
    b. **Challenging worldviews** and **relational rules** that support and maintain the problem.

Closing Phase of Treatment (Last Four or More Sessions)
Closing Phase Counseling Tasks

1. *Develop aftercare plan and maintain gains. Diversity note:* Reassess functioning in all areas before ending counseling to ensure problem has not shifted to another aspect of system.
    Intervention:
    a. Reinforce new **epistemology and relational rules** and use **circular questions** to apply new skills to future challenges.

Closing Phase Client Goals (*One to Two Goals*)*:* Determined by theory's definition of health and normalcy

1. *Increase* **satisfying interactions** in intimate, social, and/or work relationships (whichever were not already addressed in working phase) to reduce feelings of hopelessness, anxiety, fear, and so on.
    Interventions:
    a. **Shaping competency** to transfer strengths from one area to another.
    b. **Circular questions** to capitalize on strengths and expand to new areas.

2. *Increase* **flexibility in worldview and relational interactions** to reduce potential for new problems to develop.
    Interventions:
    a. **Challenge rigid rules for relating and responding.**
    b. **Circular questions** to enable client to discover limits of worldview.

Snapshot: Bowen's Intergenerational Family Approach

Murray Bowen's (1976, 1985) intergenerational family approach combines a psychoanalytically grounded multigenerational approach with systems theory, resulting in a distinct and fascinating approach that traces relational patterns *across generations*. Bowen's theory posits that healthy adult functioning is characterized by *differentiation*, the ability to separate thought from feeling and self from others. Differentiation is critical because of the evolutionary process that has made humans *emotionally interdependent* due to an inherent *chronic anxiety* related to survival. Each family system develops patterns for managing closeness and distance and regulating anxiety; these patterns are passed down from one generation to the next. The more the family allows for differentiation between members, the less pathology its members experience. Intergenerational counselors are quick to distinguish between *emotional cutoff* and healthy differentiation. Emotional cutoff is a sign of low levels of differentiation that require a person to stop relating to a family member because of high levels of anxiety and fusion; in contrast, healthy differentiation is marked by high levels of emotional intimacy counterbalanced with autonomy. Another problematic means of managing chronic anxiety, *triangulation* (see the discussion of triangulation), refers to pulling in a third person to stabilize tension in a dyad, such as a mother who becomes close to a child to make up for intimacy she is not experiencing in the marriage.

The primary goals of intergenerational counseling are to (a) increase differentiation and (b) reduce emotional reactivity and chronic anxiety. Intergenerational counselors use *genograms*, a graphic representation of three or more generations that is similar to a family tree, to identify intergenerational patterns, such as emotional cutoff and triangulation. In addition, genograms can be used to identify other family patterns related to gender, death, personality, illness, mental health, substance abuse, sexual abuse, occupation, and so on. In session, intergenerational counselors relate to clients using a differentiated, *nonanxious presence* that role models differentiation, reduces triangulation, and encourages clients' differentiation. The techniques of intergenerational counseling focus on encouraging client differentiation using process questions that help clients become more aware of intergenerational patterns.

Snapshot: Satir's Human Growth Model

One of the most influential women in the field of mental health, Virginia Satir (1972, 1983, 1988) developed a comprehensive family counseling model that integrated humanism and system theory. Her theory is based on four primary assumptions:

1. People tend naturally towards positive growth (humanistic principle).
2. All people possess the resources for positive growth (humanistic principle).
3. Every person and every thing or situation impact and are impacted by everyone and everything else (systemic principle).
4. Therapy is a process, which involves interaction between therapist and client; and, in this relationship, each person is responsible for himself/herself (systemic and humanistic principle). (Satir, Banmen, Gerber, & Gomori, 1991, pp. 14–15)

Similar to other experiential counselors (see Chapters 6–8), Satir used the person of the counselor to develop a warm, empathetic, and encouraging relationship with clients. In addition to using the systemic assessment ideas outlined above in this chapter, Satir also conceptualized family interactions in terms of the *communication* or *survival stances*. Survival stances refer to communication patterns a person adopts as a child to cope with difficult family interactions. She identified four different communication stances and one health stance:

- *Placating:* The person manages interpersonal stress by recognizing the needs of *others* and the *context* but not the *self*.
- *Blaming:* The inverse of placators, the person manages interpersonal stress by recognizing the needs of *self* and the *context* but not *others*.
- *Superreasonable:* The person manages interpersonal stress by recognizing *contextual rules* but not more subjective needs of *self* and *others*.
- *Irrelevant:* This person manages interpersonal stress by not acknowledging *contextual demands*, *personal needs*, or the *needs of others*.
- *Congruent:* A person using a congruent stance is able to simultaneously honor the needs of self and respect the needs of others while responding appropriately to context.

The goals of Satir's approach are twofold: (a) to communicate congruently in all relationships and (b) to self-actualize (similar to other humanistic approaches). Satir uses an active style that includes having the family visually arrange each other to depict family dynamics using a technique called *family sculpting*. She also used communication coaching to help clients learn how to communicate congruently. Another common intervention helps clients identify the *ingredients of an interaction*, helping them separate out (a) what is heard and said, (b) what meanings are made, (c) what feelings are felt about the meanings, (d) feelings about the feelings, (e) defenses that are used to manage feelings, (f) rules for communicating about the feelings, and, finally, (g) the outward response to the situation.

Snapshot: Research and the Evidence Base

Quick Summary: Good research support, especially for newer empirically supported treatments.

Systemic counseling has a strong and growing evidence base for its effectiveness with a wide range of issues, including conduct disorder, substance abuse, childhood disorders, marital problems, couple enrichment, domestic violence, severe mental illness, mood disorders, and physical disorders (Sprenkle, 2002, 2011). In fact, the empirically supported treatments for youth diagnosed with substance abusing and/or conduct disorders are some of the best researched and supported treatments in all of mental health. Similarly, evidence-based treatments for distressed couples—emotionally focused therapy and integrated behavioral couples therapy—have been refined through research for over three decades. Some of the better-known empirically supported treatments include the following:

- *Brief strategic family therapy* (structural ecosystemic therapy and structural ecodevelopmental preventive interventions; Szapocznik, Hervis, & Schwartz, 2003; Szapocznik & Williams, 2000)
- *Ecosystemic structural family therapy* (Lindblad-Goldberg, Dore, & Stern, 1998)
- *Emotionally focused therapy* (Johnson, 2004)
- *Family psychoeducation* (McFarlane, 2004)
- *Functional family therapy* (Sexton, 2009)
- *Integrative couples therapy* (Jacobson & Christensen, 1996)
- *Multisystemic family therapy* (Henggeler, Schoenwald, Borduin, Rowland, & Cunningham, 1998)
- *Multidimensional family therapy* (Liddle, Dakof, & Diamond, 1991)

Snapshot: Evidence-Based Therapy: Emotionally Focused Therapy

In a Nutshell: The Least You Need to Know

Emotionally focused therapy (EFT) is one of the most thoroughly researched approaches in the field and is an empirically validated treatment for treating couples (Johnson, 2004). Sue Johnson and Les Greenberg (1985, 1994) developed the model using a combination of (a) attachment theory, (b) experiential theory (specifically, Carl Rogers's person-centered therapy), and (c) systems theory (specifically, systemic-structural therapies; Johnson, 2004). Emotionally focused therapists focus on the motional system of the couple and use affect heightening to help couples restructure their interactional patterns to increase emotional intimacy and to address their attachment needs.

Attachment and Adult Love

Johnson (2004, pp. 25–32) uses Bowlby's theory of attachment to conceptualize adult love, identifying 10 tenets of this theory:

1. *Attachment is an innate motivating force:* The desire to be connected to others is intrinsic.
2. *Secure dependence complements dependency:* Neither complete independence nor overdependence is possible, only effective or ineffective dependency.
3. *Attachment offers an essential safe haven:* Secure attachment provides a buffer for stress and uncertainty.
4. *Attachment offers a secure base:* A secure base allows for exploration, innovation, and openness.
5. *Emotional accessibility and responsiveness build bonds:* Secure attachment is established by being emotionally accessible and responsive.
6. *Fear and uncertainly activate attachment needs:* When threatened, a person experiences a strong emotional need for comfort and connection.

7. *The process of separation distress is predictable:* If attachment needs are not met, the person experiences predictable responses of anger, clinging, depression, and despair.
8. There are a finite number of insecure attachment styles:
   - *Anxious/hyperactivated:* When needs are not met, the person becomes anxiously clingy and relentlessly pursues connection and may become aggressive, blaming, and critical.
   - *Avoidance:* When needs are not met, the person suppresses attachment needs and instead focuses on tasks or other distractions.
   - *Combination anxious and avoidant:* In this style, the person pursues closeness and then avoids it once offered.
9. *Attachment involves working models of self and other:* People use the quality of attachments to define themselves and others as lovable, worthy, and competent.
10. *Isolation and loss are inherently traumatizing:* Isolation and loss of connection are inherently traumatic experiences.

EFT Tasks and Stages

Johnson (2004) identifies *three primary therapeutic tasks* of EFT:

Task 1: Creation and maintenance of alliance

Task 2: Assessing and formulating emotion

Task 3: Restructuring interactions

She also identifies *three stages with nine steps* that describe the progression of therapy (Johnson, 2004):

Stage 1: De-escalation of Negative Cycles

Step 1: Create an alliance and delineate conflict in the attachment struggle.

Step 2: Identify the negative interaction cycle.

Step 3: Access unacknowledged emotions and underlying interactional positions.

Step 4: Reframe problem in terms of negative cycle and attachment needs with the cycle being the common enemy.

Stage 2: Change Interactional Patterns

Step 5: Promote identification of disowned attachment needs and aspects of self, integrating these into relational interactions.

Step 6: Promote acceptance of the partner's experience along with new interaction sequences.

Step 7: Encourage expression of needs and wants while increasing emotional engagement and bonding to redefine the couple's attachment.

Stage 3: Consolidation and Integration

Step 8: Facilitate new solutions to old problems.

Step 9: Consolidate new positions and new cycles of attachment.

Snapshot: Working With Diverse Populations

"Every family has elements in their own culture, which if understood and utilized, can become levers to actualize and expand the family members' behavioral repertoire. Unfortunately, we therapists have not assimilated this axiom" (Minuchin & Fishman, 1981, p. 262).

Quick Summary: Excellent support for working with diverse, urban populations, including immigrants, single-parent families, Hispanics, and African Americans.

An action-oriented, strength-based, relational approach, systemic counseling models fit and adapt well with the values of many minority cultures. Minuchin's systemic structural approach was originally developed to work with poor, ethnically diverse, urban families because traditional insight-oriented approaches were ineffective with these populations; this approach is the foundation for many of the evidence-based treatments for minority youth (Aponte, 1994, 1996; Colapinto, 1991; Minuchin et al., 1967; Szapocznik & Williams, 2000). In addition, case conceptualization and assessment concepts, such as interaction patterns, boundaries, and hierarchy, inherently consider culture and readily adapt to a wide range of diversity issues, such as sexual orientation, religion, and economic status. Furthermore, as a nonpathologizing approach, systemic theory includes a "safety check" for unknowingly imposing counselor bias: if a behavior or dynamic is not creating symptoms, it is not a problem. Systemic counselors aim to work from *within* the client's worldview, allowing the counselor to respectfully alter language and interventions to the client's values and beliefs. In addition, several systemic counselors integrate spiritual perspectives in their work (Aponte, 1994, 1996; Walsh, 2009).

Systemic Case Study and Treatment Plan

Navid, a 22-year-old of Persian descent, has come to counseling because his parents have insisted he deal with his pot use, or they will not pay for him to finish his last semester at an elite private college. Navid admits that his grades have plummeted this last semester, but he claims that it is because his parents want him to become a doctor, and he does not want to. He says that he smokes pot only on the weekends with friends and when he is stressed and preparing for an exam; he denies other substance use except for drinking "some beers" at parties. He prefers to play music—he is an avid guitarist—but his parents say that is not a real profession. His younger sister in high school who is the "perfect one" understands his frustration but would never speak up for him in a conversation with their parents. His parents recently caught him smoking pot during a recent visit home. His uncle, a medical doctor, was called in to "educate" him about drugs. His father stopped talking to him for the rest of the visit because he was so upset by Navid's choice to "throw his life away after all I've done for him." He reports hearing his mother frequently cry over the incident. Navid said he really doesn't care about graduating but is coming because he doesn't know what else to do with his family and his life.

Systemic Case Conceptualization

This case conceptualization was developed by selecting key concepts from the "The Viewing: Case Conceptualization" section of this chapter. You can use any of the concepts in that section to develop a case conceptualization for this or other cases.

Strengths

Some of AM's (adult male) strengths include his intelligence, musical ability, and awareness of family dynamics and a willingness to come to counseling. The family's strengths include valuing and supporting AM's professional success, involvement of extended family, and caring for each other and the welfare of the family.

Family Life Cycle Stage of Development

The family is in the early phases of launching, which requires some of the most significant changes in the family life cycle and affects all parties and relationships, including the marriage, which is in the process of becoming the parent's primary relationship again. The parents are still using more authoritarian parenting methods rather than an authoritative or even mentoring style to encourage AM to learn to make good decisions without their intervention, which is more appropriate in the launching stage.

Role of Symptom in the Relational System

Although it is tempting to see AM's behavior as a type of rebellion against his family, systemic analysis reveals a different dynamic. At a systemic level, it serves to keep the parents in a parenting position and also keep AM in the child role by engaging in behaviors that—by the family's cultural and socioeconomic standards—require parental intervention, even if he is 22. Thus, his substance use serves to keep the family connected and roles stable during the difficult period of launching.

Subsystems

AM and his sister have a sibling subsystem in which they understand each other's desire to adopt more Western values, such as do what you love rather than what will best support the family, and is therefore a subsystem organized around immigration and acculturation values. Additionally, extended family members, namely, the uncle, also are part of the parenting subsystem, as is culturally common in immigrant families.

Boundaries and Hierarchy

As is common in Iranian families, there is a clear hierarchical structure with the father at the head of the household. He has always had more rigid boundaries with the children, using more authoritarian parenting approaches. The mother is more emotionally connected with the children but never counters what the husband says or does, as that would be disrespectful.

Complementarity

In this family, the father tends to play the "bad parent" and the mother the "good/nice parent," as evidenced by their reaction to the substance use. AM and his sister are playing complementary roles right now as good/bad child.

Interactional Patterns and Behavioral Sequences

AM wanting to avoid medical classes and parents' control ➡ AM gets high ➡ father becomes angry and cuts off communication ➡ women in family quietly support AM ➡ AM equally dismissive of father ➡ uncle called in to mediate ➡ AM backs down but ready for next fight.

Systemic Treatment Plan

Initial Phase of Treatment (First One to Three Sessions)
Initial Phase Counseling Tasks

1. *Develop working counseling relationship. Diversity note:* Assess for AM's level of acculturation and adapt relationship accordingly.
   Relationship building intervention:
   a. **Join** with AM using **social courtesy** and by respecting family's culture and class; maintain a neutral position when AM discusses frustration with his family, especially the father.

2. *Assess individual, systemic, and broader cultural dynamics. Diversity note:* Carefully assess level of acculturation of parents and children and consider how this impacts dynamics.
   Assessment Strategies:
   a. Obtain detailed description of **problem behavioral sequences**, encouraging nonblaming descriptions of each person's actions.
   b. Identify **boundary, subsystems, triangles, hierarchy,** and **complementary patterns** that contribute to AM's substance use and family conflict.

Initial Phase Client Goals

1. *Increase* motivation to ensure that his life is on the right track to reduce use of marijuana.
   Interventions:
   a. Directives to **interrupt escalation of substance use when stressed** and identify alternative means to manage stress.
   b. **Reframing** crisis situation to increase AM's sense of personal responsibility for life direction and reduce need to rebel against father.

(continued)

Working Phase of Treatment (Three or More Sessions)
Working Phase Counseling Tasks

1. *Monitor quality of the working alliance. Diversity note:* Ensure positive alliance with AM and family members who are not in session; adapt for level of acculturation. *Assessment Intervention:*
   a. Use Session Rating Scale; verbally ask AM about alliance.

Working Phase Client Goals

1. *Increase* AM's ability to **interrupt problem interaction cycle** and do something different to reduce stress related to father and motivation to use substances. *Interventions:*
   a. **Directive** to do one small thing different on his part to interrupt problem interaction pattern, such as writing a thank-you to uncle.
   b. **Systemic reframing** that frames his substance use as a way his father is *still* controlling him because he is simply being the antithesis of what father wants rather than own person.
   c. **Ordeal and paradoxical directions** that require AM to engage in unappealing ordeal before substance use in order to reduce use.

2. *Increase* **clear boundaries with parents** that allow for better communication of personal needs and wishes to reduce self-sabotaging substance use. *Interventions:*
   a. **Enactments** adapted for individual to help AM practice alternative ways of responding to parents.
   b. **Circular questions** to increase AM's understanding of the covert family dynamics and his role in perpetuating them.

3. *Increase* developmental and cultural appropriateness of AM's **rules for relating** to reduce his use of substances and increase responsibility for life direction. *Interventions:*
   a. **Circular questions** to increase awareness of relational assumptions that underlie family conflict and AM's substance use.
   b. **Challenging worldviews and relational rules** that support and maintain the problem while remaining respectful of cultural norms.

Closing Phase of Treatment (Last Four or More Sessions)
Closing Phase Counseling Tasks

1. *Develop aftercare plan and maintain gains. Diversity note:* Reassess functioning in all areas before ending counseling to ensure problem has not shifted to another aspect of system. *Intervention:*
   a. Reinforce new **epistemology and relational rules** and use **circular questions** to apply new skills to future challenges.

Closing Phase Client Goals

1. *Increase* **satisfying interactions** with nuclear and extended to reduce feelings of hopelessness. *Interventions:*
   a. **Shaping competency** to transfer strengths from relating to father to relating to all family members.
   b. **Circular questions** to capitalize on strengths and expand to new areas.

2. *Increase* effective **development transition** to young adult who makes good life decisions without parents' intervention to reduce substance abuse and self-sabotage. *Interventions:*
   a. **Challenge rigid definitions of self** based on old role in system as child.
   b. **Circular questions** to increase AM's ability to see the responsibilities and possibilities of his new development stage more clearly.

ONLINE RESOURCES

Associations and Institutes

American Association of Brief and Strategic Therapists
www.aabst.org

American Association for Marriage and Family Therapy
www.aamft.org

Brief Strategic and Systemic World Network
www.bsst.org

Brief Strategic Family Therapy Training
www.brief-strategic-family-therapy.com

BSFT Training Manual
www.nida.nih.gov/TXManuals/bsft

International Association of Marriage and Family Counselors
www.iamfconline.com

Functional Family Therapy
www.fftinc.com

Mental Research Institute
www.mri.org

Multisystemic Therapy
www.mstservices.com

Philadelphia Child and Family Therapy Training Center
www.philafamily.com

Journals

Family Process
www.familyprocess.org

Journal of Marital and Family Therapy
www.jmft.net

Journal of Systemic Therapies
www.guilford.com

References

*Asterisk indicates recommended introductory readings.

Aponte, H. J. (1994). *Bread and spirit: Therapy with the new poor: Diversity of race, culture, and values.* New York: Norton.

Aponte, H. J. (1996). Political bias, moral values, and spirituality in the training of psychotherapists. *Bulletin of the Menninger Clinic, 60*(4), 488–502.

*Bateson, G. (1972). *Steps to an ecology of mind: Collected essays in anthropology, psychiatry, evolution, and epistemology.* San Francisco: Chandler.

Bateson, G. (1979). *Mind and nature: A necessary unity.* New York: Dutton.

*Boscolo, L., Cecchin, G., Hoffman, L., & Penn, P. (1987). *Milan systemic family therapy: Conversations in theory and practice* New York: Basic Books.

Bowen, M. (1976). Theory in practice of psychotherapy. In P. J. Guerin (Ed.), *Family therapy: Theory and practice* (pp. 42–90). New York: Gardner Press.

*Bowen, M. (1985). *Family therapy in clinical practice.* New York: Jason Aronson.

Campbell, D., Draper, R., & Crutchley, E. (1991). The Milan systemic approach to family therapy. In A. S. Gurman & D. P. Knishern (Eds.), *Handbook of family therapy* (pp. 325–362). New York: Brunner/Mazel.

Carter, B., & McGoldrick, M. (Eds.). (2005). *The expanded family life cycle: Individuals, families, and social perspectives* (3rd ed.) New York: Allyn and Bacon.

*Cecchin, G. (1987). Hypothesizing, circularity, and neutrality revisited: An invitation to curiosity. *Family Process, 26*(4), 405–413.

*Colapinto, J. (1991). Structural family therapy. In A. S. Gurman & D. P. Kniskern (Eds.), *Handbook of family therapy* (Vol. 2, pp. 417–443). New York: Brunner/Mazel.

Fisch, R., & Schlanger, K. (1999). *Brief therapy with intimidating cases: Changing the unchangeable.* New York: Jossey-Bass.

*Fisch, R., Weakland, J., & Segal, L. (1982). *The tactics of change: Doing therapy briefly.* New York: Jossey-Bass.

Gehart, D. R. (2010). *Mastering competencies in family therapy: A practical approach to theories and clinical case documentation.* Belmont, CA: Brooks/Cole.

Haley, J. (1963). *Strategies of psychotherapy.* New York: Grune & Stratton.

Haley, J. (1973). *Uncommon therapy: The psychiatric techniques of Milton H. Erickson, M.D.* New York: Norton.

Haley, J. (1976). *Problem-solving therapy: New strategies for effective family therapy.* San Francisco: Jossey-Bass.

Haley, J. (1980). *Leaving home: The therapy of disturbed young people.* New York: McGraw-Hill.

Haley, J. (1981). *Reflections on therapy.* Chevy Chase, MD: Family Therapy Institute of Washington, DC.

Haley, J. (1984). *Ordeal therapy.* San Francisco: Jossey-Bass.

*Haley, J. (1987). *Problem-solving therapy* (2nd ed.). San Francisco: Jossey-Bass.

Haley, J. (1996). *Learning and teaching therapy.* New York: Guilford.

Haley, J., & Richeport-Haley, M. (2007). *Directive family therapy.* New York: Hawthorne.

Henggeler, S. W., Schoenwald, S. K., Borduin, C. M., Rowland, M. D., & Cunningham, P. B. (1998). *Multisystemic treatment of antisocial behavior in children and adolescents.* New York: Guilford.

Jackson, D.D. (1967). The myth of normality. *Medical Opinion and Review, 3,* 28–33.

Jacobson, N. S., & Christensen, (1996). *Integrative couple therapy.* New York: Norton.

Johnson, S. M. (2004). *The practice of emotionally focused marital therapy: Creating connection* (2nd ed.). New York: Brunner-Routledge.

Johnson, S. M., & Greenberg, L. S. (1985). The differential effects of experiential and problem solving interventions in resolving marital conflicts. *Journal of Consulting and Clinical Psychology, 53,* 175–184.

Johnson, S. M., & Greenberg, L. S. (Eds.). (1994). *The heart of the matter: Perspectives on emotion in marital therapy.* New York: Brunner/Mazel.

Liddle, H. A., Dakof, G. A., & Diamond, G. (1991). Adolescent substance abuse: Multidimensional family therapy in action. In E. Daufman & P. Kaufman (Eds.), *Family therapy of drug and alcohol abuse* (pp. 120–171). Boston: Allyn and Bacon.

Lindblad-Goldberg, M., Dore, M., & Stern, L. (1998). *Creating competence from chaos.* New York: Norton.

Madanes, C. (1981). *Strategic family therapy.* San Francisco: Jossey-Bass.

Madanes, C. (1990). *Sex, love, and violence: Strategies for transformation.* New York: Norton.

Madanes, C. (1991). Strategic family therapy. In A. S. Gurman & D. P. Knishern (Eds.), *Handbook of family therapy* (pp. 396–416). New York: Brunner/Mazel

Madanes, C. (1993). Strategic humanism. *Journal of Systemic Therapies, 12*(4), 69–75.

McFarlane, W. R. (2004). *Multifamily groups in the treatment of severe psychiatric illness.* New York: Guilford.

Mental Research Institute. (2002). *On the shoulder of giants.* Palo Alto, CA: Author.

Minuchin, S. (1974). *Families and family therapy.* Cambridge, MA: Harvard University Press.

*Minuchin, S., & Fishman, H. C. (1981). *Family therapy techniques.* Cambridge, MA: Harvard University Press.

Minuchin, S., Montalvo, B., Guerney, B. G., Rosman, B., & Schumer, F. (1967). *Families of the slums: An exploration of their structure and treatment.* New York: Basic Books.

Minuchin, S., & Nichols, M. P. (1993). *Family healing: Tales of hope and renewal from family therapy.* New York: Free Press.

Minuchin, S., Nichols, M. P., & Lee, W. Y. (2007). *Assessing families and couples: From symptom to system.* Boston: Allyn and Bacon.

*Nardone, G., & Watzlawick, P. (1993). *The art of change: Strategic therapy and hypnotherapy without trance.* San Francisco: Jossey-Bass.

Satir, V. (1972). *Peoplemaking.* Palo Alto, CA: Science and Behavior Books.

Satir, V. (1983). *Conjoint family therapy* (3rd rev. ed.). Palo Alto, CA: Science and Behavior Books.

Satir, V. (1988). *The new peoplemaking.* Palo Alto, CA: Science and Behavior Books.

Satir, V., Banmen, J., Gerber, J., & Gomori, M. (1991). *The Satir model: Family therapy and beyond.* Palo Alto, CA: Science and Behavior Books.

Segal, L. (1991). Brief therapy: The MRI approach. In A. A. Gurman & D. P. Knishern (Eds.), *Handbook of family therapy* (pp. 171–199). New York: Brunner/Mazel.

Selvini Palazzoli, M. (Ed.). (1988). *The work of Mara Selvini Palazzoli.* New York: Jason Aronson.

*Selvini Palazzoli, M., Boscolo, L., Cecchin, G., & Prata, G. (1980). Hypothesizing-circularity-neutrality: Three guidelines for the conductor of the session. *Family Process, 19*(1), 3–12.

Selvini Palazzoli, M., Cecchin, G., Prata, G., & Boscolo, L. (1978). *Paradox and counterparadox: A new model in the therapy of the family in schizophrenic transaction.* New York: Jason Aronson.

Sexton, T. (2009). *Functional family therapy: An evidence-based clinical model for working with troubled adolescents and their families.* New York: Routledge.

Sprenkle, D. H. (Ed.). (2002). *Effectiveness research in marriage and family therapy.* Alexandria, VA: American Association for Marriage and Family Therapy.

Sprenkle, D. H. (Ed.). (2011). *Effectiveness research in marriage and family therapy* (2nd ed.). Alexandria, VA: American Association for Marriage and Family Therapy.

Szapocznik, J., Hervis, O. E., & Schwartz, S. (2003). *Brief stategic family therapy for adolescent drug abuse* (NIH Publication No. 03-4751). NIDA Therapy Manuals for Drug Addiction. Rockville, MD: National Institute for Drug Abuse.

Szapocznik, J., & Williams, R. A. (2000). Brief strategic family therapy: Twenty-five years of interplay among theory, research and practice in adolescent behavior problems and drug abuse. *Clinical Child and Family Psychology Review, 3*(2), 117–134.

von Bertalanffy, L. (1968). *General system theory: Foundations, development, applications.* New York: George Braziller.

Walsh, F. (Ed.). (2009). *Spiritual resources in family therapy* (2nd ed.). New York: Guilford.

Watzlawick, P. (1977). *How real is real? Confusion, disinformation, communication.* New York: Random House.

Watzlawick, P. (Ed.). (1984). *The invented reality: How do we know what we believe we know?* New York: Norton.

Watzlawick, P. (1988). *Ultra solutions: How to fail most successfully.* New York: Norton.

Watzlawick, P. (1990). *Munchhausen's pigtail or psychotherapy and "reality" essays and lectures.* New York: Norton.

Watzlawick, P. (1993a). *The language of change: Elements of therapeutic conversation.* New York: Norton.

Watzlawick, P. (1993b). *The situation is hopeless but not serious: The pursuit of unhappiness.* New York: Norton.

Watzlawick, P., Bavelas, J. B., & Jackson, D. D. (1967). *Pragmatics of human communication: A study of interactional patterns, pathologies, and paradoxes.* New York: Norton.

Watzlawick, P., & Weakland, J. H. (1977). *The interactional view: Studies at the Mental Research Institute, Palo Alto, 1965–1974.* New York: Norton.

*Watzlawick, P., Weakland, J., & Fisch, R. (1974). *Change: Principles of problem formation and problem resolution.* New York: Norton.

Weakland, J., & Ray, W. (Eds.). (1995). *Propagations: Thirty years of influence from the Mental Research Institute.* Binghamton, NY: Haworth.

CHAPTER

11

Solution-Based Approaches

One of the most important aspects of SFBT [solution-focused brief therapy] is the general tenor and stance that is taken by the therapist. The overall attitude is positive, respectful, and hopeful. There is a general assumption that people have within them strong resiliencies, and can utilize these to make changes. Further, there is a core belief that most people have the strength, wisdom, and experiences to effect change.

(de Shazer et al., 2007, p. 4)

Lay of the Land

If you have been waiting for an upbeat and eminently practical theory in this book, you may enjoy meeting this optimist group of counselors. The quintessential strength-based approach, solution-based counseling is a positive, future-focused, and active approach that helps clients take small, consistent steps toward enacting their solutions. Broadly speaking, there are three strands of practice, which share more similarities than differences:

- *Solution-focused brief therapy (SFBT)*, developed by Steve de Shazer (1985, 1988, 1994) and Insoo Berg at the Milwaukee Brief Family Therapy Center, emphasizes a future focus with minimal discussion of the presenting problem or the past; interventions target small steps in the direction of the solution.
- *Solution-oriented therapy* (O'Hanlon & Weiner-Davis, 1989) and the related approach *possibility therapy* (O'Hanlon & Beadle, 1999), developed by Bill O'Hanlon and colleagues, share many tenets and practices with SFBT, adding more language-based techniques as well as more interventions that draw from the past and present to identify potential solutions.
- *Solution-focused school counseling* has been widely used in school contexts because of its brief and strengths-based characteristics (Cooley, 2009; Davis & Osborn, 2000; Kelly, Kim, & Franklin, 2008; Metcalf, 2003, 2007; Murphy, 2008; Parsons, 2009; Sklare, 2004). Solution-focused school counselors work with individual students, teachers, staff, and administrators to improve individual student and entire classroom performance and behavior.

Because of the numerous commonalities, I will present brief solution-focused and solution-oriented approaches together in this chapter; special applications for school counseling are presented in a separate section at the end.

Solution-Based Counseling

In a Nutshell: The Least You Need to Know

Solution-based counseling evolved from systemic family counseling (see Chapter 10) and the work of the Mental Research Institute (MRI) as well as Milton Erickson's brief therapy and trance work (de Shazer, 1985, 1988, 1994; O'Hanlon & Weiner-Davis, 1989). Both Steve de Shazer and his wife Insoo Kim Berg collaborated with the colleagues at MRI, who conceptualized interventions around problem formation and problem resolution. In contrast, de Shazer and Berg based their work on solutions, boldly proclaiming that the *solution is not necessarily related to the problem* (de Shazer, 1988). They developed their work around the miracle question, which invites clients to describe what they would notice happening differently (not what would *not* be happening) if the problem were miraculously solved overnight without their knowledge. This concrete, behavioral description of the solution is then used to develop interventions to help clients take small, consistent steps toward change. In addition to the miracle questions, solution-based counselors use exception questions to identify times without the problems and scaling questions to break the solution down into small, easily achievable steps. Rather than being "solution givers," solution-based counselors collaborate with the client to envision potential solutions based on the client's experience and values. If ever the process seems to get stuck, the counselor does not blame the client's lack of effort but instead works with the client to identify more appropriate and viable routes to change. As this approach is goal focused and emphasizes measurable change, it tends to be brief, making it a favorite approach in managed care environments, schools, and other time-limited contexts.

Common Solution-Based Therapy Myths

More so than others, solution-based counselors are haunted by myths and misconceptions about what actually happens in session. So let's straighten these out before we go any further.

Myth:	Solution-based counselors propose solutions to clients (which amounts to advice giving).
Closer to the truth:	Solution-based counselors do not suggest logical solutions to clients (O'Hanlon & Beadle, 1999). Instead, it is primarily the job of the client to identify solutions with the help of the counselor, who identifies *exceptions* to the problem, descriptions of what is already working, and client resources to help the client envision potential solutions. Once a clear, behavioral goal is identified, the counselor works with the client to take small steps in this direction.
Myth:	Solution-based counselors *never* talk about the problem.
Closer to the truth:	Solution-based counselors are not psychic and therefore, like all counselors, must spend some time talking about the problem. However, they spend *less* time talking about the problem than most other counselors, especially SFBT counselors (De Jong & Berg, 2002). Solution-based counselors typically follow the lead of clients in determining how much and how often they need to talk about the problem versus the solution. To add further myth-busting evidence, hallmark techniques, such as *exception questions*, require talking about the problem as part of identifying the solution.
Myth:	Solution-based counselors *never* talk about the past.
Closer to the truth:	Again, solution-based counselors are not psychic and actually have numerous techniques that are grounded in talking about the past. However, when they talk about the past, they focus on the strengths as well as the problem (Bertolino & O'Hanlon, 2002). Talking about the past is one of the most important means of identifying exceptions, strengths, and solutions. The past is talked about in ways that facilitate the enactment of solutions.

Myth: Emotions are not discussed in solution-based counseling.

Closer to the truth: Emotions cannot be avoided in therapy, even by solution-based counselors. However, solution-based counselors do not view emotions as inherently within an individual or consider the expression of emotions curative, as is often assumed in psychodynamic and humanistic approaches (Lipchick, 2002). Instead, emotions are viewed as intimately connected with context, having idiosyncratic meaning, and are used as clues as to what works and where clients want to go.

The Juice: Significant Contributions to the Field

If you remember one thing from this chapter, it should be …

Scaling Questions and the Miracle Scale

If I were challenged to use only one technique to work with clients from start to finish, scaling questions would have to top the list of possibilities, as they are arguably one of the most versatile and comprehensive interventions. Counselors can use scaling questions to (a) assess strengths and solutions, (b) set goals, (c) design homework tasks, (d) measure progress, and (e) manage crises with safety plans (see "Scaling for Safety" in Gehart, 2010). They can be used in the first session and can be reused weekly until the last. Like many modern-day miracle, all-in-one products—such as shampoo-conditioners, moisturizer-sunscreen-foundations, and car wash-and-waxes—this technique is likely to be one of your go-to techniques for years to come.

As the name indicates, *scaling questions* involve asking clients to define their goals and rate their progress toward them using a scale, most often a 10-point scale, but sometimes percentages or shorter, nonnumeric versions are used with children (Bertolino, 2010; de Shazer, 1994; O'Hanlon & Weiner-Davis, 1989; Selekman, 1997). De Shazer et al. (2007) recommend having 0 represent "when you decided to seek help" rather than when things are "at their worst." When scaling 0 to mean "at their worst," this can refer to decades earlier or have different meanings to different people. Instead, scaling from "when you decided to seek help" allows for a clearer system for measuring progress from the beginning to end of counseling; they refer to these as "miracle scales" and use these scales to follow up with the miracle question (see "The Viewing: Case Conceptualization" section). Others use 0 or 1 to represent things at their *worst* (Bertolino, 2010).

Two Approaches to Scaling

Miracle Scale: Measures Progress From Beginning of Counseling

When You Decided to Seek Help   *Miracle Situation*

0----------1---------- 2---------- 3---------- 4---------- 5---------- 6---------- 7---------- 8---------- 9---------- 10

Worst-to-Solution Scale: Measures Progress in General

Things at Their Worst   *Solution*

0----------1---------- 2---------- 3---------- 4---------- 5---------- 6---------- 7---------- 8---------- 9---------- 10

Scaling questions can be used early in the counseling process to help identify meaningful long-term goals, much the way the miracle question is used (see the following box):

Scaling Question for Long-Term Goal Setting
(assessing solutions and setting goals)

If you were to put your situation on a scale from 1 to 10 with 0 being where you were when you decided to seek help (or at their worst) and 10 being where you'd like them to be, can you describe to me what you would be doing (*not* what you would *not* be doing) if things were at a 10? Where are you today? What was happening, and what were you doing at a 0?

As the client responds, the counselor listens for clear, specific descriptions of what life would be like at a 10, helping the client to paint a clear, behavioral picture: what is the client doing, what are others doing, and how does the day go? Once a clear description of the 10 scenario is developed, the counselor can then ask where things are today and obtain a behavioral description of the current situation. A concrete description of when things were at the point the client decided to seek help or at their worst (0 or 1) can also be useful assessment information. Once the big picture is assessed, the same scale can be used to identify *what works*.

Scaling Question for Assessing What Works

If 0 is where you were when you decided to seek help and 10 is where you would be if the problem you came here for was resolved, where are you today? [If above a 0] What are you doing or what is happening that tells us you are at a 3 and not 0? How did you get from a 0 to here?

This next set of questions helps identify what works, exceptions, and potential solutions that need to be assessed before more specific interventions can be developed. If the client gets stuck answering any of these questions, it can be helpful to ask what significant others might rate them on the scale. After exploring where a client is this week, where he or she was when deciding to seek counseling, and where he or she would like to be, it is time to use scaling to identify the next step.

Scaling Question for Designing Week-to-Week Interventions and Tasks

On a scale from 0 to 10 with 10 being your desired goal, where are you this week? [Client responds and rates: e.g., 3]. If you are at a 3 this week, what things would need to be different in your life for you to come in and say you were at a 4, one step higher (or *half* a step higher if client tends toward pessimism or needs to keep goal smaller)?

This is not an easy question to answer. Often clients rush ahead and describe an 8, 9, or 10 when the next step is really a 4. In such cases, the counselor needs to help clients identify more realistic expectations. In other cases, clients say, "I don't know"; when this happens, counselors need to practice patience, silence, and encouragement to help clients identify ministeps toward their goal, which is a critical part of the process. The client—not the counselor—is the only person who can answer this question in any meaningful way. Remember, the counselor is *not* a solution giver.

Once a clear description of the next step is developed, this information is used to identify specific, small tasks the client can take during the next week to move one step higher on the scale. It generally takes an entire session to fully flesh out concrete steps that are (a) realistic and meaningful and (b) something that the client is motivated to try. For the intervention to work, the counselor and client need to develop microsteps that take into account the client's motivation, willingness, schedule, variations in the schedule, reactions of others, and so on. The counselor asks questions to identify and listens for potential barriers and pitfalls as well as helpful resources, working with the client to find ways to negotiate these. Together, the clients and counselors work to develop specific homework tasks that clients believe will help move them toward their goals.

For example, if the client's initial response is that "At a 4, I would feel less anxious," the counselor needs to ask follow-up questions, such as "How would you know you were less anxious?" "What would you be doing differently?" "How would your days be different?" "What changes would other people notice in you?" These questions help the client identify one or two specific, small steps to be taken over the week, such as "invite a friend over," "go to the mall alone," "watch a funny movie," and so on. The steps need to be small enough that the client thinks the steps are easily attainable, especially early in the process.

> ### Scaling Question for Measuring Progress
> Last week you said you were at a 3. Where would you say you are this week and why? [If things got better] What did *you do* that helped move you up the scale? [If things stayed the same or got worse] What happened that kept things the same (or made them worse)?

The counselor follows up the next week to see if the homework tasks helped move clients closer to their goals. If so, they explore what helped and how to do more of it. If clients don't report progress or report that things got worse (with or without doing the homework), the counselor does not despair but simply goes back to more carefully assess whether (a) the solution has been meaningfully assessed and concretely identified and (b) whether the task was small enough, concrete enough, and motivating enough. This scale can be used to measure progress from the beginning to the end of the counseling process. In the case study at the end of this chapter, scaling questions are used throughout treatment to help Marcella cope with the death of the brother who abused her and resurfacing memories of the abuse; in the early stages, scaling questions are used to help manage cutting (Selekman, 2006) and in the later phases to help her take action to resolve issues related to the abuse.

Rumor Has It: The People and Their Stories
Behind-the-Scenes Inspiration:
Milton Erickson A physician and psychiatrist, Milton Erickson was a master clinician, well known for his brief, rapid, and creative interventions whose work greatly influenced the solution-based work of Steve de Shazer and Bill O'Hanlon (Erickson & Keeney, 2006; Haley, 1993; O'Hanlon & Martin, 1992). Erickson did not follow a specific theory but instead relied on keen observation while listening with an open mind to each patient's unique story. Erickson frequently employed *light trance* to evoke patient strengths and latent abilities (Haley, 1993; O'Hanlon & Martin, 1992). At a time when most forms of psychotherapy focused on the past, Erickson directed his clients to focus on the present and future, often *envisioning future times without the problem*, a frequent goal of solution-based techniques. Although others have meticulously studied his work, there has been no consensus or singular definition of Ericksonian therapy. The influence of his trance work is clearly evident in intervention such as the *miracle question* and *crystal ball technique*, which rely on a *pseudo-orientation to time* as well as the *implicit assumption* that change *will* occur.

Solution-Focused Brief Therapy: Milwaukee Brief Family Therapy Center
Steve de Shazer Steve de Shazer was a theorist, clinician, philosopher, and prolific writer (de Shazer, 1985, 1988, 1994; de Shazer et al., 2007), laying much of the philosophical and theoretical foundations for the solution-focused approach. After his early work at MRI with Jay Haley, Paul Watzlawick, John Weakland, and Virginia Satir, the late Steve de Shazer developed with his wife Insoo Kim Berg solution-focused brief therapy. His early work was influenced by the trance work of Milton Erickson (de Shazer, 1985, 1988) and his later work by the Ludwig Wittegenstein's philosophy of language, who viewed language as inextricably woven into the fabric of life (de Shazer et al., 2007). With Insoo Kim Berg, he founded the Milwaukee Brief Family Therapy Center and the Solution-Focused Brief Therapy Association, where they taught until their deaths in 2005 (Steve) and 2007 (Insoo). He is remembered thusly: "An iconoclast and creative genius known for his minimalist philosophy and view of the process of change as an inevitable and dynamic part of everyday life, he was known for reversing the traditional psychotherapy interview process by asking clients to describe a detailed resolution of the problem that brought them into therapy, shifting the focus of treatment from problems to solutions" (Trepper, Dolan, McCollum, & Nelson, 2006, p. 133).

Insoo Kim Berg Warm and exuberant, the late Insoo Kim Berg was an energetic developer and leading practitioner of SFBT, cofounding the Milwaukee Brief Family Therapy

Center and the Solution-Focused Therapy Association with her husband, Steve de Shazer (Dolan, 2007). She was an outstanding clinician who furthered the development of SFBT, developing solution-focused approaches to working with drinking issues (Berg & Miller, 1992), substance abuse (Berg & Reuss, 2007), family-based services (Berg, 1994), child protective services (Berg & Kelly, 2000), children (Berg & Steiner, 2003), and personal coaching (Berg & Szabo, 2005).

Scott Miller, Barry Duncan, and Mark Hubble   Originally trained in a brief solution-focused therapy approach, Scott Miller, Barry Duncan, and Mark Hubble have been strong proponents of the *common factors* movement (see Chapter 2; Miller, Duncan, & Hubble, 1997) and client-centered, outcome-informed therapy. Their recent works emphasize using client feedback to improve outcomes and activate common factors in everyday practice.

Yvonne Dolan   Yvonne Dolan studied and worked with de Shazer and Berg at the Milwaukee Brief Family Therapy Center, specializing in sexual abuse and trauma treatment (Dolan, 1991, 2000). Her work represents one of the first hopeful strength-based approaches to working with sexual abuse.

Solution-Oriented Therapy

Bill O'Hanlon   A former student of Milton Erickson, Bill O'Hanlon is an energetic and popular leader in solution-oriented, strength-based counseling, including solution-oriented therapy and possibility therapy (O'Hanlon & Beadle, 1999; O'Hanlon & Weiner-Davis, 1989). A prolific and highly accessible writer and speaker, O'Hanlon's solution-oriented approach emphasizes the significance of language, using subtle shifts in language to spark change. His work aims to transform client *viewing* as well as *doing* of the problem while attending to broader *contextual* issues that impact the client's situation (Bertolino & O'Hanlon, 2002). He has written extensively on numerous topics, including solution-oriented couples therapy (Hudson & O'Hanlon, 1991), solution-oriented approaches to treating sexual abuse (O'Hanlon & Bertolino, 2002), solution-oriented hypnosis (O'Hanlon & Martin, 1992), solution-oriented therapy with children and teens (Bertolino & O'Hanlon, 1998), and spirituality in therapy (O'Hanlon, 2006), as well as books for clients and popular audiences (O'Hanlon, 2000, 2005, 2006).

Michelle Weiner-Davis   Michelle Weiner-Davis developed a highly successful solution-oriented approach to working with divorce that she calls *divorce busting* (Weiner-Davis, 1992). She uses a brief, solution-oriented self-help approach to help couples wanting to prevent divorce.

Solution-Focused Approaches in Schools

Michael Kelly, Johnny Kim, and Cynthia Franklin   Michael Kelly, Johnny Kim, and Cynthia Franklin (Kelly et al., 2008) use solution-focused brief therapy in school contexts and have developed a classroom consulting method, "Working on What Works," to improve classroom culture.

Linda Metcalf   Linda Metcalf applies solution-focused counseling in school contexts, including solution-focused school counseling (Metcalf, 2008), solution-focused children's groups (Metcalf, 2007), solution-focused parenting (Metcalf, 1998), and solution-focused teaching (Metcalf, 2003).

John Murphy   A former high school teacher with training as a school psychologist, John Murphy (2008) trained with Barry Duncan and eventually developed his approach for using solution-focused therapy ideas in school contexts.

Big Picture: Overview of Counseling Process

Solution Building

The process of solution-based counseling is described as *solution building* rather than problem solving, highlighting that the problem is not necessarily related to the solution

(De Jong & Berg, 2002). By design, the solution-building process is brief and forward focused. "Brief" can mean as few as 1 to 10 sessions or a year or more, depending on the severity of the problem, client resources, and numerous other factors (O'Hanlon & Weiner-Davis, 1989). The process focuses on identifying where the client wants to go (the solution) rather than trying to analyze and troubleshoot the problem. For example, rather than identify the cause of depression, the focus is on identifying what life would look like without depression and start taking steps to move in that direction.

After a relatively brief assessment phase, solution-based counselors quickly move to helping clients take *small action steps* between sessions to help clients move toward their identified solutions. These steps are practical and small enough to be achievable between sessions, such as call a friend to go to lunch, exercise three days a week, or go on a date night with a partner. Thus, most weeks, clients leave with some sort of homework assignment or task that involves taking action toward the identified solutions. An important part of the counselor's role is to help motivate the client to take these action steps, and this requires working closely with the client to develop meaningful goals and tasks. A less obvious part of this process is that in session counselors ask questions and offer observations that shift *how* clients think about their situation so that they move from a problem focus to a perspective that emphasizes resources, strengths, abilities, possibilities, and the future. In general, counselors maintain an upbeat, hopeful attitude in session. In the closing phase of the counseling process, counselors work with clients to identify strategies for managing future problems using the newly acquired resources and strategies.

Making Connection: The Counseling Relationship
Optimism and Hope

Signature characteristics, optimism and hope are immediately and undeniably palpable in solution-based counseling (Miller, Duncan, & Hubble, 1996; Miller et al., 1997). Solution-based counselors assume that change is inevitable and that improvement—in some form—is always possible, and they clearly communicate this verbally and nonverbally to clients (O'Hanlon & Weiner-Davis, 1989). Their optimism and hope do not stem from naïveté but rather is grounded in their ontology and epistemology: their theory of what it means to be human and how people learn. Because change is always happening—moods, relationships, emotions, and behaviors are in constant flux—*change is inevitable* (Walter & Peller, 1992). They have hope that the change will be positive because the client is in therapy to make an improvement and because over 90% of clients report positive outcomes in psychotherapy (Miller et al., 1997). Hope is cultivated early in therapy to develop motivation and momentum (Bertolino & O'Hanlon, 2002).

Carl Rogers With a Twist: Channeling Language

O'Hanlon and Beadle (1999) describe how they build counseling relationships by reflecting feelings, similar to Carl Rogers but with a twist. The solution-oriented twist is that their reflections *delimit* the difficult feeling, behavior, or thought by reflecting on a time, context, or relational limit. Such reflections generally use one or more of three strategies for delimiting the problem:

1. *Past tense:* Rather than describe a person's mood as a chronic state or characteristic, reflect statements back to clients in the *past tense* (e.g., "You were feeling down *yesterday*").
2. *Partial:* Rather than using global descriptions of people, situations, or things, describe these as *partial* or *periodic* (e.g., "*A part of you* thinks things will never get better").
3. *Perception:* When a client makes an unhelpful global truth statement (e.g., "Life will never get better"), reflect back the sentiment as a *perception* (e.g., "Right now *it seems to you* that things will never get better").

For example, a client-centered reflection with a client who is telling a story about how her boyfriend got angry at her for "no reason" would be something like "You aren't feeling understood" (present-focused statement about client's unexpressed emotion), whereas the solution-focused twist to delimit would be "you were not feeling understood *by your boyfriend last Saturday.*" The solution-oriented twist emphasizes the limited time and relational context in order to (a) define the problem in more solvable ways and (b) engender hope. O'Hanlon and Beadle (1999) refer to this process as "channeling language." By channeling a client's language while listening to the client's story, both the client and the counselor more easily transition to identifying desired outcomes. Channeling language is actually a very difficult skill to develop because it requires a paradigm shift in how the counselor listens for problems and strengths, but with practice it becomes habit.

Beginner's Mind

O'Hanlon and Weiner-Davis (1989) use *beginner's mind* when forming a relationship, referring to the classic Zen saying, "In the beginner's mind there are many possibilities; in the expert's mind there are few" (p. 8). Assuming a position of beginner's mind involves listening to each client's story as if you are listening for the first time, not filling in blanks with personal or professional knowledge. Most counselors underestimate how hard this is to do. When a client starts talking about "feeling depressed," most clinicians believe they have useful diagnostic information, unthinkingly assuming that clients have read diagnostic manuals and use the term as a professional would. In contrast, solution-oriented counselors bring a beginner's mind to the conversation and are curious about *how this person experiences his or her unique depression.* If you get in the habit of asking, you will find that every depression is surprisingly "one of a kind." Thus, solution-oriented counselors make no assumptions when they are listening, asking to hear more about clients' unique experiences and understandings.

Echoing Client's Key Words

Solution-based counselors carefully attend to *client word choice* and echo their key words whenever possible (De Jong & Berg, 2002). For example, rather than teaching clients to use psychiatric terms such as "depression" or "hallucinations" to describe their experience, the counselor prefers to use the client's own language, such as "feeling blue" or "schizos." Using client language often makes the problem more "solvable" and engenders greater hope. For many, "ending the blahs" or "getting back to my old self" is a more attainable goal than treating a psychiatrically defined problem of "296.22 Major Depressive Disorder, Single Episode, Moderate."

The Viewing: Case Conceptualization

Introduction to Solution-Based Case Conceptualization

Unlike most forms of counseling, solution-based counseling primarily involves conceptualizing *where to go from here* (i.e., the solution) rather than where the client has been (i.e., the problem). A basic tenet of solution-based counseling is that *the solution is not necessarily related to the problem,* and thus the solution—where to go—is the focus of assessment (de Shazer et al., 2007). This does not mean that the past is ignored; instead, it is discussed only as long as is necessary to better understand the potential solution. Outside of exceptions (see "Exceptions, Previous Solutions, and 'What Works'"), the past is not the focus of the assessment and case conceptualization process.

The Miracle and Other Solution-Generating Questions

The original solution-generating question, the *miracle question* serves to both (a) conceptualize and assess and (b) set goals in solution-based counseling. Legend (and good authority) has it that Insoo Kim Berg developed the miracle question based on a client's desperate and exasperated claim to Insoo that "maybe only a miracle will help." So, Insoo, using the clients' language and worldview, played with the idea and had clients describe how life would be if there were a miracle (de Shazer, 1988; de Shazer et al., 2007). The intervention was so successful that it was crafted into a hallmark intervention that is frequently used early in treatment to identify the focus of treatment. Since then, several variations have been developed, including the crystal ball technique (de Shazer, 1985), magic wand questions (Selekman, 1997), and the time machine

(Bertolino & O'Hanlon, 2002). When successfully delivered, these questions help clients envision a future without the problem, generating hope, motivation, and goals.

- *Miracle question:* Imagine that you go home tonight, and during the middle of the night a miracle happens: all the problems you came here to resolve are miraculously resolved. However, when you wake up, you have no idea a miracle has occurred. What are some of the first things you would notice that would be different? How would you know that the problems that brought you here were resolved?

- *Crystal ball question:* Imagine I had a crystal ball that allowed us to look into the future to a time when the problems you came here for are already resolved. I hold it up to you, and you look in. What do you see?

- *Magic wand question:* Imagine we had a magic wand (or imagine that this magic wand I have here actually works), and you could wave it and all of the problems you came here for are miraculously resolved. What would be different?

- *Time machine:* Imagine I had a time machine that could propel you into the future to the point in time when the problems you came to see me for are totally resolved. Imagine you stepped in: Where do you end up? Who is with you? What is happening? How is your life different? How did your problems go away?

Successfully delivering one of these solution-generating questions is far more difficult than it appears. As you can imagine, if done poorly, these hit the floor like a lead balloon. To avoid such humiliation, de Shazer et al. (2007, pp. 42–43) describe seven steps for successfully delivering the miracle question:

1. *Obtain client agreement (wait for nod #1):* The first and most critical step is to prepare clients by changing their state of mind so that they are willing to engage in an atypical conversation. By asking, "Is it okay if I ask you a strange question?" or "Would you be willing to play along if I ask a somewhat odd question?," the counselor signals clients to change their frame of mind so that they are better able to enter a more fanciful, creative conversation. The counselor waits for the client to say "yes" or nod in agreement.

2. *Custom tailor initial setup (wait for nod #2):* After the client agrees to the odd question, begin delivering the question but customize it to include numerous little details from the client's everyday life to get him or her fully engaged in the story and enable him or her to better visualize the miracle. For example, you might say, "Let's imagine that after we are done talking here, you get in your car and drive home; you make dinner for the family like you usually do; you clean up dishes like you usually do; and check the kids' homework like you usually do." *Continue until the client starts to nod.*

3. *Setup for miracle (wait for nod #3):* Once the client nods, continue with, "Then you get the kids to bed, maybe do some minor chores or watch television, and then you finally get to bed and fall asleep." Up to this point, you have only asked the client to imagine a regular day, but this is very important. The client needs to mentally leave the therapy office and vividly imagine being at home where the miracle is to occur. *Wait for the confirmatory nod or "yea" before moving on to the miracle.*

4. *Introduce the miracle (wait for pause):* "Then, during the night … while you are sleeping … a miracle happens." Pause. Pause and wait for a reaction: a smile, lifted eyebrow, laugh, or questioning look. Insoo says she often looks intently at the client and smiles, but Steve warns that if pause for too long, the client is likely to respond with, "I don't believe in miracles"; so keep moving.

5. *Specifically and clearly define the terms of the miracle:* "And it's not just any miracle. This miracle makes the *problems that brought you here* today disappear … just like that" (snapping your fingers at this point is optional but adds flair). The most common mistakes counselors make with the miracle question is to leave out the "problems that brought you here" part of the question. Without this limit on the

miracle, clients will spend a lot of time exploring vague and unrelated goals, and the counselor will have to do a lot of repair work by later asking follow-up questions to get this information.

6. *Add the mystery (nod #4, optional)*: "But since the miracle happens while you are asleep, you won't know it has happened." If delivered well, most clients nod at this point, stare **off in**to space, and begin to behave as if they were thinking about the proposition.

7. *Ask what is different*: "So, you wake up the morning after the miracle happens during the night. All the problems that brought you here are gone—poof—just like that. What is the very first thing you notice after you wake up? What are the little changes you start to notice that tell you the problem is gone?" At this point, many clients take a moment to think about their answer, often becoming quiet and still as their breath slows. The counselor needs to quietly and patiently *wait* for the response.

Once the client begins to describe what is different, the counselor helps focus the answer by asking about behavioral changes in the client and others. In typical solution-focused style, the counselor is interested not in what the client is *not* doing but instead in what the client *is doing*. For example, if the client says, "I will not be depressed any more," the counselor responds with, "What will you be doing instead?" Once the client identifies one new behavior, the counselor asks for more: "What else would be different?" The counselor continues until several (three or more) concrete miracle behaviors are identified that can be useful for developing goals and clear direction for change. In the case study at the end of this chapter, the counselor uses the miracle question with Marcella to identify what "getting over" sexual abuse will look like for her, which included having a relationship with her parents and pursing her dream to become a pediatrician.

Exceptions, Previous Solutions, and "What Works"

Successful solution-based counseling requires developing an uncanny, sleuthlike ability to detect even the minutest exceptions to problems (this is generally an endearing quality in personal relations by the way, so it is worth cultivating). Solution-based counselors assess for *exceptions*, *previous* (helpful) *solutions*, and examples of *what works* in three different ways: (a) as part of the follow-up to the miracle question, (b) listening for spontaneous descriptions of exceptions, and (c) directly asking about exceptions (de Shazer, 1985, 1988; de Shazer et al., 2007; O'Hanlon & Weiner-Davis, 1989). First, if the miracle or other solution-generating question has been used, exceptions can be identified by asking, "What elements of the miracle are happening now, even just a little?" This prompt often results in a heartening description for both client and counselor of what elements of the miracle are already there; most are thrilled to think that half (or 25%) of the work is already done. Alternatively, the finely tuned solution-focused ear attends to clients' spontaneously offered descriptions of exceptions and examples of what works: "Except for when I am on my boat, I am always depressed" or "The only time I don't worry is when I am playing with my kids" or "Suzy is the only one who cares about me." These seemingly minor exceptions provide clues as to what works and therefore what clients need to do more frequently. Additionally, solution-based counselors directly ask about exceptions to gather more information about what works:

Examples of Exception Questions

- Are there any times when the problem is less likely to occur or be less severe?
- Can you think of a time when you expected the problem to occur but didn't?
- Are there any people who seem to make things easier?
- Are there places or times when the problem is not as bad?

The vast majority of clients will be able to identify exceptions with questions such as these: note that the assumption underlying most of these questions is that the problem varies in *intensity*; the times when the problem is *less severe* is considered a type of exception and generally provides clues as to what works (de Shazer, 1985; O'Hanlon & Weiner-Davis, 1989). Especially true with diagnoses such as depression that are experienced most of the time most days, counselors need to focus on identifying the varying of intensity rather than the absence of the symptom to identify exceptions.

Pre-session Change

Solution-based counselors pay careful attention to *pre-session change*: change that occurs *after* the initial phone call to make an appointment and *before* the first session (de Shazer et al., 2007). Counselors can assess this by asking, "Since we spoke on the phone (or you made the appointment), what changes have you noticed that have happened or started to happen?" In early research surveys, Weiner-Davis, de Shazer, and Gingerich (1987) reported that the majority of clients reported *some* positive changes *before* the first changes, leading them to hypothesize that simply the anticipation of change and making a commitment to change (i.e., an appointment with a professional) mobilizes clients resources and begins the change process. This question is asked *very early* in the first session to assess for what works, strengths, and resources.

Assessing Client Strengths

Assessing client strengths is one of the key areas of assessment in solution-based counseling (Bertolino & O'Hanlon, 2002; De Jong & Berg, 2002; O'Hanlon & Weiner-Davis, 1989). Strengths include resources in a person's life, personally, relationally, financially, socially, or spiritually and may include family support, positive relationships, and religious faith. Most counselors *underestimate* the difficulty of identifying strengths. In fact, identifying client strengths is often *harder* than diagnosing pathology because clients come in with a long list of problems they want fixed and are thus prepared to discuss pathology. Surprisingly, many clients, especially those with depressive or anxious tendencies (the majority of outpatient cases), have great difficulty identifying areas without problems in their lives. Similarly, many couples who have been distressed and arguing for long periods of time have difficulty identifying positive characteristics in their partners, happy times in the marriage, and, in the most desperate of cases, the reasons they got together in the first place. Therefore, counselors often have to ask more subtle questions and attend to vague clues in order to assess strengths well.

Solution-based counselors assess strengths in two ways: (a) by directly asking about strengths, hobbies, and areas of life that are going well and (b) by listening carefully for *exceptions* to problems and for areas of unnoticed strength (Bertolino & O'Hanlon, 2002; De Jong & Berg, 2002). Furthermore, I have found that any strength in one context has the potential to be a liability in another context and that the inverse is also true: any weakness in one area is generally a *strength* in another area (see the section "Assessment of Strengths and Diversity" in Chapter 15). Therefore, if a client has difficulty identifying strengths and more readily discusses weaknesses and problems, a fine-tuned solution-focused ear will be able to identify potential areas in which the weakness is a strength. For example, a person who is critical, anxious, and/or negative in a relational context typically excels at detailed or meticulous work and tasks. This insight can be useful in identifying ways for clients to move toward their goals.

Solution-based counselors have been on the vanguard of a larger movement within mental health that emphasizes identifying and utilizing client strengths to promote better clinical outcomes (Bertolino & O'Hanlon, 2002). Increasingly, county mental health and insurance companies are requiring assessment of strengths as part of initial intake assessments. The key to successfully assessing strengths is the unshakable belief that *all* clients have significant and meaningful strengths no matter how dire and severe their situations appear in the moment. It is helpful for counselors to remember that we see people typically in their worst moments; therefore, even if we are not seeing strengths in the moment, they are undoubtedly there. Solution-based counselors maintain that all people have strengths and resources and make it their job to help identify and utilize them toward achieving client goals.

Client Motivation: Visitor, Complainant, and Customers

Steve de Shazer (1988) assessed client motivation for change using three categories: visitors, complainant, and customers. These categories are used to understand the type of *relationship* the counselor has with the client rather than labeling the client (De Jong & Berg, 2002):

- *Visitor-type relationship:* In this relationship, the client does not have a complaint, but generally others have a complaint against him or her. These clients are typically brought to therapy by an outside other, such as courts, parents, or spouse. They are often most motivated to get the third party "off their back"; thus, the counselor should honor this and quickly identify the specific goals that would achieve this end, making class to probation officers and social workers as necessary.
- *Complainant-type relationship:* In this type of relationship, the client identifies a problem but expects the counselor or some other person to be the primary source of change. Rather than try to convince these clients to change their perspectives, the solution-focused counselor works with these clients to identify small ways they can positively affect the situation.
- *Customer-type relationships:* In this type of relationship, the client and counselor jointly define a problem and solution picture, and the client is motivated to take action toward the solution.

	Visitor Type	Complainant Type	Customers Type
Motivation	Low	Moderate to high	High
Source of problem or solution	Outside other (spouse, parent, court) thinks client has a problem.	Problem generally related to outside cause or person; expect counselor or another to be source of solution.	Self as part of problem and active agent in solution.
View of who needs to change	Outside other needs to see there is no problem.	Outside other needs to change and/or fix it.	Self needs to take action to fix things.
Building therapeutic alliance	Identify areas where client sees problem willing to work on to make them a customer for change.	Honoring client's view of the situation while identifying specific instances where client can make a difference.	Join with client by complimenting readiness for change.
Focus of interventions	Building alliance; understanding client perspective; framing outside request for change as the problem.	Observation-oriented tasks (e.g., identifying exceptions over week; Selekman, 1997, 2010).	Reframing; identifying what does not work; action-oriented tasks.
Readiness for action	Not ready for making active changes in life until client believes there is a problem and is motivated for change.	Not ready for action until open to the idea that their actions can make a difference.	Ready to take action to make changes.

Assessing clients' motivation is helpful in knowing how to build relationships with the client as well as how to proceed. Many new counselors assume that all clients are customers for change: ready to take action to improve their situation simply because they showed up for a therapy session. However, this is often not the case. People come to therapy with mixed emotions and varying levels of motivation. Generally, most mandated clients are "visitors," and counselors need to find a way to connect with their agenda while still working with the referring party's agenda. This same dynamic is often the case with children, teens, and even one-half of a couple. In complainant relationships, counselors need to either find ways that the client can contribute to making a difference or help shift the viewing of the problem to increase client willingness to take action. In the case study at the end of this chapter, Marcella begins as a complainant, feeling as though the problem was her brother's death and sexual abuse; however, she is quickly able to identify changes she wants and can make, making her a customer for change.

Details, Details, Juicy Details

Throughout the assessment and case conceptualization process, solution-focused counselors are continually asking about the *details*: who, what, where, why, and when. Effective "solution building requires getting details, details, and more details" (De Jong & Berg, 2002, p. 24). By learning more about when symptoms are better or worse, who is around when things are better or worse, and what happens step-by-step when things get a little better, counselors become well provisioned for helping to build solutions. For example, when a client reports that the depressed feelings are reduce at work or when busy (very common), the counselor asks about the details of what happens in these contexts to identify potential elements of solutions, such as being around people or away from people, having a purpose, being outside, avoiding thinking about another problem, and so on.

Targeting Change: Goal Setting

Goal Language: Positive and Concrete

Solution-based counselors state their goals in positive, observable terms (De Jong & Berg, 2002). Positive goal descriptions emphasize what the client is *going to be doing* rather than focusing symptom reduction, which is typical in pathology-focused counseling approaches. Observable descriptions include clear, specific behavioral indicators of the desired change.

Positive, Observable Goal Example	Negative (Symptom Reducing), Nonobservable Goal Examples
Increase periods of engaging in hobbies and enjoyable activities	Reduce depression
Increase sense of confidence and calm in social situations	Reduce panic attacks
Increase frequency of choosing healthy foods and healthy portions	Reduce binging and purging

You may have noticed that simply reading the left column generates more hope and provides greater direction for clinical intervention than the right column. Positive, observable goals provide a constant reminder to the counselor and client of the goal and reinforce a solution-focused and solution-oriented perspective. Many solution-based techniques, such as scaling questions (see "Scaling Questions"), invite the client to measure goal progress weekly; thus, carefully crafted goal language is particularly critical to success in solution-based counseling.

Additional qualities of solution-based goals include the following (Bertolino & O'Hanlon, 2002; De Jong & Berg, 2002):

- *Meaningful to client:* Goals must be *personally* important to the client, not just a "good idea."
- *Interactional:* Rather than reflect a general feeling (e.g., "feeling better"), the goals should describe how interactions with others will change.
- *Situational:* Rather than global terms, goals are stated in situational terms (e.g., improved mood at work).
- *Small steps:* Goals should be short term and with identifiable small steps.
- *Clear role for client:* Goals should identify a clear role for the client rather than for others.
- *Realistic:* Goals need to be realistic for this client at this time.
- *Legal and ethical:* Goals should be legal and adhere to client, counselor, and professional ethics.

One Thing Different

In the beginning, goals should focus on doing one small thing differently rather than target broad, lofty goals (e.g., call a friend this week rather than visit with someone everyday; de Shazer, 1985, 1988; O'Hanlon, 2000; O'Hanlon & Weiner-Davis, 1989). Similarly, a goal such as "get up and exercise one day this week" rather than every day this week is more likely to generate change and motivation for further action. In most cases, making this *one small change* starts a cascade of change events that are inspired from client's *own* motivation rather than the prescription of the counselor (or even cocreated solution with the counselor). Ideas generated in therapy are not viewed as the "best," "only," or "correct" solution but rather as activities that will spark clients to identify what works for them.

The Doing: Interventions
Solution-Focused Tenants for Intervention

De Shazer et al. (2007, p. 2) identify basic tenets of solution-focused intervention that counselors can use to guide their work:

1. *If it isn't broken, don't fix it:* Don't use therapeutic theory to determine areas of intervention.
2. *If it works, do more of it:* Amplify and build on things that are currently working.
3. *If it's not working, do something different:* Even if it's a good idea, if it's not working, find another solution.
4. *Small steps can lead to big changes:* Begin with small doable changes; these typically happen and quickly lead to more change.
5. *The solution is not necessarily related to the problem:* Focus on moving forward, not understanding why there is a problem.
6. *The language for solution development is different from that needed to describe a problem:* Problem talk is negative and past focused; solution talk is hopeful, positive, and future focused.
7. *No problem happens all the time; there are always exceptions that can be utilized:* Even the smallest exception is useful for identifying potential solutions.
8. *The future is both created and negotiable:* Clients have a significant role in designing their future.

Scaling and Miracle Questions

Described in "The Juice", scaling and miracle questions are the bread-and-butter techniques for week-to-week interventions. They can be used to (a) assess whether the last week's tasks were helpful, (b) identify potential areas for change, and (c) develop specific homework tasks for the following week.

Formula First Session Task

As the name implies, the *formula first session task* (de Shazer, 1985) is typically used in the first session with all clients, regardless of issue, to increase client hope in the therapy process and motivation for change.

> *Formula First Session Task:* "Between now and the next time we meet, we [I] would like you to observe, so that you can describe to us [me] next time, what happens in your [pick one: family, life, marriage, relationship] that you want to continue to have happen" (de Shazer, 1985, p. 137).
>
> *Formula First Session Task (Paraphrased with introduction):* "As we are starting therapy, many things are going to change. However, I am sure that there are many things in your life and relationships that you do *not* want to have change. Over the next week, I want you to generate a list of the things in your life and relationships that you *do not* want to have changed by therapy. Notice small things as well as big things that are working right now."

This directive stimulates clients to notice what is working and to identify their strengths and resources and helps generate hope and agency.

Presuppositional Questions and Assuming Future Solution

Presuppositional questions and talk that assume future change help clients envision a future without the problem, generating hope and motivation (O'Hanlon & Beadle, 1999; O'Hanlon & Weiner-Davis, 1989). Solution-focused counselors assume change based on the observation that all things change: a client's situation *cannot not* change. Knowing that change is inevitable and that most clients benefit from therapy, counselors can be confident when they ask presuppositional questions such as the following:

- What will you be doing differently once we resolve these issues?
- Do you think there are other concerns you will want to address once we resolve these issues?
- When the problem is resolved, what is one of the first things you will do to celebrate?

Questions such as these can be very helpful in cases where clients feel hopeless or have difficulty imagining a future without the problem.

Videotalk

Videotalk is a technique that distinguishes between two basic levels of experience: (a) *facts* and (b) *stories and experience* (Hudson & O'Hanlon, 1991). The *facts* are a behavioral description of what was done and said—what would be recorded on videotape (hence the name). The *story* is the interpretation and meaning that a person associates with the behaviors and words, while the *experience* is a person's internal thoughts and feelings. The overarching goal of videotalk is to separate out facts (what behavioral happened) from interpretation (stories and subjective experience in response to what happened). By separating what happened to how clients interpret the events, counselors and clients can closely examine how meanings were made and responses created, allowing new understandings and responses.

> ### Anatomy of Videotalk: Facts Versus Interpretation
>
> - *Facts:* What is captured by video camera; *behavioral description* of what was said and done.
>
> *Examples:*
>
> "If I had a video camera, what would I see you do or say when you are feeling depressed?"

(*continued*)

> "If I had a video camera, what would I see you do or hear you say the day of your miracle?"
>
> - *Interpretations*: Description of the *stories* (interpretations) and subjective *experiences* (what was thought and felt)
>
> *Examples*:
>
> "When you are laying in bed not wanting to get up, what are you thinking and feeling? What type of meaning do you make of this situation and who you are because of it?"
>
> "When you are getting up before the alarm rings and going for a run, what are you thinking and feeling? What type of meanings are you making about your self and your choice to get up and run before the alarm goes off? How do you feel about yourself?"

When a client reports vague feelings or goals, counselors can help them bring greater clarity to and descriptions of the problem and solution by using videotalk. These descriptions are used to define the problem behaviorally and identify potential solutions using small weekly behavioral tasks. In addition, solution-oriented counselors prefer to use the descriptive language of videotalk to describe problems and solutions (e.g., "wanting to sleep in" or "when you are running in the mornings again") rather than vague interpretation or experience labels, such as "depressed" or "feeling better." When counselors consistently use videotalk to separate the *behaviors* from *interpretation of the behaviors*, clients are better able to identify where and how to make changes. For example, in the case study at the end of this chapter, the counselor uses videotalk to help Marcella to identify how she can more effectively interact with her parents who disapprove of her sexual orientation.

Utilization

Based on the hypnotic work of Milton Erickson, de Shazer (1988) employed *utilization* techniques to help clients identify and enact solutions. Utilization refers to finding a way to use and leverage whatever the client presents as a strength, interest, proclivity, or habit to develop meaningful actions and plans that will lead in the direction of solutions. For example, if a client has difficulty making friends and close relations but has numerous pets, the counselor would utilize the client's interest in animals to develop more human connections, perhaps by taking a dog for a walk in public places, joining a dog agility class, or volunteering at a pet shelter.

Coping Questions

Coping questions generate hope, agency, and motivation, especially when clients are feeling overwhelmed (De Jong & Berg, 2002; de Shazer et al., 2007). They are used when the client is not reporting progress, describing an acute crisis, or otherwise feeling hopeless. Coping questions direct clients to identify how they have been coping through a current or past difficult situation:

> - "This sounds hard—how have you managed to cope with this to the degree that you are?" (de Shazer et al., 2007, p. 10)
> - "How have you managed to prevent the situation from getting worse?" (p. 10)

Compliments and Encouragement

Solution-based counselors use compliments and encouragement to motivate clients and highlight strengths (De Jong & Berg, 2002). The key with compliments is to compliment *only* when clients are making steps toward goals *that they have set or compliment specific strengths that relate to the problem*. This is so important that I am going to say it again and put it in a special box so you don't forget:

> ## How to Compliment Clients
>
> *Compliment only when clients are making steps toward goals that* they *have set or compliment specific strengths that relate to the problem; compliment their progress, not their personhood.*
>
> Basic therapeutic compliment:
>
> - "Wow. You made real progress toward your goal this week."
>
> Even better therapeutic compliment:
>
> - "I am impressed; you not only followed through on the chart idea we developed last week but you came up with your own additional strategies—setting up a weekend outing with his friend—to improve your relationship with your son." (compliment specific behavior toward goal)
>
> Not-so-therapeutic compliments:
>
> - "I really admire what you have done with your life." (too personal and does not clearly relate to the problem; sounds like you are "buttering up" client)
> - "You really are a great mom." (nonspecific; evaluating mothering skills globally; not allowing client to reflect on and evaluate his or her own behavior)

When you compliment on anything else, you are setting up a situation where you are rendering judgment, albeit a positive one, on the client and/or his or her life. Compliments should not be used to be nice to clients (De Jong & Berg, 2002). Instead, compliments should be used to reinforce progress toward goals that clients have set for themselves and stated in such a way that it encourages clients to validate themselves rather than rely on an outside authority figure to do so. When clients can set goals and make progress toward them, they develop a greater sense of *self-efficacy*, which is a greater predictor of happiness than self-esteem (Seligman, 2004).

Homework and Experiments

Just in case it hasn't been obvious, almost every week solution-based counselors assign a homework assignment or task that requires the clients to take small, concrete steps toward their desired goals. These tasks are collaboratively identified during session using any number of techniques listed earlier. The counselor's role is to help concretely define the task so that the client (a) knows exactly what to do, (b) is motivated to do it, and (c) is likely to succeed. To ensure success, counselors should also identify potential obstacles, including weekends, holidays, visitors, schedule changes, and so on or anything that might keep clients from attaining their goals.

Interventions for Specific Problems
Sexual Abuse

Dolan (1991) and O'Hanlon and Bertolino (2002) use solution-based counseling with child and adult survivors of childhood sexual abuse. Solution-based approaches stand out from traditional approaches to sexual abuse treatment in their optimistic and hopeful stance that emphasizes the resiliencies of survivors. Given that survivors of sexual abuse have *survived* such a difficult trauma, solution-oriented counselors harness those strengths in new ways to help them resolve current issues. Some of the distinctive qualities of solution-oriented approaches to treating sexual abuse include the following:

Honoring the Agency of Survivors More so than traditional approaches, solution-based counselors honor the agency of survivors, allowing them to decide whether to tell their abuse stories and determine the pacing of their treatment (Dolan, 1991; O'Hanlon & Bertolino, 2002). Although many counselors insist that a survivor cannot heal without sharing the details of their abuse to their counselors, solution-based counselors would not readily agree. Instead, solution-based counselors work with clients to identify if, when, how, and to whom it is best to tell their stories. By fully honoring their agency, counselors create a relationship in which survivors reclaim full authority over the private aspects of their lives, reclaiming autonomy that was lost through the abuse. Counselors who play a more directive role in working with a survivor may unintentionally replicate the abuse pattern by forcing clients to reveal parts of their sexual life in the name of "treatment" before the client is ready, leaving the client feeling violated and retraumatized.

The Recovery Scale: Focusing on Strengths and Abilities   Dolan (1991, p. 32) uses the *Solution-Focused Recovery Scale* to identify areas of the client's life that were not affected by the abuse, reducing the sense that the client's whole life and self have been affected. The success strategies in these areas are used to address areas that are affected by the abuse. Questions from this scale are rated "not at all," "just a little," "pretty much," and "very much" and include questions such as the following:

- Able to think/talk about the trauma
- Feels part of family
- Goes to work
- Cares for pets, plants
- Holds hands with loved one
- Able to relax without drugs or alcohol
- Accepts praise well
- Shows healthy appetite

3-D Model: Dissociate, Disown, and Devalue   O'Hanlon and Bertolino (2002) conceptualize the aftereffects of abuse and trauma using the *3-D Model*, which postulates that abuse leads people to *dissociate*, *disown*, and *devalue* aspects of the self. The goal of counseling is to reconnect people with these disowned parts, parts that tend to either inhibit experience (e.g., lack of sexual response, lack of memories, or lack of anger) or create intrusive experiences (e.g., flashbacks, sexual compulsions, or rage). O'Hanlon and Bertolino (2002) note that many of the symptoms related to sexual abuse are experienced as a sort of *negative trance*, feeling as though the experience is uncontrollable and involving only a part of the self. Solution-oriented counselors use *permission* (i.e., allowing clients to express and feel undesirable feelings), *validating* (i.e., helping clients acknowledge difficult or unwanted feelings), and *inclusive language* (i.e., creating space for contradictory parts or feelings to be simultaneously recognized) to encourage clients to revalue and include the devalued aspects of self that were disowned through the abuse.

Constructive Questions   Dolan (1991, pp. 37–38) uses constructive questions to construct solutions by identifying the specifics of clients' unique solutions:

- What will be the first (smallest) sign that things are getting better, that this (the sexual abuse) is having less of an impact on your current life?
- What will you be doing differently when this (sexual abuse trauma) is less of a current problem in your life?
- What will you be doing differently with your time?
- What will you be thinking about (doing) *instead* of thinking about the past?
- Are there times when the above is already happening to some (even a small) extent? What is different about those times? What is helpful about those differences?
- What differences will the above healing changes make when they have been present in your life over extended time (days, weeks, months, or years)?
- What do you think your (significant other) would say would be the first sign that things are getting better? What do you think your significant other will notice first?
- What do you think your (friends, boss, significant other, etc.) will notice about you as you heal even more?
- What differences will these healing changes you've identified make in future generations of your family? (p. 37-38)

Videotalk (Action Terms) With Abuse and Trauma Survivors   Because of the intense emotions that characterize abuse and trauma, survivors often have difficulty identifying the current effects of abuse in their present life. O'Hanlon and Bertolino (2002) use videotalk (see preceding text) with survivors to help identify specific actions and patterns of behavior that recreate the traumatic experience, including the sequence of events, antecedents, consequences, invariant actions, repetitive actions, and body responses. Once these recurrent patterns are identified, counselors help clients either change one part of the context to interrupt the cycle and create space for new responses or, if the client feels a certain degree of control over the symptoms, identify new, alternative solution-generating actions. For example, if a client gets flashbacks when watching sexual scenes in movies, the counselor helps identify the behaviors before and after the flashbacks as well as the thoughts, feelings, and interpretations of these events. Using this information, such as the client's anxiety building as the suspense builds in the movie, the counselor can help the client identify ways to interrupt the cycle by hitting the mute button, turning on the lights, or going for a bathroom break.

Putting It All Together: Solution-Based Treatment Plan Template

Use this treatment plan template for developing a plan for clients with depressive, anxious, or compulsive types of presenting problems. Depending on the specific client, presenting problem, and clinical context, the goals and interventions in this template may need to be modified only slightly or significantly; you are encouraged to significantly revise the plan as needed. For the plan to be useful, goals and techniques should be written to target specific beliefs, behaviors, and emotions that the client is experiencing. The more specific, the more useful it will be to you.

Treatment Plan

Initial Phase of Treatment (First One to Three Sessions)
Initial Phase Counseling Tasks

1. *Develop working counseling relationship. Diversity note:* Attend to diversity issues.
   Relationship building intervention:
   a. Build rapport by identifying **strengths, resources,** and **channeling language** to delimit **problem,** identify areas of **functioning,** and generate **hope.**

2. *Assess individual, systemic, and broader cultural dynamics. Diversity note:* Identify **resources** related to diversity.
   Assessment Strategies:
   a. **Miracle question** to obtain behavioral description of solutions and motivate clients.
   b. **Identify exceptions, previous solutions, "what works," presession change,** and **strengths.**

Initial Phase Client Goals* *(One to Two Goals):* Manage crisis issues and/or reduce most distressing symptoms

1. *Increase* safety and ability to **use resources** to prevent crisis situations (personal/relational dynamic) to reduce [crisis-related behavior] (symptom).
   Interventions:
   a. Motivate client to use **scaling for safety** to generate **step-by-step safety plan.**
   b. Identify personal, relational, and community **resources** to provide immediate support for client.
   c. **Formula first session task** to identify what *is* working well right now and to generate hope.

*Note: Solution-based treatment plans will have *only* goals that begin with "increase" as they use positively stated goals.

(continued)

Working Phase of Treatment (Three or More Sessions)
Working Phase Counseling Task

1. *Monitor quality of the working alliance. Diversity note:* Address diversity issues.
    Assessment Intervention:
    a. Session Rating Scale; adjust alliance based on client level of **motivation** (visitor, complainant, or customer); if intervention does not work, **do something different**.

Working Phase Client Goals *(Two to Three Goals).* Target individual and relational dynamics using theoretical language (e.g., decrease avoidance of intimacy, increase awareness of emotion, increase agency)

1. *Increase* [behaviors derived from **"exceptions," "what works,"** and/or **"previous solutions"**] (personal/relational dynamic) to reduce depressed mood, anxiety, problem behaviors, and so on (symptom).
    Interventions:
    a. **Scaling questions** to identify specific behavioral tasks each week to generate incremental improvement.
    b. **Coping questions** to augment areas of strength and resource utilization.

2. *Increase* [one set of behaviors identified **in miracle question**] (personal/relational dynamic) to reduce depressed mood, anxiety, problem behaviors, and so on (symptom).
    Interventions:
    a. **Scaling questions** to identify specific behavioral tasks each week to generate incremental improvement.
    b. **Videotalk** to identify specific behaviors and how they inform client's personal and relational identities.

3. *Increase* [another set of behaviors identified in **miracle question**] (personal/relational dynamic) to reduce depressed mood, anxiety, problem behaviors, and so on (symptom).
    Interventions:
    a. **Scaling questions** to identify specific behavioral tasks each week to generate incremental improvement.
    b. **Presuppositional questions** to help client envision solution and build hope.

Closing Phase of Treatment (Last Two or More Sessions)
Closing Phase Counseling Tasks

1. *Develop aftercare plan and maintain gains. Diversity note:* Include individual, family, and community resources to support client.
    Intervention:
    a. Adapt **miracle question** to have client envision future problem and how he or she used resources learned in counseling to handle it.

Closing Phase Client Goals *(One to Two Goals):* Determined by theory's definition of health and normalcy

1. *Increase* confidence and solidify **new identity** related to living the solution (personal/relational dynamic) to reduce depressed mood, anxiety, problem behaviors, and so on (symptom).
    Interventions:
    a. **Compliments and encouragement** to build new identity based on solution behaviors, choices, and so on.
    b. **Scaling questions** to reflect on progress and what worked; discuss how to maintain.

(continued)

2. Increase use of new skills to **build solutions** in personal, family, interpersonal, and occupational situations (personal/relational dynamic) to reduce depressed mood, anxiety, problem behaviors, and so on (symptom).
   Interventions:
   a. **Compliments and encouragement** of new skills and ability to adapt them to new situations.
   b. **Scaling into the future** to anticipate ups and downs and how to manage.

Source: Metcalf, Parenting Toward Solutions, 1st Edition, © 1998. Reprinted by permission of Pearson Education, Inc., Upper Saddle River, NJ.

Solution-Focused School Counseling

Of all the areas of specialty, school counselors have been most enthusiastic about solution-focused counseling (Cooley, 2009; Davis & Osborn, 2000; Kelly et al., 2008; Metcalf, 2003, 2007; Murphy, 2008; Parsons, 2009; Sklare, 2004). The potential to be brief makes solution-focused counseling ideal for implementation in school contexts where counselors often have 5- to 20-minute windows of time in which to do their work. Furthermore, for decades research has shown that students live up (or down) to teacher *expectations*: if a teacher believes a child to be smart and well behaved, more often than not the child lives up to this perception. Thus, if solution-focused methods are used to increase the ability of teachers, students, parents, and administrators to see the strengths of students, this approach can have powerful, long-term, and widespread effects on students in schools (Kelly et al., 2008). Research over the past decade provides support for solution-focused school counseling as a promising approach, particularly to help students reduce the intensity of negative emotions, conduct problems, and externalizing behaviors (Kim & Franklin, 2009).

Assumptions in Solution-Focused School Counseling

Murphy (2008) identifies five assumptions in solution-focused school counseling:

1. If it works, do more of it. If it doesn't work, do something different.
2. Every client is unique, resourceful, and capable of changing.
3. Cooperative relationships enhance solutions.
4. No problem is constant.
5. Big problems do not always require big solutions.

Solution-Focused Viewing in School Contexts

Metcalf (2008) describes a five-step approach to viewing and assessing situations in school contexts that helps counselors identify helpful action steps:

1. *Problem:* The problem is defined in nonpathological, nonblaming terms and languaged to emphasize ways in which the persons involved can effect change.
   Example: A seventh grader, Jose's grades have dropped over the past 3 months; he has been withdrawn in classes and hangs out with fewer friends. (Note: Attitude, personality, and mood are not described; instead, behavioral and neutral depictions are used to define the problem.)
2. *Goals:* Using the principles of solution-focused goal development, goals are jointly developed with the family, teachers, and client, using their preferred language.
   Example: Jose will get his grades back where they used to be: a 3.5 grade-point average; increase Jose's classroom participation and engagement with peers during lunchtime. (Note: Specific, concrete, and doable.)
3. *Problem maintenance:* The counselor, parents, teacher, and student identify what actions are helping to maintain the problem while minimizing blame. Counselors should explore how *each person* may in some small way collude with the problem, intentionally or unintentionally, to perpetuate the life of the problem.
   Example: Jose watches television rather than doing homework when he gets home.

His mother repeatedly tells him to do his homework until he does.

Jose says he never had to work this hard in sixth grade, when his grades were good (may need study skills).

Jose has fewer classes with his friends this year.

Jose's teachers say he's a nice kid but doesn't seem to study or have friends.

4. *Exceptions:* The counselor helps students, teachers, and parents identify exceptions or when the problem is less of a problem.
   Example: Jose does a good job finishing homework and getting points for that; he has a harder time studying for tests and doing well on tests.
   Jose likes doing hands-on science projects and enjoys these most.
   Jose has lunch with a friend some days at school.
   Jose will talk to other kids in class if he has to for a group assignment.
   Jose enjoys playing soccer and plays well with siblings.

5. *Task:* Working with those involved, the counselor helps to identify things that the student, teacher, and/or parents can do differently to improve the situation.
   Example: Jose's parents and teacher will help him with study skills for the next test, perhaps by making flash cards or some other action-based study skills.
   Jose will say "hi" when he walks in the class (if the bell hasn't already rung) to his last science partner that he sort of liked even on days when they aren't working on a project.
   Jose will find a friend to have lunch with every day.

Solution-Focused Groups in School Contexts

Increasingly, school counselors are asked to create groups for students with particular problems, such as anger, study skills, divorcing parents, and so on. Groups are highly efficient means of providing counseling services, saving both time and money. Metcalf (2008) provides a generic template for how to organize a solution-focused group session in a school context:

1. *Set the mood for focusing on solutions:* Since students aren't always sent to counseling groups under the best of circumstances, counselors should establish an upbeat, nonblaming, positive atmosphere. The counselor can ask, "What brings you here today?" or "Why do you think X sent you here? What are your thoughts on this?"

2. *Goal setting:* Next, the counselor helps each group member define goals in positive terms, such as "How will you know when things are better for you?" If the student angrily responds, "When my teacher or parent think I am done" or something similar, the counselor goes with it in solution-focused style and asks, "What will you need to be doing for person X to believe you don't need to be here?" Counselors can also use scaling questions to establish goals and measure progress from week to week. If the group has met before, the counselor should also follow up on homework tasks and explore where students are on the scale this week.

3. *Identifying exceptions and strengths:* Using the miracle question, exception question, strengths assessment, and input from group members who know each other or the situation, the counselor helps identify exceptions to help with building solutions. Also, the counselor can point out exceptions and strengths in the group setting, such as noting how the boy who says he is shy and has no friends seems to be making friends and talking quite a bit in the group.

4. *Encouraging motivation:* Using the group for support and positive encouragement, the counselor helps to motivate students to make one small change. A positive group environment can be a remarkable motivator for students to make a turn around.

5. *Developing tasks:* Finally, each student should leave with one clear task for the upcoming week to take a step toward their solutions.

6. *Conclusion:* At the end, the counselor can ask what was helpful in the session today that students would like to do more of next time the group meets; this allows the counselor to tailor the group to meet student needs while giving students a sense of ownership and investment.

Kelly et al. (2008, pp. 109–110) describe an eight-session template for organizing middle and high school groups to address a specific topic, such as anxiety, divorce adjustment, or grades:

Session 1: Getting Started

- Introductions, informed consent, and group expectations.
- Discuss goals of the group.

Session 2: Goal Setting

- "What do you hope to achieve by participating in this group for 8 weeks?"
- Miracle question to identify solutions (if appropriate for age, have students draw miracle).

Session 3: Scaling

- "On a scale from 0 to 10, with 10 being where you want be at the end of this group and 0 being where you were when someone first had the idea to have you join the group, where are you today? What would have to happen for you to move one point up the scale before the next time we meet?"
- Identify specific tasks and behaviors for each student to help them move up the scale.

Session 4: Signs of Success

- Review Session 3 homework assignment, having students identify "signs of success."
- Use relational questions to motivate for next week, "If I asked your teacher, Mr./Ms._____ what signs of success he or she noticed, what do you think he or she would say?"
- Homework to include *writing down* signs of success.

Session 5: Elicit, Amplify, and Reinforce Change

- Follow up on homework, looking for opportunities to elicit descriptions of success, amplify change, and reinforce new behaviors; use exception questions.
- Homework and tasks to continue moving up the scale.

Session 6: Older, Wiser Self

- Follow up on progress with scaling question.
- Instruct students to write a letter to themselves from their older, wiser self (Dolan, 1995): "Imagine that you have grown to be a healthy, wise old man or woman and you are looking back on this period of your life. What would this older and wiser person suggest to you to help you reach your goals?"

Session 7: New Self

- Review letters from older, wiser self.
- Discuss how "new self" is starting to emerge and how others are responding to it.

Session 8: Prepare for Setbacks; Celebrate Success

- Discuss achievements using scaling questions.
- Normalize and create a plan for dealing with setbacks.
- Distribute certificates to celebrate success.

Working on What Works: Coaching Classrooms

Originally developed by Insoo Kim Berg and Lee Shilts when consulting in Florida in 2002, Working on What Works (WOWW; Kelly & Bluestone-Miller, 2009; Kelly et al., 2008) is a solution-focused technique that school counselors use to help teachers and their classrooms improve behaviorally and academically. Serving as more of a consultant or coach, the school counselor uses strengths assessment and scaling to help teachers and students wok together to improve classroom performance and culture. Preliminary pilot research is promising, with positive increases in teachers' perception of student behavior, teachers' view of self as effective classroom managers, and students' perception of themselves and their behavior.

The WOWW coaching process involves three phases:

Phase 1: Observation and compliments (weeks 1–3): In this phase, the school counselor introduces the process to the class: "I'm going to be visiting your room to watch for all the things the class does that are good and helpful. I will report back to you what I see" (Kelly & Bluestone-Miller, 2009, p. 65). The counselor visits for about an hour, the first 45 minutes spent observing and the last 15 minutes reporting back by complimenting behaviors of individual students and groups of students.

Phase 2: Create goals and rating (scaling) system (weeks 4–6): Using a variation on scaling questions, the school counselor begins by having the class identify in *positive, behavioral* terms what the "best class" would be doing (e.g., raising their hands to speak, doing class work quietly, speaking kindly to each other). The counselor is careful that all descriptions of the best class are in terms of what the class *is doing*, not what they are not doing. Over one or more weeks, the counselor and class develop a rubric using a 1–5, 1–10, or smiley-face scale that the class will use for self-assessment, defining behaviors for each possible score.

Phase 3: Goal setting and amplifying change (remaining sessions): After the class has developed their goals and scale, the counselor coaches them on selecting one or two (no more) goals that the class is going to work on for the following week. The teachers are encouraged to scale progress *daily* and to do so on a chart that is always readily visible. The counselor's role is to notice and amplify strengths with each visit. Once one set of goals has been reached, new goals are set for the class to work toward.

Snapshot: Research and the Evidence Base

Quick Summary: Strong, growing evidence base for the solution-based counseling in a wide range of contexts.

Solution-focused therapy has a quickly growing foundation of empirical support. In 2000, Gingerich and Eisengart published the first critical review of solution-focused outcome research, listing 15 controlled studies. Of the five well-controlled studies, four showed that solution-focused therapy was *better* than both treatment as usual and a no-treatment control group; one study found solution-focused to be as effective as treatment as usual. The other 10 studies, which were moderately or poorly controlled, all supported the effectiveness of solution-focused therapy, providing promising support for the effectiveness of solution-focused therapy. As of November 2007, Gingerich and Patterson (2007) have identified 150 controlled outcome studies on the effectiveness of solution-focused therapy, a dramatic increase over 7 years that attests to the increasing interest in establishing solution-focused therapy as an evidence-supported approach.

In his introduction to a special issue of the *Journal of Family Psychotherapy*, McCollum (2007) identifies three key practical and philosophical challenges of establishing solution-focused therapy as an evidence-based approach. First, it is difficult to adequately manualize solution-focused therapy and capture not only the techniques, which are more easily quantified, but also the spirit and epistemological positioning that is the essence of the model. A rigid or shallow adherence to solution-focused techniques without grounding in the collaborative, strength-based mind-set of the theory results in a pushy or Pollyanna approach that is not an accurate enactment of solution-focused therapy. Second, McCollum advocates for "streams" of studies that address particular populations or problems in greater depth. Finally, certain solution-focused philosophical principles, namely, the honoring of each client's uniqueness and recognizing change processes outside of therapy, are at odds with the broader research project that aims to make global assessments of the effectiveness of this approach, thereby obscuring client uniqueness and extratherapeutic factors that contribute to change.

Snapshot: Working With Diverse Populations

Quick Summary: Widely used with diverse populations in the United States, Canada, and internationally; easily adapted for a wide range of value systems and communication styles.

As an approach that does not use a theory of health to predefine client goals (de Shazer et al., 2007; O'Hanlon & Weiner-Davis, 1989), solution-focused therapy is appropriate for working with a wide range of diverse populations because it is readily adapted to the client's value and meaning systems. Solution-focused therapy is widely used with diverse populations in the North America, South America, Europe, the Middle East, East Asia, and Australia (Gingerich & Patterson, 2007). Solution-focused therapy has been studied with a range of client ethnicities, including immigrants, African Americans, Hispanics, Saudi Arabians, Chinese, Koreans, and in a wide range of contexts, such as schools, prisons, hospitals, business, and colleges (Gingerich & Patterson, 2007). When working with diverse clients, counselors can use the solution-focused approach to identifying strengths to access the unique emotional, cognitive, and/or social resources that are inherent with the client's experience of diversity.

Solution-Based Study and Treatment Plan

Marcella, a 32-year-old nurse practitioner, is seeking treatment after her brother was killed in a car accident. On the one hand, she is saddened by his tragic death, but on the other, she feels a smug sense of vindication because she feels that God has finally punished him for sexually abusing her when she was 12 or 13. She has been feeling depressed since his death, partially because of the grief and partially because his death has brought up memories of the abuse for which she never sought treatment because although her parents intervened to stop her brother when she finally told, they never sought outside assistance to avoid shaming the family. Her parents simply encouraged her to forgive him and to pray to Mary when she needed comfort. However, during that time, she cut herself to cope with the pain and has started doing so again. After coming out in college, Marcella has not been close to her parents or family, who are strict Catholics. Marcella's partner has been very supportive of her but increasingly bitter toward Marcella's family, whom she sees as not supporting Marcella like they should have. Marcella says that the loss of her brother makes her want to be closer to her family again, who has been more connected since the death, as well as regain the self-confidence she feels she lost after the abuse. Her long-term goal is to be a pediatrician, but she has never felt she was good enough to be a doctor. AF (Adult Female) finds her greatest peace when horseback riding, a hobby she has had since childhood.

Solution-Based Case Conceptualization

This case conceptualization was developed by selecting key concepts from "The Viewing: Case Conceptualization" section of this chapter. You can use any of the concepts in that section to develop a case conceptualization for this or other cases.

The Miracle Question

AF's (adult female) miracle involves having a good relationship with her family, who accepts her as she is; regaining her self-confidence; feeling at peace with the loss of her brother who abused her; and pursuing her dream to become a pediatrician.

Exceptions, Previous Solutions, and "What Works"

AF feels most at peace while horseback riding, which provides periods when she does not feel overwhelmed by her brother's death or memories of the abuse. She also describes a supportive partner and some regular connection with her family since the death, thus lessening the distance that had been created when she came out. Identify the times when she could cut but does not.

Assessing Client Strengths

AF was brave and confident enough to come out to her family, who she knew would not be supportive of her. She was raised with strong religious faith, which she still possesses and is using to help make sense of her brother's death and her healing from the abuse. She has been professionally successful and has clear goals for her next career move. Although she cuts, she does not report suicidal thoughts; explore these strengths further with her.

Client Motivation: Visitor, Complainant, and Customers

AF initially presents as a complainant, seeing the problem as her brother's death and abuse, but seems to be ready to be a customer for change, as evidenced by her goals to want a closer connection to her family, feel confident again, and pursue advanced career goals.

Details, Details, Details

Rather than assume generic symptoms typically associated with sexual abuse, the solution-focused counselor focuses specifically on the unique symptoms that AF sees as a result of her abuse, such as loss of confidence, not pursuing her career goals, ruminating about the abuse, and so on.

Solution-Based

Initial Phase of Treatment (First One to Three Sessions)
Initial Phase Counseling Tasks

1. *Develop working counseling relationship. Diversity note:* Ensure that AF feels that her sexual orientation and ethnicity are respected in the counseling relationship.
   Relationship building intervention:
   a. Build rapport by identifying **strengths** and **resources** and **channeling language to delimit problem**, identify areas of **functioning despite the abuse**, and generate **hope** for full recovery.

2. *Assess individual, systemic, and broader cultural dynamics. Diversity note:* Identify **resources** related to diversity.
   Assessment Strategies:
   a. **Miracle question** to obtain behavioral description of solutions and motivate AF to make specific changes; ask question to emphasize what will be different in relation to the problem and what she will be doing differently.
   b. **Identify exceptions, previous solutions, "what works," presession change,** and **strengths**.

Initial Phase Client Goals

1. *Increase* safety and ability to **use resources** when feeling overwhelmed by emotions to stop cutting.
   Interventions:
   a. Motivate client to use **scaling for safety** to generate **step-by-step safety plan;** involve partner if possible.
   b. Identify personal, relational, and community **resources** to provide immediate support for client when feeling as though she wants to self harm.
   c. **Formula first session task** to identify what *is* working well right now and to generate hope between the first and second sessions.

(continued)

Working Phase of Treatment (Two or More Sessions)
Working Phase Counseling Tasks

1. *Monitor quality of the working alliance. Diversity note:* Continue to ensure that AF feels safe in the counseling relationship and that her sexual orientation, ethnicity, and religious beliefs are respected.
   Assessment Intervention:
   a. Session Rating Scale; adjust alliance as she becomes more of a customer for change; if intervention does not work, **do something different.**

Working Phase Client Goals

1. *Increase* proactive behaviors that build sense of confidence to reduce depressed mood related to abuse.
   Interventions:
   a. **Scaling questions** to identify specific behavioral tasks that represent an increase in self-confidence each week to generate incremental improvement.
   b. **Coping questions** to help AF identify all the ways she has coped with the abuse and alienation from family because of her sexual orientation.

2. *Increase* satisfying contact with family of origin to reduce depressed mood.
   Interventions:
   a. **Scaling questions** to identify specific behavioral tasks each week that are likely to lead to improved relations with her family.
   b. **Videotalk** to identify specific behaviors she can use to improve relationship with family.

3. *Increase* ability to effectively manage strong emotions to reduce desire to cut and grief feelings.
   Interventions:
   a. **Scaling questions** to identify specific things she can do to (a) avoid emotions from becoming overwhelming and (b) effectively manage them as they first arise.
   b. **Presuppositional questions** to help client envision herself as able to handle strong emotions effectively.

Closing Phase of Treatment (Last Two or More Sessions)
Closing Phase Counseling Tasks

1. *Develop aftercare plan and maintain gains. Diversity note:* Involve partner in identifying early signs of relapse and return to cutting.
   Intervention:
   a. Adapt **miracle question** to have AF envision future problems and how she can use resources learned in counseling to handle them.

Closing Phase Client Goals

1. *Increase* confidence and solidify **new identity** as someone who has worked through sexual abuse and loss of brother to reduce depressed mood.
   Interventions:
   a. **Compliments and encouragement** to build confidence and identity as someone who has developed numerous resources and discovered great personal strength through her ordeals.
   b. **Scaling questions** to reflect on progress and what worked; discuss how to maintain these gains in the years ahead.

2. *Increase* proactive behavior to reach professional goals (personal/relational dynamic) to reduce sense of hopelessness.
   Interventions:
   a. **Compliments and encouragement** to develop confidence and resolve to follow her life dreams.
   b. **Scaling into the future** to anticipate ups and downs in pursuing MD and how to manage.

ONLINE RESOURCES

Associations

Milton H. Erickson Foundation
www.erickson-foundation.org

Solution-Focused Brief Therapy Association
www.sfbta.org

Solution-Oriented, Possibility Therapy
www.billohanlon.com

Divorce Busting
www.divorcebusting.com

European Brief Therapy Association
www.ebta.nu

Review of Solution-Focused Therapy Research
http://gingerich.net/SFBT/2007_review.htm

References

*Asterisk indicates recommended introductory books

Berg, I. K. (1994). *Family based services: A solution-focused approach*. New York: Norton.

Berg, I. K., & Kelly, S. (2000). *Building solutions in child protective services*. New York: Norton.

Berg, I. K., & Miller, S. (1992). *Working with the problem drinker: A solution-focused approach*. New York: Norton.

Berg, I. K., & Reuss, N. H. (2007). *Solutions step by step: A substance abuse treatment manual*. New York: Norton.

Berg, I. K., Steiner, T. (2003). *Children's solution work*. New York: Norton.

Berg, I. K., & Szabo, P. (2005). *Brief coaching for last solutions*. New York: Norton.

Bertolino, B. (2010). *Strength-based engagement and practice: Creating effective helping relationships*. New York: Allyn and Bacon.

Bertolino, B., & O'Hanlon, B. (1998). *Therapy with troubled teenagers: Rewriting young lives in progress*. New York: Wiley.

*Bertolino, B., & O'Hanlon, B. (2002). *Collaborative, competency-based counseling and therapy*. New York: Allyn and Bacon.

Cooley, L. A. (2009). *The power of groups: Solution-focused group counseling in schools*. Thousand Oaks, CA: Corwin.

Davis, T. E., & Osborn, C. J. (2000). *Solution-focused school counseling: Shaping professional practice*. New York: Routledge.

*De Jong, P., & Berg, I. K. (2002). *Interviewing for solutions* (2nd ed.). New York: Brooks/Cole.

*de Shazer, S. (1985). *Keys to solution in brief therapy*. New York: Norton.

*de Shazer, S. (1988). *Clues: Investigating solutions in brief therapy*. New York: Norton.

de Shazer, S. (1994). *Words were originally magic*. New York: Norton.

*de Shazer, S., Dolan, Y., Korman, H., Trepper, T., McCollum, & Berg, I. K. (2007). *More than miracles: The state of the art of solution-focused brief therapy*. New York: Haworth.

*Dolan, Y. (1991). *Resolving sexual abuse: Solution-focused therapy and Ericksonian hypnosis for survivors*. New York: Norton.

Dolan, Y. (2000). *One small step: Moving beyond trauma and thearapy into a life of joy*. New York: Excel Press.

Dolan, Y. (2007). Tribute to Insoo Kim Berg. *Journal of Marital and Family Therapy, 33*, 129–131.

Erickson, B. A., & Keeney, B. (Eds). (2006). *Milton Erickson, M.D.: An American healer*. Sedona, AZ: Leete Island Books.

Gehart, D. R. (2010). *Mastering competencies in family therapy: A practical approach to theories and clinical case documentation*. Belmont, CA: Brooks/Cole.

Gingerich, W. J., & Eisengart, S (2000). Solution-focused brief therapy: A review of the outcome studies. *Family Process, 39*, 477–498.

Gingerich, W. J., & Patterson, L. (2007). *The 2007 SFBT effectiveness project*. Retrieved March 20, 2008, from http://gingerich.net/SFBT/2007_review.htm

Haley, J. (1993). *Uncommon therapy: The psychiatric techniques of Milton H. Erikson, M.D.* New York: Norton.

Hudson, P. O., & O'Hanlon, W. H. (1991). *Rewriting love stories: Brief marital therapy*. New York: Norton.

Kelly, M., & Bluestone-Miller, R. (2009). Working on What Works (WOWW): Coaching teachers to do more of what's working. *Children and Schools, 31*(1), 35–38.

Kelly, M. S., Kim, J. S., & Franklin, C. (2008). *Solution-focused brief therapy in schools: A 360-degree view of research and practice*. New York: Oxford University Press.

Kim, J., & Franklin, C. (2009). Solution-focused brief therapy in schools: A review of the outcome literature. *Children and Youth Services Review, 31*(4), 464–470. doi: 10.1016/j.childyouth.2008.10.002

Lipchick, E. (2002). *Beyond technique in solution-focused therapy: Working with emotions and the therapeutic relationship*. New York: Guilford.

McCollum, E. (2007). Introduction to special issue. *Journal of Family Psychotherapy, 18*(3), 1–9.

Metcalf, L. (1998). *Parenting towards solutions*. Paramus, NJ: Prentice Hall.

Metcalf, L. (2003). *Teaching towards solutions* (2nd ed.). Carmethen: Crown House Publishing.

Metcalf, L. (2007). *Solution-focused group therapy.* New York: Free Press.

Metcalf, L. (2008). *Counseling towards solutions: A practical solution-focused program for working with students, teachers, and parents* (2nd ed.). New York: Jossey-Basss.

Miller, S. D., Duncan, B. L., & Hubble, M.A. (1997). *Escape from Babel: Towards a unifying language for psychotherapy practice.* New York: Norton

Miller, S. D., Duncan, B. L., & Hubble, M. (Eds.). (1996). *Handbook of solution-focused brief therapy.* San Francisco: Jossey-Bass.

Murphy, J. J. (2008). *Solution-focused counseling in schools.* Alexandria, VA: American Counseling Association.

O'Hanlon, B. (2000). *Do one thing different: Ten simple ways to change your life.* New York: Harper.

O'Hanlon, B. (2005). *Thriving through crisis: Turn tragedy and trauma into growth and change.* New York: Penguin/Perigee.

O'Hanlon, B. (2006). *Pathways to spirituality: Connection, wholeness, and possibility for therapist and client.* New York: Norton Professional.

*O'Hanlon, B., & Beadle, S. (1999). *A guide to possibilityland: Possibility therapy methods.* Omaha, NE: Possibility Press.

O'Hanlon, B., & Bertolino, B. (2002). *Even from a broken web: Brief and respectful solution-oriented therapy for resolving sexual abuse.* New York: Norton.

O'Hanlon, W. H., & Martin, M. (1992). *Solution-oriented hypnosis: An Ericksonian approach.* New York: Norton.

*O'Hanlon, W. H., & Weiner-Davis, M. (1989). *In search of solutions: A new direction in psychotherapy.* New York: Norton.

Parsons, R. (2009). *Thinking and acting like a solution-focused school counselor.* Thousand Oaks, CA: Corwin Press.

Selekman, M. D. (1997). *Solution-focused therapy with children: Harnessing family strengths for systemic change.* New York: Guilford.

*Selekman, M. (2006). *Working with self-harming adolescents: A collaborative, strength-oriented therapy approach.* New York: Norton.

*Selekman, M. D. (2010). *Collaborative brief therapy with children.* New York: Guilford.

Seligman, M. (2004). *Authentic happiness.* New York: Free Press.

Sklare, G. B. (2004). *Brief counseling that works: A solution-focused approach for school counselors and administrators* (2nd ed.). Thousand Oaks, CA: Corwin Press.

Trepper, T. S., Dolan, Y., McCollum, E. E., & Nelson, T. (2006). Steve de Shazer and the future of solution-focused therapy. *Journal of Marital and Family Therapy, 32,* 133–140.

Walter, J. L., & Peller, J. E. (1992). *Becoming solution-focused in brief therapy.* New York: Brunner/Mazel.

Weiner-Davis, M. (1992). *Divorce busting.* New York: Summit Books.

Weiner-Davis, M., de Shazer, S., & Gingerich, W. J. (1987), Building on pretreatment change to construct the therapeutic solution: An exploratory study, *Journal of Marital and Family Therapy, 13,* 359–363. doi:10.1111/j.1752-0606.1987.tb00717.x

CHAPTER
12

Narrative
and Collaborative
Approaches

Lay of the Land

If you thought that systemic ideas were challenging to how we normally perceive the world (i.e., I am totally separate from you), the postmodernists really shake things up, calling into question unquestionable assumptions, such the self, coherent identity, and independent thought. The newest kids on the block, postmodern counseling approaches are grounded in social constructionist theories that examine how societal discourses (e.g., "talk of the town," media images, movie plots, etc.) about gender, culture, race, religion, and economic status affect a person's sense of personhood and the development of problems. Much like systemic approaches, these theories place an emphasis on interpersonal relationships and how they shape a person's understanding and experience of self. In fact, they radically posit that one's sense of self is constructed in and through relationships rather than being independently thought up in one's head. These approaches can be broadly divided into two streams of practice:

- *Narrative counseling*: Based on the work of Australia- and New Zealand–based practitioners Michael White and David Epston (1990), narrative counselors help separate people from their problems by exploring the sociocultural influences and language habits that maintain problems.
- *Collaborative approaches*: Developed by Harlene Anderson and Harry Goolishian (1988, 1992) in Texas and Tom Andersen in Norway (1991), collaborative approaches focus on facilitating dialogical conversations that "dissolve" problems with conversations and relationships that allow for the cocreation of new meaning related to problems.

Similar to solution-based counselors (see Chapter 11), postmodernists optimistically focus on client strengths and abilities. Despite many philosophical similarities, these approaches differ in significant ways, most notably their philosophical foundations, the stance of the counselor, the role of interventions, and the emphasis on political issues.

	Narrative	Collaborative
Primary philosophical foundations	Foucault's philosophical writings; critical theory; social constructionism	Postmodernism, social constructionism; hermeneutics (the study of interpretation)
Counseling relationship	Active role as "coeditor" or "coauthor"	Facilitative role; democratic; "client is the expert"
Counseling process	Uses structured interventions; focus on various forms oppression	Avoid formal interventions; counselor focuses on facilitating dialogical process
Politics and social justice	Social justice issues regularly included in counseling conversations	Political issues raised tentatively for client consideration

Narrative Approaches

In a Nutshell: The Least You Need to Know

Developed by Michael White and David Epston in Australia and New Zealand, narrative counseling is based on the premise that we "story" and create meaning of life events using available *dominant discourses*—broad societal stories, sociocultural practices, assumptions, and expectations about how we should live. People experience "problems" when their personal lives do not fit with these dominant societal discourses and expectations. The process of narrative counseling involves *separating the person from their problem* by critically examining the assumptions that inform how the person evaluates himself or herself and his or her life. Through this process, clients identify alternative ways to view, act, and interact in daily life. Narrative counselors assume that all people are resourceful and have strengths, and they do not see "people" as having problems but rather see people as being imposed on by unhelpful or harmful societal cultural practices.

The Juice: Significant Contributions to the Field

If you remember one thing from this chapter, it should be …

Understanding Oppression: Dominant Versus Local Discourses

Like feminist approaches, narrative counseling is one of the few theories that integrates societal and cultural issues into its core conceptualization of how problems form and are resolved. Narrative counselors maintain that problems do not exist separate from their sociocultural contexts, which are broadly constituted in what philosopher Michel Foucault referred to as *dominant discourses* (Foucault, 1980; White & Epston, 1990). *Dominant discourses* are culturally generated stories about how life should go that are used to coordinate social behavior, such as how married people should act, what happiness looks like, and how to be successful. These dominant discourses organize social groups at all levels: large cultural groups down to individual couple and family stories about how life should go. These discourses are described as *dominant* because they are foundational to how each of us behaves and evaluates our lives, yet we are rarely conscious of their impact or origins.

Foucault contrasts *dominant discourses* with *local discourses*, which occur in our heads, our closer relationships, and marginalized (not mainstream) communities. Local discourses have different "goods" and "shoulds" than dominant discourses. A classic example is women's valuing of relationship compared to men's valuing of outcome in typical work environments. Both discourses have a value they are working toward; however, men's is generally privileged over women's and thus is considered a dominant discourse, while women's is local. Narrative counselors closely attend to the fluid interactions of local and dominant discourses and how these different stories of what is "good" and valued collide in our web of social relationships, creating problems and difficulties. By attending to this level of social interaction, narrative counselors help clients become aware of how these different discourses are impacting their lives; this awareness serves to increase clients' sense of agency in their struggles, allowing them to find ways to more successfully resolve their issues.

Rumor Has It: The People and Their Stories

Michael White

A pioneer in narrative counseling and the first to write about the process of *externalizing* problems, Michael White was based at the Dulwich Centre in Adelaide, Australia. Along with David Epston, he wrote the first book on narrative counseling, *Narrative Means to Therapeutic Ends* (White & Epston, 1990). His last publication, *Maps to Narrative Practice* (White, 2007), describes his later work before his death in 2008.

David Epston

From Auckland, New Zealand, David Epston worked closely with Michael White in developing the foundational framework for narrative counseling. His work emphasized creating unique sources of support for clients, such as writing letters to clients to solidify the emerging narratives and developing communities of concern or *leagues* (see section "Leagues") in which clients provide support to each other.

Jill Freedman and Gene Combs

Based in the United States, husband-and-wife team Jill Freedman and Gene Combs (1996) have developed the narrative approach emphasizing the process of the social construction of realities and further developed the narrative metaphor for conceptualizing counseling intervention. They are the codirectors of the Evanston Family Therapy Center in Evanston, Illinois.

Gerald Monk and John Winslade

Beginning their work in New Zealand and now working in the United States, Gerald Monk and John Winslade have developed narrative approaches for schools counseling, multicultural counseling, mediation, and consultation (Monk, Winslade, Crocket, & Epston, 1997; Monk, Winslade, Sinclair, 2008; Winslade & Monk, 2000, 2007, 2009).

Big Picture: Overview of Counseling Process

The process of narrative counseling involves helping clients find new ways to view, interact with, and respond to problems in their lives by redefining the role of problems in their lives (White, 2007). From a narrative perspective, "persons are not the problem; problems are the problem." Although there is variety among practitioners, narrative counseling broadly involves the following phases (Freedman & Combs, 1996; White & Epson, 1990):

- *Meeting the person:* Getting to know people separate from their problems by learning about hobbies, values, and everyday aspects of their lives
- *Listening:* Listening for the effects of dominant discourses and identifying times without the problems
- *Separating persons from problems:* Externalizing and separating people from their problems to create space for new identities and life stories to emerge
- *Enacting preferred narratives:* Identifying new ways to relate to problems that reduce their negative effects on the lives of all involved and to "thicken" their identity and problem stories (see section "Thickening Descriptions")
- *Solidifying:* Strengthening preferred stories and identities by having them witnessed by significant others in a person's life

Thickening Descriptions

Narrative counseling process is a *thickening* and enriching of the person's identity and life accounts rather than a "story-ectomy," the replacing of a problem story with problem-free one. Instead, narrative counselors *add* new strands of identity to the problem-saturated descriptions with which clients enter counseling. In a given day, there are an infinite number of events that can be storied into our accounts of the day and who we are. When people begin to experience problems, they tend to notice *only* those events that fit with the problem narrative. For example, if a person is feeling hopeless, he or she tends to notice when things do not go his or her way during the day and does not give much weight to the good things that happened. Similarly, when couples start a period of fighting, they start to notice only what the other person is doing that confirms their position in the fight and ignore and/or forget other events. In narrative counseling, the counselor helps clients create more *balanced* descriptions of the events of their lives to enable clients to build more accurate and appreciative descriptions of themselves and others, helping clients build successful and enjoyable lives.

Making Connection: The Counseling Relationship
Meeting the Person Apart From the Problem

Narrative counselors generally begin their first session with clients by *meeting the person apart from the problem*: meeting clients as everyday people before learning about the problem (Freedman & Combs, 1996). When meeting a client apart from the problem, narrative counselors ask questions such as the following to familiarize themselves with clients' everyday lives:

Questions for Meeting the Person Apart From the Problem

- What do you do for fun? Do you have hobbies?
- What do you like about living here? What don't you like?
- Tell me about your friends and family.
- What is important to you in life?
- What is a typical weekday like? Weekend?

The answers to these questions enable narrative counselors to know and view their clients much in the same way that clients view themselves: as an everyday person. This brief and seemingly mundane intervention can have profound effects in terms of developing an effective counseling relationship and informing meaningful interventions. In the case study at the end of this chapter, the counselor makes a concerted effort to meet Elan apart from his role in the death of his friend and his alcohol use, both of which have strong, negative social stereotypes, thus helping Elan to feel accepted and valued as a person from the beginning of their relationship.

Separating People From Problems: The Problem Is the Problem

In narrative counseling, the motto is, "The problem is the problem. The person is not the problem" (Winslade & Monk, 1999, p. 2). Once counselors have gotten to know the client apart from the problem and have a clear sense of who the client is as a person, they begin to "meet" the problem in much the same way, keeping their identities separate. The problem—whether depression, anxiety, marital conflict, attention-deficit/hyperactivity disorder, defiance, loneliness, or a breakup—is viewed as a separate entity or situation that is *not* inherent to the person of the client. The attitude is again one of a polite, social "getting-to-know-you" feel.

Questions for "Meeting" the Problem

- When did the problem first enter your life?
- What was going on with you then?
- What were your first impressions of the problem? How have they changed?
- How has your relationship with the problem evolved over time?
- Who else has been affected by the problem?

Narrative counselors can take an adversarial stance (wanting to outwit, outsmart, or evict the problem; White, 2007) or a more compassionate stance (wanting to understand its message and concerns; Gehart & McCollum, 2007) toward the problem.

Optimism and Hope

Because narrative counselors view problems as problems and people as people, they have a deep, abiding optimism and hope for their clients (Monk et al., 1997; Winslade & Monk, 1999). Their hope and optimism are not a sugarcoated, naive wish but instead are derived from their understanding of how problems are formed—through language, relationship, and social discourse—having confidence that their approach can make a difference. Furthermore, by separating people from their problems, they quickly connect with the "best" in the client, reinforcing a sense of hope and optimism.

Coauthor/Coeditor

The role of the counselor is often described as a *coauthor* or *coeditor*, emphasizing that the counselor and client engage in a joint process of constructing meaning (Freedman & Combs, 1996; Monk et al., 1997; White & Epston, 1990). Rather than attempting to offer a "better story," the counselor works alongside the client to generate a more useful narrative. The degree and quality of input on the part of the counselor vary greatly among narrative counselors, and there is a tendency to focus on the sociopolitical aspects of a client's life. In fact, some narrative counselors maintain that counselors should take a stance on broader sociocultural issues of injustice with all clients (Zimmerman & Dickerson, 1996), although this agenda is not shared by all narrative counselors (Monk & Gehart, 2004).

Investigative Reporter

In his later works, White (2007) describes his relationship to problems as that of an *investigative reporter*:

> The form of inquiry that is employed during externalizing conversations can be likened to investigative reporting. The primary goal of investigative reporting is to develop an exposé on the corruption associated with abuse of power and privilege. Although investigative reporters are not politically neutral, the activities of their inquiry do not take them into the domains of problem-solving, of enacting reform, or of engaging indirect power struggles ... their actions usually reflect a relatively "cool" engagement. (pp. 27–28)

Thus, the counselor uses a calm but inquisitive stance when exploring the origins of problems with clients to inspire the clients to develop a better understanding of the larger context of the problem rather than rushing in to fix it.

The Viewing: Case Conceptualization
Problem-Saturated Stories

As clients are talking, narrative counselors listen for the *problem-saturated story* (Freedman & Combs, 1996; White & Epston, 1990), the story in which the "problem" plays the leading role and the client plays a secondary role, generally that of victim. The counselor attends to the ways the problem affects the client at an *individual level* (health, emotions, thoughts, beliefs, identity, relationship with the divine, etc.) and how it affects him or her at a *relational level* (significant other, parents, friends, coworkers, teachers, etc.) as well as how it affects each of these significant others at a personal level. While listening to a client's problem-saturated story, the counselor listens closely for alternative endings and subplots in which the problem is less of a problem and the person is an effective agent in the story; these are referred to as *unique outcomes*.

Unique Outcomes and Sparkling Events

Unique outcomes (White & Epston, 1990) or *sparkling events* (Freedman & Combs, 1996) refer to stories or subplots in which the problem-saturated story does not play out in its typical way: the child cheerfully complies with a parent's request, a couple is able to stop a potential argument from erupting with a soft touch, or a teenager decides to call a friend rather than allow herself to cut. These stories often go unnoticed because they had no dramatic ending or particularly notable outcome that warrants attention, and therefore they are not "storied" in clients' or others' minds. These unique outcomes are used to help clients create the lives they prefer and to develop a more full and accurate account of their and others' identities.

Dominant Cultural and Gender Discourses (see "The Juice")

Narrative counselors listen for dominant cultural and gender themes that have informed the development and perception of a problem (Monk et al., 1997; White & Epston, 1990). The purpose of all discourses is to identify the set of "goods" and "values" that organize social interaction in a particular culture. All cultures are essentially a set of dominant discourses: social rules and values that make it possible for a group of people to meaningfully interact.

Dominant discourses are the societal stories of how life "should" go: for example, to be a "happy" and "good" person, you should get married; get a stable, high-paying job; have kids; get a nice car; buy a house; volunteer at your child's school; and build a white-picket fence. Whether you comply with this vision of happiness, rebel against it, or simply are not even in the game because of social or physical limitations that prevent it, problems can arise in relation to it. In working with clients, narrative counselors listen closely for the dominant discourses that are most directly informing the perception of a problem. In response, they inquire about *local* or *alternative discourses*.

Local and Alternative Discourses: Attending to Client Language and Meaning

Local and *alternative discourses* are those that do not conform to the dominant discourse (White & Epston, 1990): couples who choose not to have children, same-sex relationships, immigrant families wanting to preserve their roots, speaking English as a second language, teen subculture in any society, and so on. The local discourses offer a different set of "goods," "shoulds," and ethical "values" than what is portrayed in the dominant discourse. If we take the case of teens and adults in the same culture, the teens have created a subculture with a different set of "goods," beauty standards, sexual norms, vocabulary, friendship rules, and so on. The teen culture represents an alternative discourse that counselors can tap into to understand the teen's worldview and values as well as explore with the teen how this alternative discourse can successfully coexist with the dominant discourse. Thus, the local discourse provides a resource for generating new ways of viewing the self as well as talking and interacting with others around the problem.

Targeting Change: Goal Setting
Preferred Narratives and Identities

As a postmodern approach, narrative counseling does not include a set of predefined goals that can be used with all clients. Instead, goal setting in narrative counseling is unique to each client. In the broadest sense, the goal of narrative counseling is to help clients enact their *preferred narratives and identities* (Freedman & Combs, 1996). In most cases, enacting preferred narratives and identities involves increasing clients' sense of *agency*, the sense that they influence in the direction of their lives. When identifying these preferred realities, counselors work with clients to develop thoughtfully reflected goals that consider local knowledges rather than simply adopting the values of the dominant culture. During the process of counseling, clients often redefine their preferred narrative to incorporate local knowledges and lessen the influence of dominant discourses. For example, many gay men find that they prefer the gay subculture in one city more than another, highlighting that even within local cultures, there can be multiple variations of local knowledge that a person can choose to connect with. Thus, the key is defining the "preferred" narrative and identity thoughtfully and with intention after considering the impact of dominant and local discourses. This process is often a gradual shift from "make this problem go away" to "I want to create something beautiful/meaningful/great with my/our life/lives."

Examples of Working Phase: Targeting Immediate Symptoms and Presenting Problem

- Reduce frequency of allowing depression to talk client into avoiding pleasurable activities.
- Increase opportunities to interact with friends using "confident, social" self.
- Increase instances of defiance in response to anorexia's directions to not eat.

Examples of Closing Phase: Targeting Personal Identity, Relational Identity, and Expanded Community

- *Personal identity:* Solidify a sense of personal identity that derives self-worth from meaningful activities, relationship, and values rather than body size.
- *Relational identity:* Develop a family identity narrative that allows for greater expression of differences while maintaining family's sense of closeness and loyalty.
- *Expanded community:* Expand preferred "outgoing" identity to social relationships and contexts.

Interventions

Externalizing: Separating the Problem from the Person

The signature technique of narrative counseling, *externalizing* involves conceptually and linguistically separating the person from the problem (Freedman & Combs, 1996; White & Epston, 1990). To be successful, externalization requires a sincere belief that people are separate from their problems; thus, the *attitude* of externalization is key to its effectiveness (Freedman & Combs, 1996). More than a single-session intervention, externalization is an organic and evolving process of shifting the client's perception of their relationship to the problem from "having" it to seeing it outside the self. Counselors can externalize by naming the problem as an external other, switching a descriptive adjective into a noun, such as from a client being depressed to having a relationship with depression. Other times, clients respond better talking about "sides" of themselves or a relationship, such as "the little girl in me who is afraid" or "the competitive side of our relationship."

For externalization to work, it cannot be forced on to the client; rather, it needs to emerge from the dialogue or be introduced as a possibility for how to think about the situation. In most cases, using techniques such as *mapping the influence of persons and problem* (see below) invites a natural, comfortable process for externalizing the problem. Periodically, clients already have a name for the problem and conceptualize the problem as a sort of external entity or very discrete part of themselves, and in such cases counselors need only to build on the externalization process the client has started.

Relative Influence Questioning: Mapping Influence of the Problem and Persons

Relative influence questioning was the first detailed method for externalization (White & Epston, 1990). Used early in counseling, relative influence questioning serves as an assessment and intervention simultaneously and is composed of two parts: (a) mapping the influence of the problem and (b) mapping the influence of persons.

Mapping the Influence of Problems   When mapping the influence of problems, counselors inquire about the ways the problem has affected the life of the client and significant others in the client's life, often *expanding* the reach of the problem beyond how the client generally thinks of it; thus, it is critical that this is followed up by *mapping the influence of person* questions to ensure that the client does not feel worse afterward. Mapping the influence of problems involves asking about how the problem has affected the following:

Mapping the Influence of the Problem

Examine all the ways the problem has affected the client.

- The client at a physical, emotional, and psychological level
- The client's identity story and what he or she tells oneself about his or her worth and who he or she is
- The client's closest relationships: partner, children, parents
- Other relationships in the client's life: friendships, social groups, work/school colleagues, and so on
- The health, identity, emotions, and other relationships of significant people in the client's life (e.g., how parents may pull away from friends because they are embarrassed about a child's problem)

Mapping the Influence of Persons   Mapping the influence of persons begins the external-ization process more explicitly. In this phase of questioning, which should immediately follow *mapping the influence of problems*, involves identifying how the person has affected the life of the problem, reversing the logic of the first series of questions:

Mapping the Influence of Persons

Examine how the client has affected the problem.

- When have the persons involved kept the problem from affecting their mood or how they value themselves as people?
- When have the persons involved kept the problem from allowing them to enjoy special and/or casual relationships in their lives?
- When have the persons involved kept the problem from interrupting their work or school lives?
- When have the persons involved been able to keep the problem from taking over when it was starting?

White and Epston (1990) report the following benefits to externalization:

- Decreases unproductive conflict and blame between family members
- Undermines sense of failure in relation to the problem by highlighting times the persons have had influence over it
- Invites people to unite in a struggle against the problem and reduce its influence
- Identifies new opportunities for reducing the influence of the problem
- Encourages a lighter, less stressed approach to interacting with the problem
- Increases interactive dialogue rather than repetitive monologue about the problem

Externalizing Conversations: The Statement of Position Map

White (2007) describes his more recently developed process for facilitating externalizing conversations, *the statement of position map*. This map includes four categories of inquiry that are used multiple times throughout a session and across sessions to shift the client's relationship with the problem and open new possibilities for action:

Inquiry category 1: Negotiating a particular, experience-near definition of the prob-lem: White begins by defining the problem using the client's language (experience-near) rather than professional or global terms (e.g., a diagnosis). Thus, "feeling blue" is preferred to "depressed."

Inquiry category 2: Mapping the effects of the problem: Similar to his early work (White and Epston, 1990), mapping the effects of problems involves identifying how the problem has affected the various domains of the client's life: home, work, school, and social contexts; relationships with family, friends, and oneself; and one's identity and future possibilities.

Inquiry category 3: Evaluating the effects of the problem's activities: After identifying the effects of the problem, the counselor asks the client to evaluate these effects (White, 2007, p. 44):

- Are these activities okay with you?
- How do you feel about these developments?
- Where do you stand on these outcomes?
- Is the development positive or negative—or both, or neither, or something in between?

Inquiry category 4: Justifying the evaluation: In the final phase, the counselor asks about how and why clients have evaluated the situation the way they did (White, 2007, p. 48):

- Why is/isn't this okay for you?
- Why do you feel this way about this development?
- Why are you taking this stand/position on this development?

These why questions must be offered in a spirit of allowing clients to give voice to what is important to them rather than creating a sense of moral judgment (cont. These questions should open up conversations about what is important to clients, what motivates them, and how they want to shape their identities and futures.

When externalizing using the four above categories, White (2007, p. 32) employs various metaphors for relating to problems:

- Walking out on the problem
- Going on strike against the problem
- Defying the problem's requirements
- Disempowering the problem
- Educating the problem
- Escaping the problem
- Recovering or reclaiming territory from the problem

- Refusing invitations from the problem
- Disproving the problem's claims
- Resigning from the problem's service
- Stealing their lives from the problem
- Taming the problem
- Harnessing the problem
- Undermining the problem

Avoid Totalizing and Dualistic Thinking

White (2007) avoids totalizing descriptions of the problem—the problem being all bad—because such descriptions promote dualistic, either/or thinking, which can be invalidating to the client and/or obscure the problem's broader context. In the case study at the end of this chapter, the counselor uses statement of position maps to enable Elan to clearly define a healthy and desired relationship to alcohol and the accident that killed his friend rather than directly confront him on these issues.

Externalizing Questions

Narrative counselors use *externalizing questions* to help clients build different relationships with their problems (Freedman & Combs, 1996). In most cases, externalizing questions involve changing *adjectives* (e.g., depressed, anxious, angry, etc.) to *nouns* (e.g., Depression, Anxiety, Anger, etc.; capitalization is used to emphasize that the problem is viewed as a separate entity). Externalizing questions *presume* that the person is separate from the problem and that the person has a two-way relationship with the problem: it affects them, and they affect it.

To experience the liberating effects of externalizing, Freedman and Combs (1996, pp. 49–50) have developed the following two set questions: one representing conventional counseling questions and the other externalizing. To do this exercise, choose a quality or trait that you or others find problematic, usually an adjective; substitute this for X in the following questions. Then find a noun form of that trait; substitute this for Y in the following questions. Examples include X = depressed/Y = Depression, X = critical/Y = Criticism, and X = angry/Y = Anger.

Conventional questions (Insert problem description as *adjective* for X)	*Externalizing questions* (Insert problem description as *noun* for Y)
When did you first become X?	What made you vulnerable to the Y so that it was able to dominate your life?
What are you most X about?	In what contexts is the Y most likely to take over?
What kinds of things happen that typically lead to your being X?	What kinds of things happened that typically lead to the Y taking over?
When you are X, what do you do that you wouldn't do if you weren't X?	What has the Y gotten you to do that is against your better judgment?
What are the consequences for your life and relationships of being X?	What effects does the Y have on your life and relationship?
How is your self-image different when you are X?	How has the Y lead you into the difficulties you are now experiencing?

(continued)

If by some miracle you woke up some morning and were not X anymore, how, specifically, would your life be different?	Does the Y blind you from noticing your resources, or can you see them through it?
Are there times when you are not X?	Have there been times when you have been able to get the best of the Y? Times when the Y could have taken over, but you kept it out of the picture?

Problem Deconstruction: Deconstructive Listening and Questions

Based on the philosophical work of Jacques Derrida, narrative counselors use deconstructive listening and questions to help clients trace the effects of dominant discourses and to empower clients to make more conscious choices about which discourses they allow to affect their lives (Freedman & Combs, 1996). *Deconstructive listening* involves the counselor listening for "gaps" in their understanding and asking people to fill in the details or having them explain the ambiguities in their stores. For example, if a client reports feeling rejected because friends did not call when they said they would, the counselor would listen for the meanings that lead to the sense of feeling "rejected."

Deconstructive questions help clients to further "unpack" their stories to see how they have been constructed, identifying the influence of dominant and local discourses. Typically used in externalizing conversations, these questions target problematic beliefs, practices, feelings, and attitudes by asking clients to identify the following:

- The *history of their relationship* with the problematic belief, practice, feeling, or attitude ("When and where did you first encounter the problem?")
- *The contextual influences* on the problematic belief, practice, feeling, or attitude ("When is it most likely to be present?")
- *The effects or results* of the problematic belief, practice, feeling, or attitude ("What effects has this had on you and your relationship?")
- *The interrelationship with other* beliefs, practices, feelings, or attitudes ("Are there other problems that feed this problem?")
- *Tactics and strategies* used by the problem belief, practice, feeling, or attitude ("How does it go about influencing you?")

Mapping in Landscapes of Action and Identity/Consciousness

Based on the narrative theory of Jerome Bruner (1986), "mapping the problem in the landscape of action and identity" (White, 2007) or "consciousness" (Freedman & Combs, 1996) refers to a specific technique for harnessing unique outcomes to promote desired change. Mapping in the landscapes of action and identity generally involves the following steps:

1. *Identify a unique outcome:* Listen for and ask about times when the problem could have been a problem but it was not.
2. *Ensure that the unique outcome is preferred:* Rather than assume, ask clients about whether the unique outcome is a preferred outcome: is this something you want to do or have happen more often?
3. *Map in landscape of action:* First, the counselor begins by mapping the unique outcome in the landscape of action, identifying what actions were taken by whom in which order. The counselor does this by asking specific details: What did you do first? How did the other person respond? What did you do next? The counselor carefully plots the events until there is a step-by-step picture of the actions of the client and involved others, gathering details about the following:
   - Critical events
   - Circumstances surrounding events
   - Sequence of events

- Timing of events
- Overall plot

4. *Mapping in the landscape of identity/consciousness:* After obtaining a clear picture of what happened during the unique outcome, the counselor begins a process of mapping in the landscape of identity. This phase of mapping *thickens the plot* associated with the successful outcome, thus directly strengthening the connection of the preferred outcome with the client's personal identity. Mapping in the landscape of identity focuses on the psychological and relational implications of the unique outcomes. Areas of impact include the following:

- What do you believe this says about you as a person? About your relationship?
- What were your intentions behind these actions?
- What do you value most about your actions here?
- What, if anything, did you learn or realize from this?
- Does this change how you see life/God/your purpose/your life goals?
- Does this affect how you see the problem?

Intentional Versus Internal State Questions

White (2007) privileges *intentional* state questions (questions about a person's intentions in a given situation: "What were your intentions?") over *internal* state questions (questions about how a person was feeling or thinking: "What were you feeling?") because intentional state questions promote a sense of *personal agency*, whereas internal state questions can have the effect of diminishing one's sense of agency, increasing one's sense of isolation, and discouraging diversity.

Scaffolding Conversations

White (2007) uses *scaffolding conversations* to move clients from that which is familiar to that which is novel using developmental psychologist Vygotsky's concept of *zones of proximal development*. Vygotsky emphasized that learning is inherently relational, requiring adults to structure the child's learning in ways that make it possible for them to interact with new information. The "zone of proximal development" is the distance between what the child can do independently and what the child can do in collaboration with others. "Scaffolding" is a term that White developed to describe five incremental and progress movements across this zone of learning with clients:

- *Low-level distancing tasks: Characterizing a unique outcome:* Tasks that are at a low level of distance and very close to what is familiar to the client, encouraging the attribution of meanings to events that have gone unnoticed
- *Medium-level distancing tasks: Unique outcomes taken into a chain of association:* Tasks that introduce greater "newness," encouraging greater comparison and categorization of difference and similarity
- *Medium- to high-level distancing tasks: Reflection on chain of associations:* Tasks that encourage clients to reflect on, evaluate, and learn from the differences and similarities
- *High-level distancing tasks: Abstract learning and realizations:* Tasks that require clients to assume a high level of distance from their immediate experience, promoting increased abstract conceptualization of life and identity
- *Very high-level distancing tasks: Plans for action:* Tasks that promote a high-level distancing from immediate experience to enable clients to identify ways of enacting their newly developed concepts about life and identity.

Over the course of a conversation, counselor move back and forth between various levels of distancing tasks, progressively moving to higher levels of action planning. In the case study at the end of this chapter, scaffolding questions are used to gently move Elan from noticing one exception of not drinking to developing concrete and motivating action plans for managing his drinking.

Permission Questions

Narrative counselors use permission questions to emphasize the democratic nature of the counseling relationship and to encourage clients to maintain a strong and clear sense of agency when talking with the counselor. Quite simply, permission questions are questions that counselors use to ask permission to ask a question. This goes against the prevailing assumptions that counselors can ask any question they want to gather information they purportedly need to be helpful to the client. Socially, counselors are exempt from the prevailing social norms of polite conversation topics and **are free to** bring up taboo subjects such as sex, past abuse, relationship problems, death, **fears, and** weaknesses. Many clients feel compelled to answer these questions even if they are **not** comfortable doing so. Narrative counselors are sensitive to the power dynamic related to taboo and difficult subjects and therefore *ask for client's permission* before asking questions that are generally taboo or that the counselor anticipates will make this particular client feel uncomfortable. For example, "Would it be okay if I ask you some questions about your sex life?"

In addition, permission questions are used throughout the interview related to *what* is being discussed and *how* to ensure that the conversation is meaningful and comfortable for the client. For example, often when starting a session, the counselor may briefly outline his ideas for how to use the time, asking for client input and permission to continue with a particular topic or line of questioning. Similarly, in a situation when the counselor finds herself asking one person more questions than the others in a family session, she would pause to ask permission to continue to ensure that everyone was okay with what was going on.

Situating Comments

Similar to permission questions, *situating comments* are used to maintain a more democratic counseling relationship and reinforce client agency by ensuring that comments from the counselor are not taken as a "higher" or "more valid" truth than the client's (Zimmerman & Dickerson, 1996). Drawing on the distinction between dominant and local discourses, narrative counselors are keenly aware that any comment made by the counselor is often considered more "valid" than anything the client might say. Thus, counselors *situate* their comments by revealing the source of the perspective they are offering, emphasizing that it is only one perspective among others. By revealing the source and context of a comment, a client is less likely to overprivilege counselor comments.

Counselor Comment Without Situating	Situating Counselor Comment
I am noticing that you tend to ...	Having grown up on a farm, my attention is of course drawn to ...
Research indicates that ...	There is one counselor who has developed a theory/done a study that suggests ... Does this sound like something that would be true for you?
I suggest that you ...	Since you are asking me for a suggestion, I can only tell you what I think as someone who believes that action is more productive than talk ...

Narrative Reflecting Team Practices

Based on Tom Andersen's collaborative practice of reflecting teams (see Tom Andersen), narrative counselors have developed similar practice that supports their work. Using Andersen's format, Freedman and Combs (1996) assign the team the *three primary tasks*:

1. Develop a thorough understanding by closely attending to details of the story
2. Listen for differences and events that do not fit the dominant problem-saturated narrative
3. Notice beliefs, ideas, or contexts that support the problem-saturated descriptions

In addition, they propose the following *guidelines* for the team:

1. During the reflecting process, the reflecting team members participate together in a back-and-forth conversation rather than in a monologue.
2. Team members should not talk to each other while observing the interview.
3. Comments should be offered in a tentative manner (e.g., "perhaps," "could," "might," etc.).
4. Comments are based on what actually occurs in the room (e.g., "At one point Mom got very quiet; I was wondering what was going on for her at that moment").
5. Comments are situated in the speaker's personal experience when appropriate (e.g., "Having been a teacher, I may have been the only one who focused on this ...").
6. All family members should be responded to in some way.
7. Reflections should be kept short.

Leagues

As a means of solidifying the new narrative and identities, narrative counselors have created *leagues* (or clubs, associations, teams, etc.), membership to which signifies an accomplishment in a particular area. In most cases, leagues are virtual communities of concern (e.g., giving a child a membership certificate to the Temper Tamer's Club), although some meet face-to-face or interact via the Internet (Anti-Anorexia/Anti-Bulima League; see www.narrativetherapy.com).

Letters and Certificates

Narrative letters are used to develop and solidify preferred narratives and identities (White & Epston, 1990). Counselors can write *letters* detailing a client's emerging story after sessions in lieu of doing case notes (unless you work in a practice environment that requires a specific format). Narrative letters use the same techniques used in session to reinforce the emerging narrative and are characterized by the following:

- *Emphasizing client agency:* Highlighting client agency in their lives, including small steps in becoming proactive.
- *Taking observer position:* The counselor clearly takes the role of *observing* the changes the client is making, citing specific, concrete examples whenever possible.
- *Highlighting temporality:* The time dimension is used to plot the emerging story: where clients began, where they are now, and where they are likely to go.
- *Encouraging polysemy:* Rather than propose singular interpretations, multiple meanings are entertained and encouraged.

Letters can be used early in counseling to engage clients, during counseling to reinforce the emerging narrative and reinforce new preferred behaviors, or at the end of counseling to consolidate gains by narrating the change process.

Sample Letter   White and Epston (1990) offer numerous sample letters, such as the following:

> Dear Rick and Harriet,
>
> I'm sure that you are familiar with the fact that the best ideas have the habit of presenting themselves after the event. So it will come as no surprise to you that I often think of the most important questions after the end of an interview.... Anyway, I thought I would share a couple of important questions that came to me after you left our last meeting: Rick, how did you decline Helen's [the daughter] invitation to you to do the reasoning for her? And how do you think this could have the effect of inviting her to reason with herself? Do you think this could help her to become more responsible? Harriet, how did you decline Helen's invitations to you to be dependable for her? And how do you think this could have the effect of inviting her to depend upon herself more? Do you think that this could have the effect of helping her to take better care of her life? What does this increased vulnerability to Helen's invitations to have life for her reflect in you both as people? By the way, what ideas occurred to you after our last meeting? M.W. (pp. 109–110)

Certificates

Certificates are used often with children to recognize the changes they have made and to reinforce their new "reputation" as a "temper tamer," "cooperative child," and so on.

Certified Temper Tamer

This is to certify that

_____

has proven himself as a skilled Tamer of Tempers,

having gone two months without temper problems at home or school

using the following taming techniques that he developed for himself:

1. Asking for help when confused

2. Taking three deep breathes when the scent of Temper appears

3. Using soft words to talk about anger and frustration

Date of award: _____

Witnessed by: _____ (counselor)

_____ (parents)

_____ (teacher)

Putting It All Together: Narrative Treatment Plan Template

Use this treatment plan template for developing a plan for clients with depressive, anxious, or compulsive types of presenting problems. Depending on the specific client, presenting problem, and clinical context, the goals and interventions in this template may need to be modified only slightly or significantly; you are encouraged to significantly revise the plan as needed. For the plan to be useful, goals and techniques should be written to target specific beliefs, behaviors, and emotions that the client is experiencing. The more specific, the more useful it will be to you.

Treatment Plan

Initial Phase of Treatment (First One to Three Sessions)
Initial Phase Counseling Tasks

1. *Develop working counseling relationship. Diversity note:* Include significant persons in client's life, including friends, family, and so on.
   Relationship building intervention:
   a. Meet the **person apart from the problem** to generate **hope**.

2. *Assess individual, systemic, and broader cultural dynamics. Diversity note:* Invite significant friends and family for assessment session(s).
   Assessment Strategies:
   a. **Relative influence questioning** and **deconstructive questions** to identify effects of problem and effects of person, noting key **dominant** and **local discourses**.

(continued)

b. Identify **unique outcomes** and **sparkling moments** that do not conform to problem-saturated narrative.

Initial Phase Client Goals *(One to Two Goals):* Manage crisis issues and/or reduce most distressing symptoms

1. *Increase* the client's ability **resist invitations** to engage in [crisis behavior] to reduce [crisis symptom(s)].
    Interventions:
    a. **Relative influence questioning** to identify how client is "enticed" to engage in crisis behavior as well as times when the client resists these invitations.
    b. **Statement of position map** to identify client's desired "position" in relation to crisis behaviors; identify strategies, persons, and contexts that support the desired position.

Working Phase of Treatment (Two or More Sessions)
Working Phase Counseling Task

1. *Monitor quality of the working alliance. Diversity note:* Adapt alliance to meet client's needs.
    Assessment Intervention:
    a. Use **situating comments** and **permission questions** to situate counselor as **coeditor/investigative reporter**; regularly check in with client about alliance; use Session Rating Scale.

Working Phase Client Goals *(Two to Three Goals).* Target individual and relational dynamics using theoretical language (e.g., decrease avoidance of intimacy, increase awareness of emotion, increase agency, etc.)

1. *Increase* client's sense of **separation from** and **agency in relation to [the problem]** to reduce [specific symptoms: depression, anxiety, etc.].
    Interventions:
    a. **Externalizing questions** to separate client's identity from problem-saturated story.
    b. **Statement of position map** and **relative influence questioning** to externalize problem.

2. *Increase* frequency of [specific behavior] that supports the client's **preferred reality** to reduce [specific symptoms: depression, anxiety, etc.].
    Interventions:
    a. **Mapping in the landscapes of action and consciousness** to identify specific behaviors that support change.
    b. **Scaffolding questions** to help client move toward a new relationship with the problem.

3. *Increase* frequency of [specific behavior] that supports the client's **preferred reality** to reduce [specific symptoms: depression, anxiety, etc.].
    Interventions:
    a. **Mapping in the landscapes of action and consciousness** to identify specific behaviors that support change.
    b. **Scaffolding questions** to help client move toward a new relationship with the problem.

Closing Phase of Treatment (Last Two or More Sessions)
Closing Phase Counseling Task

1. *Develop aftercare plan and maintain gains. Diversity note:* Involve significant others when possible.
    Intervention:
    a. Use **mapping in the landscape of action and consciousness** questions to help clients identify how they can resist invitations from the presenting problem and similar problems in the future.

(continued)

Closing Phase Client Goals *(One to Two Goals):* Determined by theory's definition of health and normalcy

1. *Increase* and **thicken the plot** around the client's **new sense of identity** and **agency** in relation to the problem to reduce [specific symptoms: depression, anxiety, etc.].
   a. **Scaffolding question** to develop action plans to bolster and sustain new identity.
   b. **Landscape of action and consciousness questions** to thicken new narratives that capture the outer and inner experience of client's preferred reality.

2. *Increase* **involvement of significant persons** in client's life to **witness and support new identity narrative** and new relationship to the problem to reduce [specific symptoms: depression, anxiety, etc.].
   Interventions:
   a. **Invite significant persons, leagues, and/or reflecting teams to session** to witness changes and identify ways to support client.
   b. **Certificates, letters, and other written documents** to solidify new identity and preferred narrative.

Collaborative Language Systems and Reflecting Teams

In a Nutshell: The Least You Need to Know

Putting postmodern, social constructionist principles into action, collaborative counseling is a two-way dialogical process in which counselors and clients coexplore and cocreate new and more useful understandings related to client problems and agency. Eschewing scripted techniques, counselors focus on the *process* of counseling, namely, *how* what is of concern and importance to the client is explored and exchanged. As clients share their concerns, counselors listen for *how* the client interprets the events of their lives, responding by asking questions that naturally emerge from the conversation to better understand how the client's story "hangs together": the values and internal logic make the client's perspective make sense. As the counselor tries to understand the client *from within the client's worldview*, the client is naturally invited to share in the counselor's curiosity, joining in a process of shared inquiry—*mutual puzzling*—as to how things came to be and how things might best move forward. By asking questions and tentatively sharing their perspectives and as counselor and client engaged in the shared inquiry, alternative views and future options emerge on the client's situation. This process of mutual exploring and wondering provides an opportunity for clients to see their situation differently, allowing them to make new interpretations and develop fresh ideas. The counselor does not try to control or direct the content of this meaning-making process; instead, they honor the client's agency in determining what to do with these new ideas.

I am guessing this process still sounds a bit vague, so perhaps it is best to offer an example. If a client says she is feeling "depressed," rather than hear concrete, diagnostic information, collaborative counselors are profoundly aware of how little they know about *this* client's unique experience of depression, thus becoming sincerely curious as to how the client came to this understanding of her experience. With no predetermined set of questions, the counselor asks questions that emerge from a genuine desire to better understand, such as Does she cry often about something? About nothing? Has life gone to gray and nothing seems interesting anymore? Is her heart broken? Does she feel like a failure? There are as many unique depression stories as there are people who say they are depressed. As the counselor explores the client's view, asking questions such as the ones above, the client is invited to join in the curiosity about her depression. Each new understanding related to depression informs alternative actions, thoughts, and feelings, thus shifting experience on multiple levels until the client has found a way to manage or resolve her initial concern.

The Juice: Significant Contributions to the Field

If you remember one thing from this chapter, it should be …

Not Knowing and Knowing With

Goolishian and Anderson (1987) first introduced the idea of not knowing perhaps one of the most frequently misunderstood concepts in the collaborative approach (Anderson, 2005), in 1988. At first blush, the *not-knowing stance* sounds ironic: how can a paid professional like a counselor "not know"? Isn't that what they are paid for? What do you do with all that you have learned? Does this mean you don't have to study for the final exam? Unfortunately, no.

Not knowing refers to how counselors think about what they (think they) know and the intent with which they introduce this knowing (expertise, truths, etc.) to the client. Obviously, collaborative counselors have a very particular type of knowing they are avoiding, what Anderson refers to as "pre-knowing" (Anderson, 2007). It's the type of knowing that in the vernacular is called *assuming*, believing that you can fill in the gaps or that you have enough information without sufficient evidence. Based on a postmodern social constructionist epistemology, collaborative counselors maintain that clients with apparently similar experiences, such as "psychosis," "mania," or "sexual abuse," have unique understandings of their situations (Anderson, 1997). Each client's understanding has evolved through conversations with significant others, acquaintances, professionals, strangers, as well as the larger societal discourse and stories in the media and literature. Counselors choose to *know with* and *alongside* clients as they engage in a process of better understanding clients' lives (Anderson, 2007). Counselors view the client's knowledge as equally valid with their own.

This not-knowing, not-assuming stance requires the counselor ask what on the surface appear as either obvious or trivial questions: "You say you are sad about the loss of your mother; can you tell me what aspects of her loss touch you most deeply?" or "Tell me how you experience that sadness in your daily life." When clients begin to explore alongside the counselor the ideas, experiences, and influences that lead to the perception of a problem, they often hear themselves saying things they have never told anyone before. Hearing these thoughts aloud for the first time inevitably shifts their perspective of the situations, sometimes subtly and sometimes dramatically. These new perspectives inherently inform new action and identities related to the problem (e.g., from viewing her mother as an entirely separate person, the client may shift to seeing that she is part of how her mother lives on).

Rumor Has It: The People and Their Stories
Harlene Anderson and Harry Goolishian

Harlene Anderson and Harry Goolishian developed collaborative language systems with their colleagues at the University of Texas Medical Branch in Galveston and later the Houston-Galveston Institute (Anderson, 1997, 2005, 2007). Their collaborative approach has its roots in the early model developed by the Galveston group called multiple impact therapy, a multidisciplinary approach to working with hospitalized adolescents, their families, and broader social system. Initially their work at the Galveston Medical Center was based on the systemic ideas from the Mental Research Institute (MRI, see Chapter 10). However, over time they began to listen differently to what clients were saying rather than trying to learn the clients' language to use it as a strategic tool. They noticed that rather than the *family* having its own unique language, each *member* of the family seemed to have his or her own language, using words and phrases with unique meanings.

They became increasingly interested in hermeneutics, social constructionism, and postmodern ideas, including Lyotard's postmodern ideas, Berger and Luckman's social construction theory, and to the work of others, particularly Ludvig Wittgenstein, Mikhail Bahktin, Ken Gergen, and John Shotter; they began to conceptualize their work from a postmodern perspective, focusing on the construction of meaning in relationships. In addition, they had a mutually influencing relationship with Tom Andersen over the years. Over time, their counseling has been referred to as collaborative language systems (Anderson, 1997) and more recently collaborative therapy (Anderson & Gehart, 2007). After Harry's death in 1991, Harlene and her colleagues at the Houston Galveston Institute have continued developing this internationally practiced approach. Ken Gergen, Harlene Anderson, Sheila McNamee, and others joined together to form the Taos Institute, an organization of collaborative practitioners working in the fields of education, business, consultation, counseling, medicine, and other disciplines. Having found that the assumptions on which collaborative language system is based have applications beyond counseling systems, Harlene currently refers to her work as collaborative practices.

Tom Andersen

No relation other than a close friend to Harlene (note the "e" vs. "o" in Andersen), Tom Andersen is a Norwegian psychiatrist who is best remembered for his gentle demeanor, his respect for client privacy, and his elegant theory. Having originally studied with the Milan team using one-way mirrors, Tom transformed the systemic practice of the observation team using postmodern sensibilities that reduced the team–client hierarchy and made the process a dialogic rather than strategic one. His description of *inner and outer dialogues* as well as *appropriately unusual comments* provide collaborative counselors with very practical concepts that can be used to facilitate counseling conversations without the use of technique.

Lynn Hoffman

Known for her keen theoretical insights and broad vision, Lynn Hoffman has worked closely with many of family therapy's most influential thinkers, including Virginia Satir, Jay Haley, Paul Watzlawick, Salvador Minuchin, Dick Auserwald, Gianfranco Cecchin, Luigi Boscolo, Tom Andersen, Harlene Anderson, and Peggy Penn. Her first book, *Foundations in Family Therapy* (Hoffman, 1981), provides one of the most comprehensive overviews of systemic family counseling available. She began learning about family approaches at MRI, serving as an editor for Satir's books. She was so inspired by the ideas that she went on to pursue a career as a social worker, training in systemic family therapies. She befriended the Milan team and along with Peggy Penn helped further their later development of the model (Boscolo, Cecchin, Hoffman, & Penn, 1987). In her later years, she became increasingly attracted to postmodern, collaborative approaches (Hoffman, 2001). She has detailed her remarkable journey in *Family Therapy: An Intimate History* (Hoffman, 2001), a favorite with my students who want to learn about the theories of family counseling yet prefer a little more "juice" and excitement than is offered in a textbook such as this.

Peggy Penn

A former training director of the Ackerman Institute and published poet (Penn, 2002), Peggy Penn has developed unique approaches to using writing in collaborative language systems (Penn, 2001; Penn & Frankfurt, 1994; Penn & Sheinberg, 1991). Like Hoffman, Peggy began her training in systemic therapies, most notably the Milan approach (Boscolo et al., 1987), but her work has since evolved to a more postmodern approach. She uses various forms of writing in counseling to help clients access multiple voices and perspectives.

Jaakko Seikkula

Psychologist Jaakko Seikkula and his colleagues (Haarakangas, Seikkula, Alakare, & Aaltonen, 2007) have developed and researched the open dialogue approach to working with patients having psychotic symptoms in Finland. Since instituting this collaborative approach for working with psychosis over 20 years ago, there are no longer chronic cases of psychosis in the Lapland region of Finland served by their hospital, with patients with psychotic symptoms needing fewer medications and returning to work at a higher rate. Jaakko's research provides some of the best empirical evidence for postmodern therapies.

Big Picture: Overview of Counseling Process

Collaborative counselors do not have set stages of counseling or an outline for how to conduct a session. Instead, they use a single guiding principle: facilitate *collaborative relationships and generative, two-way dialogical conversations*, regardless of topic and participants. In short: keep the dialogue going. The key to facilitating dialogue is avoiding monologues.

Avoiding Monologues and Impasse

Harry Goolishian often said that it is easier to identify what *not* to do as a counselor than what to do. Extending this logic, collaborative approaches are often easier to understand by identifying what is *not* a collaborative conversation, which is namely a *monologue* (Anderson, 1997, 2007). A monologue can be an out-loud conversation with others or a silent conversation with oneself or imagined other. A spoken monological conversation consists of two people trying to sell their idea to the other person: a duel of realities. In a monological conversation, participants listen only long enough to plan their next defense—they are not trying to understand the other out of genuine interest. In silent conversations, monologue refers to the same description, opinion, and so on consistently occupying one's thoughts, leaving no room for new ones or curiosity and being closed to the other.

In counseling, monological conversations lead to a *therapeutic impasse*, at which point the counseling discussion no longer generates useful meanings or understandings. For most, it is easy to identify monological conversations because there is a tension and the sense that the conversational task is to convince the other of a particular point. In addition, counselors may begin to have pejorative descriptions of clients such as "resistant." When this happens—whether between counselor and client or between any two people in the room—the counselor's job is to gently shift the conversation back to a dialogical exchange of ideas. Counselors can achieve this by shifting back into a curious stance—asking to better understand the client's perspective or to inquire if there is a particular point that the client thinks the counselor is not fully understanding. However, for a counselor to reengage others in dialogue, the counselor must be in an internal dialogic mode himself or herself. In the simplest terms, a collaborative counselor's primary job is to ensure that the conversations in the room—whether between members of the client system or between the counselor and the client—do not become dueling monologues. As long as conversations are dialogical, change and transformation are inevitable.

Making Connection: Counseling Relationship
Philosophic Stance

Collaborative counselors conceptualize counselors' position as a *philosophical stance*, which refers to their particular *way of being in relation with others*. Counselors' philosophical stance informs how they speak, think about, act with, and respond in session. The philosophical stance focuses counselors' attention on the *person* of the client, shifting attention away from roles and functions. The philosophical stance essentially encompasses a sincere embodiment of the postmodern, social constructionist ideas that inform the collaborative approach, such as viewing the client as expert and valuing the transformative process of dialogue.

Conversational Partners: "Withness"

The counseling relationship in collaborative language systems is best described as a *conversational partnership* (Anderson, 1997). It is fundamentally a process of being *with* the client, respecting the client's knowledge and expertise, and responding in a collaborative and dialogical mode. This way of relating is sometimes referred to as "*withness*" (Hoffman, 2007), where the conversational partners "touch" one another, their understandings, and meanings *in* their responsive expressions. Withness also involves a willingness to go along for the roller-coaster "ride" (Anderson, 1993)—the ups and downs—of the client's transformational process regardless of how uncomfortable, unpredictable, or scary it may be—a palpable commitment to walk alongside the client no matter where the journey leads.

Curiosity: The Art of Not Knowing

A hallmark of the collaborative counseling stance (Anderson, 1997), "curiosity" refers to the counselor's sincere interest in client's unique life experiences and the meanings that are generated from these experiences. The curiosity of a collaborative counselor is fueled by a *social constructionist epistemology* (assumptions about knowledge and how we know what we know), which posits that each person constructs a unique reality formed in the webs of relationships and conversations in which they are engaged. Thus, no two people experience marriage, parenting, depression, psychosis, or anxiety the same: each has unique experiences and meanings that constitute his or her lived reality of the situation.

Client and Counselor Expertise

In 1992, Anderson and Goolishian radically proposed, "The client is the expert." Although sometimes misunderstood to mean that the counselor has no opinion and no role in the process whatsoever, the concept of "client as expert" helps focus the counselor's attention on sincerely valuing the clients' thoughts, ideas, and opinions about their lives. Clients are viewed as being the experts on their lives because counselors ultimately have very limited information about the fullness and complexity of clients' lives, whereas clients have a more complete history and "insider" perspective that counselors can never acquire to the same degree (Anderson, 1997). Thus, the concept of "client as expert" is more about the general attitude of deep, personal respect for the client than a description of how the counseling process is conducted.

In terms of in-session process, the counselor is considered to have the greater expertise, meaning that the counselor is responsible for ensuring that an effective and respectful dialogical conversation is conducted. The counselor is responsible for the quality of the dialogue, relying on the generative quality of the conversation to support client transformation rather than the counselor dictating the content, direction, or outcome of the conversation.

In broad strokes (which are always inaccurate), it may be helpful in the beginning to think of the client as holding more expertise in the area of *content* (what needs to be talked about) and the counselor as holding more expertise in the area *process* (how things are talked about); however, as a *collaborative process*, both counselor and client have input on both content and process. If the counselor believes that the client is not addressing an important area of content, a collaborative counselor would nonhierarchically raise the issue: "I know you prefer not to talk about the past, but I wonder if it might not be worthwhile to spend a little time exploring how your childhood abuse affects your marriage today." Such a comment is offered in such a way that the client feels truly free to say yes or no, and the counselor honors the client's wishes.

Conversely, the counselor is also open to client feedback about the counseling process, allowing client input on which processes work best for them, including who is in the room, the pacing, the types of homework/suggestion, the types of questions, and so on. The counselor does not necessarily take the client's request as a dictate for how to do counseling, but the counselor thoughtfully considers the request and the need that underlies it and works to find ways to address it as best as possible. This back-and-forth exchange is a sincere partnership in which the counselor works side by side with the client to find useful ways of talking. Anderson (1997) talks about this continual openness to client feedback as "research as part of everyday practice." The counselor uses the feedback from the client and what is developed in discussion about it to fine-tune the counseling process as they go along in counseling, lessening the opportunity for a counseling impasse and ensuring that counseling is tailored to each client and his or her unique needs.

Everyday, Ordinary Language: A Democratic Relationship

Collaborative counselors listen, hear, and speak in a natural, down-to-earth way that is more congruent with the client's language and more *democratic* than hierarchical (Andersen, 1991; Anderson, 2007). Although they are responsible for facilitating a dialogical process that clients find useful, they do not approach the task from a position of leadership or expertise. Instead, they assume a more humble position, using everyday language, a relaxed style, and a willingness to learn that invites clients to join them in a joint exploration of how best to proceed.

Inner and Outer Talk

Tom Andersen conceptualized conversations as involving both *inner and outer talk* (Andersen, 2007). In a conversation, we most quickly recognize the *outer talk*, the verbally spoken conversation between the counseling participants. Andersen also recognized that there were other dialogues going on, namely, *inner talk*, the thoughts and conversations each person has within while participating in a conversation. Thus, if the counselor is working with one client, there are at least three conversations that are simultaneously occurring: (a) the client's inner dialogue, (b) the counselor's inner dialogue, and (c) the outer spoken dialogue. The counselor needs to allow space and time for each one of these conversations.

The counselor allows space for clients to engage in their inner dialogues because, as Andersen (2007) pointed out, when clients are speaking, they are speaking not only to the counselor but also, more important, *to themselves*. Often in counseling, clients are saying something aloud for the first time, and they may need time to reflect on the weight or unexpected content of what they hear themselves saying to the counselor. Andersen strongly admonished counselors to not pressure clients to share their inner dialogue, as is common in some traditional counseling approaches. Thus, if a client did not want to speak about her sexual abuse or a difficult relationship, the counselor does not force the issue but instead leaves an open invitation for the client to speak about it when ready. Rare in the field of counseling, Andersen was a champion for client privacy and autonomy *in session*, which was fueled by an abiding faith that clients have the abilities to navigate their lives in a way that works best for them.

In addition to tracking the outer dialogue with the client, Andersen encouraged counselors to track their inner dialogues: their thoughts, feelings, and reactions to the client and outer dialogue. The counselor's inner dialogue provides many forms of information that can facilitate the counseling relationship: the counselor's reaction to the client may provide information about how others are relating to the client, or it may indicate that the counselor is reacting to the client based on personal history or issues rather than professional knowledge. The counselor's inner dialogue might also include insights, ideas, or metaphors that might further the outer dialogue.

In cases where the counselor's inner dialogue is distracting from the outer conversation, the counselor is encouraged to bring up the issue with the client if doing so furthers the dialogue in useful ways (Anderson, 1997). For example, if a client is talking and continually minimizes the role of alcohol in his pattern of one-night stands and yet in each incident the counselor notices there is a clear link, the counselor can *gently* put forth her observation while verbally and nonverbally giving permission for the client to maintain his opinion without feeling as if the relationship is threatened (e.g., "I know from past conversations you don't think there is a link here, but I want to say that I keep seeing a link between your nights out partying and getting into these relationships you later regret. If you do not see alcohol as the main cause, is there a minor role it might be playing?"). The key is to offer the perspective in such a way that invites curiosity rather than defensiveness.

The Viewing: Case Conceptualization

Case conceptualization in collaborative language systems involves two key questions:

- *Who* is talking about the problem?
- *How* does each understand the problem?

Counselors answer the first by assessing who is in the *problem-organizing system*, or who is in conversation with whom and about what. The second question is approached using the counselor's *philosophical stance* to understand the client's worldview.

Who's Talking? Problem-Organizing, Problem-Dissolving Systems

Anderson and Goolishian (1988, 1992) initially conceptualized counseling systems as *linguistic systems* that organize around the identification of a problem: counselors and clients come together because someone has identified a problem, issue, or concern; the word "problem" may not always be explicitly used by the client. They referred to these systems as *problem-organizing, problem-dissolving systems.* Counseling systems are *problem organizing*, coming into being only after someone has identified a problem. Counseling systems are *problem dissolving* in that they *dissolve* when the participants—counselors, clients, and interested third parties—no longer have a problem to discuss. Additionally, "dissolving" refers to the idea that the problem often is not "solved" in the traditional sense of finding a solution. Instead, the participants' understandings *evolve* through dialogue, allowing for new thoughts, feelings, and actions. In the end, the client may not feel that the problem was "solved" as much as it dissolved. For example, if a client initially reports feeling stressed because of a recent breakup, the problem is not "solved"; rather, the client comes to interpret the situation differently and therefore acts and feels differently.

Aware that all persons talking about the problem are part of the *problem-organizing, problem-dissolving system*, collaborative counselors ask about the following:

Assessing The Problem-Organizing, Problem-Dissolving System

- Who is talking about the problem in session and outside of session?
- How does each define it?
- What does each think should be done about it?

As the understanding of the problem shifts and evolves through dialogue, the counselor continually assesses who is involved in talking about it outside of session and inquiring about the multiple perspectives about the problem, encouraging all perspectives to be heard without trying to reconcile them or identify the "truth." By allowing multiple, contradictory perspectives to constantly linger in the air, clients and counselors are most likely to generate new and more useful perspectives. Thus, in the case study at the end of this chapter, the counselor seeks to understand not only the identified patient's perspective, the teen, but also her siblings, mother, mother's girlfriend, teachers, school counselor, and friends.

Philosophical Stance: Social Constructionist Viewing

Collaborative counselors' primary "tool" in counseling is not a technique or intervention but a system of viewing, their *philosophical stance* (Anderson, 1997). Collaborative counselors work from a social constructionist, postmodern perspective, which maintains that our realities are constructed in language and through relationships. Rather than seeing identities and meanings as fixed, social constructionism describes how we engage in a constant process of revising and reinterpreting our personal identities and social realities by the way we tell ourselves about what it means to be "a good person," "happy," "successful," "cared for," "living a meaningful life," "respected," and so on. These stories are shaped by conversations with friends, news stories, fiction pieces, and any exchange of ideas, whether in person or through media. The counselor's philosophical stance informs a curiosity about how clients construct their understandings of the world rather than determining how clients are "incorrect" or "off" compared to the counselor's preferred psychological theory. Thus, the counselor's focus is always on *how clients construct meaning about the events in their lives.*

Assessing the Client's Worldview

When talking with clients, collaborative counselors focus on better understanding clients' worldview, their system for interpreting the events of their lives. Grounded in a social constructionist perspective, counselors do not approach a client's worldview looking for "errors" or even "the source of the problem"; rather, they approach clients with a gentle, nonjudging curiosity, much like a child exploring a tide pool for the first time, careful not to crush the intriguing creatures in this fascinating new world (Anderson, 1997; Hoffman, 2007). In exploring the client's worldview, the counselor is looking not for right or wrong but rather for the internal logic that makes the client's world, hopes, problems, and symptoms make sense. For example, if a woman is feeling as though her marriage is failing, how did she first get this idea? How did she respond? How did she make sense of her partner's changing behaviors and her own? What does she fear it says about her as a person? What does she think happened, and what does she see as the options from here? Why did her marriage work up until now, and what would it take to get it back to where it was or better? Such questions would not be in the counselor's tool bag; rather, they would be responses that remain congruent with the conversation at any point. "Assessment" in collaborative language systems is a continuous "coassessment." It is not separate from the conversational process and involves exploring questions and curiosities to understand how the client constructs her understanding of the issues and potentials for moving forward.

Targeting Change: Goal Setting
Self-Agency

Like other postmodern approaches, collaborative counselors do not have a predefined model of health to which they steer all clients in cookie-cutter fashion. Instead, the overall goal of collaborative language systems is to increase clients' sense of *agency* in their lives: the sense that they are competent and able to take meaningful action. Anderson (1997) believes that *agency* is inherent in everyone and can only be *self-accessed*, not given to by someone else, as is implied in the concept of client "empowerment"; instead, collaborative counselors see their role as participating in a process that maximizes the opportunities for agency to emerge in clients.

Transformation

Rather than conceptualizing the output of counseling as "change," collaborative counselors conceptualize the process as *transformation*, emphasizing that some "original" aspects remain while other aspects are added or diminished. In counseling, clients' narrative of self-identity, who they tell themselves they are, is transformed through the dialogical process, opening new possibilities for meaning, relating to others, and future action. This transformational process is not controlled or directed by the counselor but emerges from within clients as they listen to themselves, the counselor, and others share their ideas, thoughts, and hopes.

Similar to feminists, collaborative counselors maintain that the process of transformation through dialogue is inherently and inescapably *mutual*. When counselors participate in dialogical conversations, they risk being changed themselves because the same dialogical process that allows clients to change creates a context in which the counselor will also be transformed (Anderson, 1997). The counselor's transformation may not be as dramatic or immediately evident, but by engaging in a sincere two-way exchange of ideas, the worldview of counselors inevitably evolves and shifts as they learn from their clients about other ways to make sense of and engage life.

Setting Collaborative Goals

As the name implies, counseling goals that would be included in a treatment plan are constructed *collaboratively* with clients using their everyday language rather than professional terms. In collaborative language systems, goals are conceptualized as continually evolving as meanings and understandings change. The evolution of goals may be small—from getting out to see friends or picking up painting again—or dramatic—from stopping violent outbursts to focusing on emotionally connecting with one's parent. Counselors do not have a set of predefined goals they use with all clients. Instead, goals are negotiated with each client individually.

Examples of Working Phase Goals to Address Presenting Problems

- Increase reengagement in "old me" activities.
- Connect with friends who support and listen to me.
- Reduce "mountain-out-of-a-molehill" thinking.

Examples of Closing Phase Goals That Target Agency and Identity Narratives

- Increase sense of agency and assertiveness when relating to colleagues at work.
- Increase sense of agency and ability to prioritize where my time and energy goes.

- Develop a sense of identity that honors the difficulties of the past without living in the shadow of the past.

The Doing: Interventions and Ways of Promoting Change
Conversational Questions: Understanding From Within the Dialogue

Conversational questions refer to questions that come naturally from within the dialogue rather than from professional theory (Anderson, 1997). They are not canned or pre-planned but instead follow logically from what the client is saying and are generated from the counselor's curiosity and desire to understand more. For example, if a client reports feeling anxious, the counselor would ask questions that logically flow from the conversation in the moment, such as "When and about what do you feel most anxious? How long have you worried about such things?" rather than using theoretically informed questions such a behavioral functional analysis (see Chapter 9), Gestalt body awareness questions (see Chapter 8), solution-focused miracle question (see Chapter 11), or externalizing questions in narrative (see following text), or systemic interaction questions in the systems approach (see Chapter 10).

Using the client's preferred words and expressions, counselors ask conversational questions to better understand the client's lived experience; by doing so, both the counselor and the client develop a better understanding of the client's lived experiences. In research on counseling process, clients reported that questions asked out of genuine curiosity are received quite differently than "conditional" or "loaded" questions, which are driven by a professional agenda to assess or intervene (Anderson, 1997). Collaborative counselors use conversational questions in a spirit of honest curiosity without a subtext or hidden professional agenda. In the case study at the end of this chapter, conversational questions are used to explore Elan's experience of his friend's death and his alcohol abuse rather than to impose professional and political views, stereotypes, and values onto his situation.

"Appropriately Unusual" Comments

Developed from his work with reflecting teams, Tom Andersen (1991, 1995) recommends counselors avoid comments and questions that are "too usual" or "too unusual" to promote collaborative conversations. Comments that are *too usual* essentially reflect back to the client's worldview, offering no possibility for generating new understanding. Thus, agreeing to or reflecting back the client's current perspective is not likely to promote change. Alternatively, comments that are *too unusual* are too different to be useful in developing new meanings. Some clients give immediate signals that a comment is too unusual by becoming "resistant," reexplaining themselves, or rejecting the comment or suggestion. Other clients will give little indication in session that the comment is too unusual but afterward will not follow up on the comment and may even lose faith in the counselor and counseling process.

With the "just right" taste of the third bowl of porridge in the Goldilocks fairy tale, *appropriately unusual* comments clearly fit within the client's worldview while inviting curiosity and perhaps offering a new perspective that is easily "digestible" to the client. For example, if a client comes in feeling overwhelmed with a new job that is more multi-faceted than the previous job, an appropriately unusual response from the counselor might be, "It sounds like your new job may require skills in multitasking and prioritizing that weren't necessary in your old job," which speaks to their current experience while offering a slightly different perspective. Such comments capture the client's attention because they are familiar enough to be safe and viable yet different enough to offer a "fresh" perspective (Anderson, 1997).

Listen for the Pause When clients hear an appropriately unusual comment, suggestion, or question, they most always have to *pause* and take time to integrate the new perspective with their current perspective: in these moments, it is most important for the counselor to allow the client time for *inner dialogue*. Sometimes a client says, "I have to think about that" or "I never thought of it that way." In response to an appropriately unusual question, a client's initial response may be, "I don't know"; given a few moments to reflect on the new idea, the client usually begins to generate a response that reflects thoughts and ideas that the client has never had before.

How Far to Go?   How unusual is appropriately unusual? The trick here is that each client needs a different level of unusualness, or, alternatively stated, each client finds a different level of difference useful for generating new ideas. I often find that when I am first working with a teen, mandated client, or someone unsure of counseling, appropriately unusual comments cannot include significant differences from the client's current worldview until he or she has developed greater trust in the counselor. Additionally, the more emotionally distraught a person is, the less useful he or she finds highly unusual comments. Some clients require and prefer that the counselor deliver comments that are quite different than their own, often in a very direct manner that verges on being socially impolite. I have had clients, particularly men, say to me, "Just tell me where you think I got it wrong" or "Just tell it to me straight—don't sugarcoat it—I hate when counselors do that." Thus, appropriately unusual depends on the client's preferred style of communication and the quality of counseling relationship. Collaborative counselors fine-tune their communication skills to deliver a range of appropriately unusual comments and carefully observe client responses to assess whether the comments are useful to clients.

Mutual Puzzling

Collaborative counselors invite their clients to join them in becoming curious about their lives in new ways: this process is referred to as *mutual puzzling* (Anderson, 1997). Anderson suggests that when the counselor's curiosity becomes contagious, clients are naturally invited into it. What begins, therefore, as the counselor's one-way inquiry shifts to a joint process. When clients join counselors in the meaning-making process, their rate of talking may slow down, there may be more pauses in the conversation, and there is an inquisitive yet hopeful air to the conversation. Often, the shift in clients is visible: their body posture softens, the head may tilt to the side, and they move more slowly or more quickly (Andersen, 2007). Mutual puzzling can occur only when counselors are successful in creating a two-way dialogical conversation in which both parties are able to sincerely take in and reflect on the contributions of the other.

For example, if a client lives in daily fear of having another psychotic episode after not having one for over 10 years and says that it is her illness that keeps her from moving forward in life, the mutual puzzling process may be sparked by a question, such as "That's interesting. You say you haven't had an episode in 10 years, so hallucinations don't seem to be plaguing you these days. But it does sound like the *worry about* hallucinations is the problem at this point. Do you think of this as part of the original problem, or is it a new problem that developed only after the first was resolved?" In this case, a new distinction is highlighted, and the client is invited to kick it around and see what, if any, new ideas emerge and to follow where they lead. The counselor does not politely insist that worrying is the new problem but rather listens for how the client made sense of the comment and continues to follow the client's thinking, kicking around the next idea that evolves from the conversation, the counselor always most curious about how the client is making sense of what is being discussed.

Being Public: Counselor's Inner Dialogue

In *being public*, counselors share their inner dialogue for two potential reasons: (a) to respect clients by honestly sharing their thoughts about significant issues affecting treatment and (b) to prevent monological conversation by offering the private thoughts into the dialogue where they are at risk for change (Anderson, 1997, 2005). When counselors make their perspectives publicly known, they do so *tentatively* and, even when discussing professional knowledge, are careful to not overshadow the client's perspective (Anderson, 2007).

This generally occurs in two situations: (a) communication about professional information with clients or outside agencies or professionals (e.g., courts, diagnosis, psychiatrists, etc.) and (b) significant differences in values, goals, purposes, and so on with the client. Importantly, being open with one's silent thoughts also helps prevent the counselor from slipping into a monological mode. The counselor's act of speaking his or her words puts him or her into the conversation for the client to respond to, and in the act of forming silent thoughts into spoken words, something different may be created for the counselor as well.

Being Public With Professional Communication Whenever collaborative counselors handle professional matters, such as making a diagnosis, speaking with a social worker, filing a report with the court, and so on, they "make public" their thoughts, rationales, and intentions by discussing them directly with clients. Openly discussing (a) what the counselor will reveal in an upcoming conversation with another professional and/or (b) recapping what happened in the last conversation goes against traditional procedures in which communications between professionals were kept confidential *from the client*, ostensibly because they could *do harm* to the client to know what professionals were thinking: the apparent "harm" was usually that the client would be angry if he or she knew what the counselors and other professionals were *actually* thinking.

In dramatic contrast, collaborative counselors have been vanguards in lifting the veil on dialogue between professionals, engaging in honest, direct conversation with clients about the contents of these conversations. Such conversations are not always easy, such as when a counselor has to tell a client that she cannot recommend unification through child protective services until x, y, and z happens (e.g., typically spelled out by the social worker or court). Rather than the past practice of the parent learning this in court or from a social worker, the counselor has an up-front conversation from the beginning, clearly laying out the types of behaviors that need to be seen for the desired recommendations and then wholeheartedly and enthusiastically working with the clients to reach this goal.

Most clients greatly respect the counselor's honesty and integrity and respond with increased motivation to make needed changes and fully understand when they are not given the report they hoped for because the counselor and client have been discussing progress—or lack thereof—consistently along the way. When working with court-mandated clients, St. George and Wulff (1998) have developed the practice of having the clients do the first draft of letters to the courts about the progress, including clinical recommendations, with the counselors then using the letter as a means to discuss their progress and goals.

Similarly, when managing dangerous situations, the counselor "makes public" concerns about safety and the potential for harm. By inviting clients—especially those not fully invested in stopping the problem behavior—into a discussion to address the counselor's concern about the client's safety, the client and counselor can work together to develop a plan that is meaningful to the client while addressing the counselor's safety concerns and following legal and ethical mandates.

Being Public With Significant Differences in Values and Goals The other situation in which collaborative counselors make public their voice is when there are significant differences in values or goals that make it hard for the counselor to move forward as an active participant in the conversation. For example, I recently had a teenager discuss his plans to meet someone who had challenged him to a fight at a park that day, saying, "Don't bring weapons or friends." The teen believed that if he didn't show up, more guys at school would gang up on him, and that could lead to more events such as this. Although I saw his point, I also saw how he was at risk for seriously being hurt, a concern I decided to make "public." I invited him to explore my concerns: the guy might come with friends or weapons, and/or there might be legal ramifications and so on. I offered my list of dangers from a place of serious concern without demanding a particular course of action on his part. Instead, I asked him how he would manage the dangers I saw; by the end of the conversation, we arrived at a place where my concerns and his were addressed and where both of us felt good about his chosen course of action, namely, to avoid the park that day and to try to find out about this person's social network. Similarly, the counselor in the case study at the end of this chapter uses being public to share his concerns about Elan's safety when using substances to develop a safety and harm reduction plan.

Accessing Multiple Voices in Writing

Peggy Penn and her associates (Penn 2001; Penn & Frankfurt, 1994; Penn & Sheinberg, 1991) access multiple, alternative voices using various forms of writing (i.e., letters, poems, and journals) to generate alternative perspectives and make room for silenced inner voices or the voices of significant persons not currently in the counseling dialogue. Penn and Frankfurt (1994) have found that "writing slows down our perceptions and reactions, making room for their thickening, their gradual layering" (p. 229). They have also found that the performative aspect, the reading aloud of letters to witnesses (the counselor, family, and others), makes things happen. Penn's writing has a different intent than writing in experiential therapies, which are meant to express repressed emotions, bring resolution to a past situation, or achieve a similar clinical aim. Instead, Penn's writing invites different voices into the conversation to generate alternative possibilities for understanding. Furthermore, writing promotes agency: "to write *gives us agency: we are not acted on by a situation, we are acting!* (Penn, 2001, p. 49; emphasis in the original). Writing in collaborative counseling may involve asking clients to write the following:

- Letters to themselves from aspects of themselves and/or from newly emerging, future, or past selves
- Letters to themselves from significant others, from the present, past, or future
- Letters to and from significant others (alive or dead) speaking from a voice/perspective that was formerly kept private
- Letters or journal entries to speak from parts of the self that are typically not expressed and/or are emerging in counseling
- Letters to the world or general audience
- Multivoiced biographies that describe one's life from various perspectives
- Poems that express inner voices and perspectives that are not readily articulated other ways

Reflecting Teams and Reflecting Process

Tom Andersen trained at the Milan Institute, where a small team of counselors would observe the counselor talking with families behind a one-way mirror, the preferred method for interviewing in early family counseling. Influenced by postmodern thinking, Andersen (1995) and his colleagues wanted to make the process more *democratic* and developed the idea of having the families listen to the team's conversation behind the mirror: thus, the reflecting team practice began. With the earliest reflecting teams, the family and team would literally switch rooms if sound could be heard in only one room or turn off the lights in the family's room and turn on the lights in the team's room, reversing the one-way mirror. In later years, the team was invited to sit in the *same room but separate from* the family and counselor having a conversation. Over the years, the practice has developed more into a general *process* of reflecting that is used for talking with clients with or without a team.

The idea behind a collaborative reflecting team is to develop *diverse* strands of conversation and for the client to choose that which resonates and that which does not. Collaborative reflecting teams avoid coming to agreement on any one description of what is going on with the client, allowing for *multiple, contradictory perspectives* to linger and promoting the development of new meanings and perspectives. Teams avoid comments that evaluate or judge the client in any way, positive or negative. Instead, the focus is on offering what are called *reflections*, observations, questions, or comments that are clearly owned by the person making it (e.g., "As I listened, I was wondering …").

General Guidelines for Reflecting Teams

Andersen (1991, 1995) provides guidelines for teams:

- *Use only with the permission of the client:* The counselor should obtain the client's permission to use a team *before* the session starts. When the counselor has a strong rapport with the client and confidently explains how the reflecting process works, most clients enthusiastically agree.

- *Give the client permission to listen or not to listen:* Andersen gives the clients *explicit* permission to listen or not listen. I find it helpful to tell clients that they will probably hear some comments that resonate deeply and others that fit less well with their experience and recommend that they focus on the comments that "strike a chord."
- *Team members should speak from something they see or hear in the family's talk with the counselor*, not *what is observed:* Comment on a specific event or statement in the conversation and then "wonder" or be "curious" about it. The wondering or curiosity statement should be *appropriately unusual* to help generate new perspectives.
- *Talk from a questioning, speculative, and tentative perspective:* Team members avoid offering opinions or interpretations and instead use "wondering" questions (e.g., "I am wondering if …") or offer a tentative perspective (e.g., "I am aware I don't know enough to know the whole story, but it seems like there might be …). If a team member offers a strong opinion, another team member may ask, "What did you see or hear in the conversation that made you think that?" to open the conversation up and invite multiple perspectives.
- *Comment on all that you hear but not all that you see:* If the family tries to cover something up, allow them the *right to not talk about* all that they think and feel. Andersen warns, "Don't confuse counseling with confession." Unlike psychodynamic and humanistic traditions, Andersen is explicit that if a client wants to hide an emotion or not say something, the client should be free to do so. He was a rare advocate for client privacy in counseling, believing that clients will share when they are ready. If a counselor notices a client getting agitated or holding back tears, he does not comment on it, allowing the client to speak about these emotions when he or she is ready to do so.
- *The team and family can be in the same room, but they should not talk to each other:* Andersen believed that an important psychological space is created by the physical space between the team and client and by the two not talking directly; later research studies supported his view (Sells, Smith, Coe, & Yoshioka, 1994). This space invites all participants to focus on their inner dialogue, stimulating new thoughts and ideas more readily.
- *Listen for what is appropriately unusual and avoid what is too usual or too unusual:* To identify useful reflections, Andersen asks himself, "Is what is going on now appropriately unusual or is it too unusual?" (Andersen, 1995, p. 21).
- *"How would you like to use this session today?"* A question that a collaborative counselor is likely to ask at the beginning of any session, this question is critical when a team is involved. If the client is nervous about using a reflecting team, the counselor can also add, "Are there particular topics you want to avoid with the team here?"

Related Reflecting Processes

Over time, the concept of the reflecting team has developed into a number of reflecting processes:

- *Reflecting team:* A team of two to four counselors observes the counselor–client conversation, sitting either in a different room using a one-way mirror (or camera) or in a separate space in the same room.
- *Single reflector:* If only one colleague is available, the counselor may turn and have a reflecting conversation with this one reflector while the client listens.
- *No outside reflector when working with a family:* When there is no outside colleague available, the counselor may choose to speak with a single family member while others listen.
- *No outside reflector when working with an individual:* In cases where the counselor is working with an individual client, a reflective process can be created by talking about issues from the perspective of someone who is not present (e.g., a parent, friend, spouse, famous person of personal significance, etc.).
- *With young children:* When working with children, reflections can include play media; a single counselor working with an individual child can create reflecting teams using puppets or other play media (Gehart, 2007a).

"As-If" Reflecting

Developed by Anderson (1997), the "as-if" reflecting processes involves having the team members or other witnesses to the conversation speak, or reflect, "as if" they are one of the people in the problem-organized system (i.e., one of the people talking about the problem), which includes the client, family members, friends, bosses, teachers, school personnel, medical professionals, probation officers, and so on. This process can be used with families or with supervisees staffing a case.

Putting It All Together: Collaborative Treatment Plan Template

Use this treatment plan template for developing a plan for clients with depressive, anxious, or compulsive types of presenting problems. Depending on the specific client, presenting problem, and clinical context, the goals and interventions in this template may need to be modified only slightly or significantly; you are encouraged to significantly revise the plan as needed. For the plan to be useful, goals and techniques should be written to target specific beliefs, behaviors, and emotions that the client is experiencing. The more specific, the more useful it will be to you.

Treatment Plan

Initial Phase of Treatment (First One to Three Sessions)
Initial Phase Counseling Tasks

1. *Develop working counseling relationship. Diversity note:* Include significant persons in client's life, including friends, family, and so on.
   Relationship building intervention:
   a. Develop **conversational partnership** and sense of **"withness"** by acknowledging **client expertise**, **being curious**, and using **everyday language**.

2. *Assess individual, systemic, and broader cultural dynamics. Diversity note:* Involve all parties who are talking about the problem.
   Assessment Strategies:
   a. Make room in the dialogue to hear the perspective of each member of **problem-determined system**, which may involve inviting persons to sessions or making out-of-session phone calls to other professionals and/or family members.
   b. **Conversational questions** to develop understanding of the problem from "within" each person's worldview.

Initial Phase Client Goals *(One to Two Goals):* Manage crisis issues and/or reduce most distressing symptoms

1. *Increase* the client's sense of **agency** related to [crisis-triggering situation] to reduce [crisis symptom(s)].
   Interventions:
   a. **Conversational questions** to understand crisis triggers, issues, and inner experience from client's perspective.
   b. **Mutual puzzling** to collaboratively identify crisis behaviors and client's preferred means for managing; use **client expertise** to develop mutually agreed-on safety plan.

Working Phase of Treatment (Three or More Sessions)
Working Phase Counseling Task

1. *Monitor quality of the working alliance. Diversity note:* Adapt conversations to meet client's needs.
   Assessment Intervention:
   a. **Mutually puzzling questions** to **publicly** reflect on quality of the relationship; use Session Rating Scale with clients who find it useful.

(continued)

Working Phase Client Goals *(Two to Three Goals)*. Target individual and relational dynamics using theoretical language (e.g., decrease avoidance of intimacy, increase awareness of emotion, increase agency)

1. *Increase* sense of available perspectives and options and expand client's understanding of [the problem] to reduce [specific symptoms: depression, anxiety, etc.].
    Interventions:
    a. **Conversational questions** to generate new understandings of problem and to generate multivoiced descriptions that include perspectives of others talking about the problem.
    b. Offer **appropriately unusual comments** to enable client to generate new inner dialogues related to the problem.

2. *Increase* frequency of [specific behavior] to support the client's **sense of agency** in relation to [the problem] to reduce [specific symptoms: depression, anxiety, etc.].
    Interventions:
    a. **Mutual puzzling** to jointly identify meaningful actions, relationships, and options that support client in reach desired goals.
    b. **Reflecting team/practices** to generate new ways of viewing and interacting in relation to the problem.

3. *Increase* frequency of [specific behavior] to support the client's **sense of agency** in relation to [another element of problem] to reduce [specific symptoms: depression, anxiety, etc.].
    Interventions:
    a. **Mutual puzzling** to jointly identify meaningful actions, relationships, and options that support client in reach desired goals.
    b. **Writing letters, poems, etc.** to generate multiple perspectives for viewing and relating to the problem.

Closing Phase of Treatment (Last Two or More Sessions)
Closing Phase Counseling Task

1. *Develop aftercare plan and maintain gains. Diversity note:* Involve significant others when possible.
    Intervention:
    a. Collaboratively identify how client can use what they have learned to prevent the future problems.

Closing Phase Client Goals *(One to Two Goals):* Determined by theory's definition of health and normalcy

1. *Increase* client's sense of **self-agency** in relation to [the problem] to reduce [specific symptoms: depression, anxiety, etc.].
    Interventions:
    a. **Appropriate unusual comments** to highlight before-during-after process of transformation.
    b. **Reflecting practices/team** to story process of transformation from multiple perspectives.
    c. **Writing letters, poems, exercises**, and so on to thicken descriptions of problem dissolution.

2. *Increase* client's agency/identity narrative as it relates to [another key area of life, such as relationship, work, etc.] to reduce [specific symptoms: depression, anxiety, etc.].
    Interventions:
    a. **Mutual puzzling questions** to explore how strengths and resources in one area of life can transfer to other areas.
    b. **Conversational questions** and using **client expertise** to identify how best to use agency in [other area of life].

Clinical Spotlight: Evidence-Based Approach: Open Dialogue
Open Dialogue and Psychosis

Jaakko Seikkula (2002) and his colleagues (Haarakangas et al., 2007) in Finland developed the open dialogue approach in their work with psychosis and other severe disorders. They report impressive outcomes in their 20 years of research, including 83% of first-episode psychosis patients returning to work and 77% with no remaining psychotic symptoms after 2 years of treatment. In comparison with standard treatment in Finland, the patients in the open dialogue treatment had more family meetings, fewer days of inpatient care, reduced use of medication, and a greater reduction in psychotic symptoms.

Using collaborative dialogue and reflecting practices, this approach includes the following:

- *Immediate intervention:* Within 24 hours of the initial call, the person who has had a psychotic break, the significant people in his or her life, and a treatment team of several professionals (e.g., for psychosis the team often includes a psychiatrist, psychotherapist, and nurse) meet to discuss the situation using collaborative dialogue.
- *Social network and support systems:* Significant persons in the client's life and other support systems are invited to participate in all phases of the process.
- *Flexibility and mobility:* Treatment is uniquely adapted to clients and their situations, with the treatment team sometimes meeting in their homes and other times in a treatment setting, depending on what is most useful.
- *Teamwork and responsibility:* The treatment team is built based on client needs; all team members are responsible for the quality of the process.
- *Psychological continuity:* The team members remain consistent throughout treatment regardless of the stage of treatment.
- *Tolerance of uncertainty:* Rather than employ set protocols, time is allowed to see how each situation will evolve and what treatment will be needed.
- *Dialogue:* The focus of each meeting is to establish an open dialogue that facilitates new meanings and possibilities. This process requires establishing a sense of safety for all participants to say what needs to be said.

Snapshot: Research and the Evidence Base

Quick Summary: With the exception of the open dialogue approach for working with clients diagnosed with psychosis, the majority of research on postmodern approaches has focused on client experiences of counseling rather than outcome.

Consistent with their philosophical, social constructionist underpinnings, postmodern counselors have conducted more qualitative than quantitative investigations about their approaches to counseling (Anderson, 1997; Gehart, Tarragona, & Bava, 2007; McLeod, 1994; Williams, 1995). Qualitative research on postmodern therapies has focused on clients' lived experience of counseling and its effects on their lives, emphasizing the clients' experience over researcher-defined measures of successful counseling (Gehart & Lyle, 1999; Levitt & Rennie, 2004; London, Ruiz, Gargollo, 1998). A notable exception, Finish psychiatrist Jaakko Seikkula (2002) and his team (Haarakangas et al., 2007) have used qualitative and quantitative methods to study their collaborative open dialogue approach to working psychosis and other severe diagnoses for the past 20 years, reporting significant evidence for their model's effectiveness (see preceding text).

Snapshot: Working With Diverse Populations

Quick Summary: Ideal for marginalized populations, these approaches focus on how the client's problems relate to the broader sociopolitical context.

Because postmodern therapies do not have preestablished theories of health, they are appropriate for working with a wide range of diverse populations because culturally defined norms are not used to assess or set goals. In fact, the broader questions of diversity and how society, its norms, and use of language affects individuals are the guiding questions in postmodern philosophical literature, making these therapies particularly suitable for clients from marginalized groups (for an in-depth discussion, see Monk et al., 2008). In particular, narrative and feminist approaches (see Chapter 13) are two of the only mental health theories that place societal issues of oppression at the heart of its counseling interventions, and most of these practitioners consider out-of-session social justice an important part of their roles as counselors (Brown, 2006; Zimmerman & Dickerson, 1996). Collaborative language systems attend more to the local level discourse, meaning that they work closely with the client and the significant people with whom they are in dialogue to determine what the problem is (for the moment, knowing its definition will continually evolve) and how best to resolve it. This focus on local knowledges ensures that the client's cultural values and beliefs are a central part of the counseling process. These approaches have international roots and are practiced in numerous countries around the world.

Despite their heavy focus on cultural issues, even postmodern counselors can encounter problems with diverse populations, reminding us of how difficult it is to really handle diversity well. The primary limitation with these approaches is that their careful attention to diversity and the unique needs of clients results in less directive approaches, which some client groups—such as immigrants—may not prefer or know how to respond well to. Additionally, narrative counselors who place a heavy and overt emphasis on social justice issues in session must be careful to maintain a strong working alliance with clients that engages them meaningfully in the process of understanding oppressive dominant discourses and inspires them to become part of the solution rather than having them feel blamed or attacked.

Postmodern Case Study and Treatment Plan

A 19-year-old of Native American descent, Elan recently lost his best friend in a drunk-driving accident. His friend was driving while under the influence on his way home from Elan's house and hit a tree; he was killed immediately on impact. Because of his extreme guilt, Elan initially did not drink for several months after the accident. Now that he has resumed drinking, he is drinking more than ever before. He says that his friend's spirit is haunting him and is considering contacting a medicine man whom his mother knows to help deal with the spirit. Elan says he is having trouble focusing in his retail job and just isn't motivated to stay in the community college classes he was enrolled in with his friend. Before his friend's death, he was socially active, played basketball, and wanted to be a computer technician, but now he hangs around the house, drinking beer and playing video games and rarely hanging out with his friends anymore because of his shame. His mother doesn't say much other than insist that he keep going to work and nag him about his drinking. His younger sister tries to reach out to him, but he keeps pushing her away.

Postmodern Case Conceptualization

This case conceptualization was developed by selecting key concepts from the "The Viewing: Case Conceptualization" sections of this chapter. You can use any of the concepts in that section to develop a case conceptualization for this or other cases.

Person Apart From the Problem

AM (adult male) describes himself before the accident as the life of the party with lots of friends, an active basketball player, and an aspiring computer technician. He also describes himself as having a "cool" family that he enjoyed hanging out with.

Problem-Saturated Stories

AM's problem-saturated story involves both personal and relational changes:

- *Personal:* Dropped out of school; stopped playing basket ball; drinking more, difficulty focusing at work; feeling too ashamed to be with friends
- *Relational:* Distant from mother; pulling away from sister and friends; feels haunted by friend's spirit

Unique Outcomes and Sparkling Events

Unique outcomes include wanting to connect with mother to find a medicine man and thereby reconnect with cultural traditions; every once in a while, agreeing to hang out with friends; and choosing not too drink so much that he is unable to go to work.

Dominant Cultural and Gender Discourses

AM's partying fits with dominant discourses about how young males, including Native Americans, "have fun." His guilt around his friend's death implies that he knew his friend was taking a risk driving home but that he probably didn't want to appear wimpy and tell him not to drink and drive.

Local and Alternative Discourses: Attending to Client Language and Meaning

AM's experience of feeling haunted by his friend's ghost is more common in Native American populations, as is his desire to seek a medicine man to help with this situation. Since no other psychotic symptoms are described, his experience of spirits should be considered within cultural norms (assuming it is not better explained by substance use).

Who's Talking? Problem-Organizing, Problem-Dissolving Systems

In terms of assessing the problem-organizing system, it is important to consider not only how AM is constructing the problem but also his mother, sister, friends, deceased friend's family, and their larger community. His mother sees the greatest problem as AM's drinking and potential to lose his job. His sister seems to see his sadness and social withdrawal as the biggest problems. His friends are also affected by his social withdrawal.

Assessing the Client's Worldview

AM sees himself as at least partially responsible for the death of his friend and seems to feel so ashamed that he does not feel entitled to pursue his life dreams, at least education and social activities, as he did before. His experience of being haunted by his friend's ghost further reinforces his sense of guilt and shame. His return to heavy drinking after not drinking initially after the accident seems to indicate that he has become increasingly hopeless and having difficulty managing his emotions.

Postmodern Treatment Plan

Initial Phase of Treatment (First One to Three Sessions)
Initial Phase Counseling Tasks

1. *Develop working counseling relationship. Diversity note:* Attend to AM's level of acculturation, especially in regard to eye contact and direct, emotionally challenging comments. *Relationship building intervention:*
   a. Meet **AM apart from the problem** (who he was before the accident) to generate **hope** and reconnect him with a sense of who he is.

2. *Assess individual, systemic, and broader cultural dynamics. Diversity note:* Consider inviting mother, sister, and/or friends.
   Assessment Strategies:
   a. **Relative influence questioning** and **deconstructive questions** to identify effects of problem and effects of person, noting key **dominant and local discourses**, carefully attending to cultural issues.
   b. Identify **unique outcomes and sparkling moments** that do not conform to problem-saturated narrative, such as times when he does not drink and/or hangs out with friends.

(continued)

Initial Phase Client Goals

1. *Increase* the client's ability **resist invitations** to engage in drinking to forget about accident to reduce alcohol abuse.
   Interventions:
   a. **Relative influence questioning** to identify how client is "enticed" to engage in problem drinking behavior as well as times when the client resists these invitations.
   b. **Statement of position map** to identify client's desired "position" in relation to crisis drinking; identify strategies, persons, and contexts that support the desired position.

Working Phase of Treatment (Two or More Sessions)
Working Phase Counseling Task

1. *Monitor quality of the working alliance. Diversity note:* Adapt alliance to acknowledge cultural norms for discussing problems and talking with a person of higher social standing.
   Assessment Intervention:
   a. Use **situating comments** and **permission questions** to situate counselor as **coeditor/investigative reporter**; regularly check in with client about alliance; use Session Rating Scale.

Working Phase Client Goals

1. *Increase* client's sense of **agency in relation** to the accident and responsibility to move forward with integrity to reduce guilt and motivation to abuse alcohol.
   Interventions:
   a. **Conversational questions** to generate new understandings of the problem and ways that the accident and loss can inform his identity moving forward.
   b. **Statement of position map** and **relative influence questioning** to externalize problem and clarify who he is, how this accident has changed him, and how best to move forward with integrity.

2. *Increase* frequency of social interactions that supports the client's **preferred reality** to reduce social withdrawal.
   Interventions:
   a. **Mutual puzzling** to identify specific behaviors that support rebuilding social connection that AM is willing to carry out.
   b. **Scaffolding questions** to help client move toward rebuilding his social network and to take responsible action within that network.

3. *Increase* motivation to return to school to pursue career goals to reduce hopelessness and depression.
   Interventions:
   a. **Mapping in the landscapes of action and consciousness** to identify specific behaviors that support successfully returning to school.
   b. **Reflecting practices** to help AM develop new meanings with returning to school in relation to the memory of his friend.

Closing Phase of Treatment (Last Two or More Sessions)
Closing Phase Counseling Task

1. *Develop aftercare plan and maintain gains. Diversity note:* Identify ways to engage support system
   Intervention:
   a. Use **mapping in the landscape of action and consciousness** questions to help AM identify how he can resist invitations from alcohol and guilt.

(continued)

Closing Phase Client Goals

1. *Increase* and **thicken the plot a**round the AM's **new sense of identity** and **agency** in relation to the accident and alcohol to reduce guilt, alcohol abuse, and loss of interest in regular activities.
   Interventions:
   a. **Mutual puzzling** to develop action plans to bolster and sustain new identity.
   b. **Landscape of action and consciousness questions** to thicken new narratives that capture AM's outer and inner experiences as he finds meaning and moves forward after this tragedy.

2. *Increase* involvement of **mother, sister, friends,** and/or **medicine man** in AM's life to **witness and support new identity narrative** and relationship to the accident to reduce social withdrawal and depression.
   Interventions:
   a. **Invite significant persons to session** to partake in an atonement or similar ceremony that helps AM story his role in the tragedy and his atonement for his part.
   b. **Letters and/or other written documents** to document atonement and solidify new identity and preferred narrative.

ONLINE RESOURCES

Institutes and Training Centres

Harlene Anderson
www.harleneanderson.org

Dulwich Centre: Michael White's Narrative Therapy
www.dulwichcenter.com

Evanston Family Therapy Center: Freedman and Combs' Narrative Therapy
www.narrativetherapychicago.com

Houston Galveston Institute: Collaborative language systems
www.talkhgi.com

Narrative Approaches
www.narrativeapproaches.com

Taos Institute: Collaborative Practices in Therapy, Consultation, Education, Business
www.taosinstitute.net

Yaletown Family Therapy: Narrative Therapy, Canada
www.yaletownfamilytherapy.com

Client site

Anti-Anorexia/Anit-Bulima League
www.narrativeapproaches.com/antianorexia%20folder/anti_anorexia_index.htm

Journal

Journal of Systemic Therapies
www.guilford.com

References

*Asterisk indicates recommended introductory readings.

*Andersen, T. (1991). *The reflecting team: Dialogues and dialogues about the dialogues.* New York: Norton.
Andersen, T. (1995). Reflecting processes; acts of informing and forming: You can borrow my eyes, but you must not take them away from me! In S. Friedman (Ed.), *The reflecting team in action: Collaborative practice in family therapy* (pp. 11–37). New York: Guilford.
*Andersen, T. (2007). Human participating: Human "being" is the step for human "becoming" in the next step. In H. Anderson & D. Gehart (Eds.), *Collaborative therapy: Relationships and conversations that make a difference* (pp. 81–97). New York: Brunner-Routledge.

Anderson, H. (1993). On a roller coaster: A collaborative language systems approach to therapy. In S. Friedman (Ed.), *The new language of change* (pp. 323–344). New York: Guilford.

*Anderson, H. (1997). *Conversations, language, and possibilities: A postmodern approach to therapy*. New York: Basic Books.

Anderson, H. (2005). Myths about "not knowing." *Family Process, 44*, 497–504.

Anderson, H. (2007). Historical influences. In H. Anderson & D. Gehart (Eds.), *Collaborative therapy: Relationships and conversations that make a difference* (pp. 21–31). New York: Brunner-Routledge.

*Anderson, H., & Gehart, D. (2007). *Collaborative therapy: Relationships and conversations that make a difference.* New York: Brunner-Routledge.

Anderson, H., & Goolishian, H. (1988). Human systems as linguistic systems: Preliminary and evolving ideas about the implications for clinical theory. *Family Process, 27*, 157–163.

*Anderson, H., & Goolishian, H. (1992). The client is the expert: A not-knowing approach to therapy. In S. McNamee & K. J. Gergen (Eds.), *Therapy as social construction* (pp. 25–39). Newbury Park, CA: Sage.

Boscolo, L., Cecchin, G., Hoffman, L., & Penn, P. (1987). *Milan systemic family therapy*. New York: Basic Books.

Brown, L. (2006). Still subversive after all these years: The relevance of feminist therapy in the age of evidence-based practice. *Psychology of Women Quarterly, 30*(1), 15–24. doi:10.1111/j.1471-6402.2006.00258.x

Foucault, M. (1980). *Power/knowledge: Selected interviews and other writings*. New York: Pantheon Books.

*Freedman, J., & Combs, G. (1996). *Narrative therapy: The social construction of preferred realities*. New York: Norton.

Gehart, D. (2007a). Creating space for children's voices: A collaborative and playful approach to working with children and families. In H. Anderson & D. Gehart (Eds.), *Collaborative therapy: Relationships and conversations that make a difference* (pp. 183–197). New York: Brunner-Routledge.

Gehart, D. R., & Lyle, R. R. (1999). Client and therapist perspectives of change in collaborative language systems: An interpretive ethnography. *Journal of Systemic Therapy, 18*(4), 78–97.

Gehart, D., & McCollum, E. (2007). Engaging suffering: Towards a mindful re-visioning of marriage and family therapy practice. *Journal of Marital and Family Therapy, 33*, 214–226.

Gehart, D., Tarragona, M., Bava, S. (2007). A collaborative approach to inquiry. In H. Anderson & D. Gehart (Eds.), *Collaborative therapy: Relationships and conversations that make a difference* (pp. 367–390). New York: Brunner-Routledge.

Goolishian, H., & Anderson, H. (1987) Language systems and therapy: An evolving idea. *Psychotherapy, 24*(3S), 529–538.

Haarakangas, K., Seikkula, J., Alakare, B., & Aaltonen, J. (2007). Open dialogue: An approach to psychotherapeutic treatment of psychosis in northern Finland. In H. Anderson & D. Gehart (Eds.), *Collaborative therapy: Relationships and conversations that make a difference* (pp. 221–233). New York: Brunner-Routledge.

*Hoffman, L. (1981). *Foundations of family therapy: A conceptual framework for systems change*. New York: Basic Books.

*Hoffman, L. (2001). *Family therapy: An intimate history*. New York: Norton.

Hoffman, L. (2007). The art of "withness": A bright new edge. In H. Anderson & D. Gehart (Eds.), *Collaborative therapy: Relationships and conversations that make a difference* (pp. 63–79). New York: Brunner-Routledge.

Levitt, H., & Rennie, D. L. (2004). Narrative activity: Clients' and therapists' intentions in the process of narration. In L. Angus & J. McLeod (Eds.), *The handbook of narrative and psychotherapy: Practice, theory, and research* (pp. 299–313). Thousand Oaks, CA: Sage.

London, S., Ruiz, G., & Gargollo, M. C. (1998). Client's voices: A collection of client's accounts. *Journal of Systemic Therapies, 17*(4), 61–71.

Monk, G., Winslade, J., Crocket, K., & Epston, D. (1997). *Narrative therapy in practice: The archaeology of hope*. San Francisco: Jossey-Bass.

Monk, G. Winslade, J., & Sinclair, S. (2008). *New horizons in multicultural counseling*. Thousand Oaks, CA: Sage.

Penn, P. (2001). Chronic illness: Trauma, language, and writing: Breaking the silence. *Family Process, 40*, 33–52.

Penn, P. (2002). *So close*. Fort Lee, NJ: Cavankerry.

Penn, P., & Frankfurt, M. (1994). Creating a participant text: Writing, multiple voices, narrative multiplicity. *Family Process, 33*, 217–231.

Penn, P., & Sheinberg, M. (1991). Stories and conversations. *Journal of Systemic Therapies, 10*(3–4), 30–37.

Seikkula, J. (2002). Open dialogues with good and poor outcomes for psychotic crises: Examples from families with violence. *Journal of Marital and Family Therapy, 28*(3), 263–274.

Sells, S., Smith, T., Coe, M., & Yoshioka, M. (1994). An ethnography of couple and therapist experiences in reflecting team practice. *Journal of Marital and Family Therapy, 20*, 247–266.

St. George, S., & Wulff, D. (1998). Integrating the client's voice within case reports. *Journal of Systemic Therapies, 17*(4), 3–13.

White, M. (1995). *Re-authoring lives: Interviews and essays*. Adelaide: Dulwich Centre Publications.

*White, M. (2007). *Maps of narrative practice*. New York: Norton.

*White, M., & Epston, D. (1990). *Narrative means to therapeutic ends*. New York: Norton.

Williams, E. F. (Ed.). (1995). *Voices in feminist therapy*. New York: Harwood Academic Press.

Winslade, J., & Monk, G. (1999). *Narrative counseling in schools: Powerful and brief*. Thousand Oaks, CA: Corwin Press.

Winslade, J., & Monk, G. (2000). *Narrative mediation*. San Francisco: Jossey-Bass.

Winslade, J., & Monk, G. (2007) *Narrative counseling in schools: Powerful and brief* (2nd ed.). Thousand Oaks, CA: Corwin Press.

Winslade, J., & Monk, G. (2009). *Practicing narrative mediation: Loosening the grip of conflict*. San Francisco: Jossey-Bass.

Zimmerman, J. L., & Dickerson, V. C. (1996). *If problems talked: Narrative therapy in action*. New York: Guilford.

Feminist and Multicultural Counseling and Psychotherapy

Lay of the Land

Rarely does anyone enjoy being stereotyped; it is never fair, accurate, or correct. Yet our brains are categorizing machines, designed to constantly separate out safe from not safe. This same mechanism that distinguishes a stick from a rattlesnake plays havoc in our social relationships and worlds. Thus, this chapter is likely to shake things up for you personally and with anyone with whom you discuss it. Raising issues such as gender, culture, race, ethnicity, and class involves stereotypes and often triggers painful moments of being ostracized, marginalized, or otherwise "less than." So, I encourage you to notice your response as you read this chapter and spend time reflecting on what comes up.

To get started, several schools of feminist and multicultural counseling have developed over the years (Worell & Johnson, 2001):

- *Liberal/reform feminisms:* Focusing on egalitarianism, liberal and reform feminists view sexism and oppression as irrational prejudices and sex role socialization; their focus is on increasing women's individual freedom, autonomy, self-fulfillment, dignity, and equality *within existing counseling and psychotherapeutic traditions.*
- *Radical/socialist feminisms:* Radical and socialist feminists view social oppression as the primary root of women's problems and therefore directly challenge patriarchy, male domination, and men's control over women's bodies. Their approach emphasizes increasing awareness of all forms of oppression, empowering women to make changes, and effecting social change.
- *Cultural/interpersonal feminisms:* Developing the popular relational-cultural and self-in-relation theories at the Stone Center, cultural feminists argue that women's experience is distinctly different than men's, constituting a unique and equally valid subculture that values relationship, cooperation, and emotionality.
- *Multicultural feminisms:* Addressing the unique needs of ethnic minority women in Western cultures, multicultural feminists attend to the various cultural contexts that impact these women's lives, including sexism within Western culture as well as their own ethnic culture. Furthermore, issues of power, status, and empowerment are different in collectivist versus individualistic cultures, creating distinct and highly complex conflicts for women of color.

- *Postmodern feminisms:* Postmodern feminists explore the construction of gender and its realities in social contexts and relationships, attending to the impact of dominant societal discourses (see "Narrative Approaches" in Chapter 12) on an individual's identity.

In a Nutshell: The Least You Need to Know

Feminist counseling theories focus on how the effects of gender, cultural, heterosexual, and other stereotypes affect an individual's identity and relationships and how these lead to the types of problems for which a person seeks counseling. Informed by cultural theory, feminist approaches are based on the premise that *humans seek, growth through, and move toward connection with others* across the life span (Jordan, 1997, 2010; Jordan, Kaplan, Miller, Stiver, & Surrey, 1991). A sense of connection and community is fundamental to an individual's sense of well-being. *Disconnection*, then, is the root cause of most forms of emotional distress, and this becomes the focus of treatment. The counseling process is characterized by egalitarianism, empathy, and mutuality; the relationship is an authentic and human encounter for both client and counselor. Through this relationship, clients learn to engage in *growth-fostering relationships*, relationships that enhance both parties' sense of well-being. The counseling process also involves analyzing the effects of oppression and social power on the client and their impact on the presenting concern. The process of counseling increases clients' awareness of sociopolitical issues in individual lives and empowers clients to make meaningful change in their personal lives, relationships, and larger community.

The Juice: Significant Contributions to the Field

If there is one thing you remember from this chapter, it should be …

Growth-Fostering Relationships and the Five Good Things

Feminists maintain that humans are primarily *relational*, that they seek, growth through, and move toward connection with others (Jordan, 2010; Jordan et al., 1991). The desire for connection is the primary motivating force, in contrast to more traditional human development models that emphasize individuation. Feminists view the idea of a separate self as a myth that is based on a spatial metaphor of separateness, with psychodynamic theories generally positing that the more separate the self, the better it functions (Jordan, 2010). In contrast, feminists use a model of human development that recognizes the inherent interdependence of humans for survival, both physical and psychological (Comstock, 2005). Rather than a stage-based model of human development, feminists describe development as a complex, multifaceted process in which people increase their abilities to be differentiated *within* relationships and increase their capacity for *mutuality*.

However, all relationships are not created equal. The type of relationships that we seek, that are good for us, and that help us to grow are different than others because they allow us to fully experience and safely explore our sense of self. Relational-cultural counselors refer to these as *growth-fostering relationships*, which are characterized by the *five good things* (Miller & Stiver, 1997; Jordan, 2010).

- Increased zest and energy
- Increased sense of self-worth
- Increased knowledge and clarity about one's own experience, the other person, and the relationship
- Increased creativity and productivity
- Increased desire for more connection without feeling helpless or needy

Feminist counselors build growth-fostering relationships with clients to (a) foster personal growth and (b) increase clients' capacity to authentically be in relationship outside of session. When assessing clients, feminist counselors listen carefully for growth-fostering relationships in clients' lives that are characterized by the five good things. Counselors help clients nurture the growth-fostering relationships that they already have, transform other relationships to be growth fostering, and/or develop new ones.

Rumor Has It: The People and Their Stories

Laura Brown

A leading feminist practitioner and author, Laura Brown (1994, 2006, 2010) is a founding member of the Feminist Therapy Institute and has written extensively on feminist ethics, the politics of diagnosis, and surviving trauma.

Carolyn Zerbe Enns

Perhaps, Carolyn Enns, an active feminist therapy theorist, focuses her work on integrating feminist and multicultural issues in everyday practice. In addition, her more recent research focuses on how to teach diversity sensitivity in the classroom (Enns, Sinacore, Ancis, & Phillips, 2004).

Carol Gilligan

Carol Gilligan's *In a Different Voice: Psychological Theory and Women's Development* (1993) is a foundational feminist work that describes women's psychosocial and moral development organized around connectedness and interdependence based on an ethic of care in contrast to traditional psychological theories based on masculine values of autonomy and individuation.

Judith Jordan

A founding member of the Stone Center (see below), Judith Jordan is the director of the Jean Baker Miller Training Institute and is a leading figure in the development of relational-cultural theory (Jordan, 2010).

Jean Baker Miller

A seminal theorist and founding member of the Stone Center (see below), Jean Baker Miller authored one of the first feminist books in the field, *Toward a New Psychology of Women* (1986), which clearly outlines an feminist alternative to the traditional understandings of the mind and relationships. Miller has been a principal figure in the development of self-in-relation and relational-cultural theories, exploring issues in practice, social action, and multiculturalism.

The Stone Center

Feminists at the Stone Center at Wellesley College have been developing cutting-edge feminist theory for over 30 years. This implies that self-in-relation and relational theory are the same. But in other occurrences in this text, it implies that they are two different theories.

Big Picture: Overview of Counseling Process

The feminist counseling process evolved around two primary themes: (a) an egalitarian counseling relationship and (b) recognition of sources of oppression. The process of counseling involves the following:

1. *Developing an egalitarian relationship:* The initial goals of the counseling process are to develop (a) a relationship in which clients feel safe and understood and (b) a sense of having a voice in shaping the process.
2. *Exploring sources of marginalization and disconnection:* Next the counselor works with the client to identify sources of relational disconnection and social marginalization that relate to and fuel the presenting problem.
3. *Fostering authenticity and empowerment:* Using the counseling relationship as a place to experience empathy and authenticity, counselors empower clients to transfer learning in session to address areas of concern in their everyday lives.
4. *Building better relationships and communities:* In the later stages of the counseling process, clients are encouraged to promote social change to reduce forms of oppression for themselves and others as a means of increasing their sense of being part of growth-fostering relationships and communities.

Making Connection: Counseling Relationship
Egalitarian

As social power is a central focus on feminist counseling, the counselor strives to make the counseling relationship *egalitarian* by closely attending to the inherent power imbalance in the relationship (Brown, 2010; Enns, 2004). How exactly do they achieve this seeming paradox? Feminist counselors have open discussions about the power dynamics and politics of counseling, such as the diagnosis process, communications with other professionals, and the counseling theories chosen. In these conversations, the counselor *demystifies* the counseling process and invites clients to share their opinions, ask questions, and do their own research, all of which is considered equally along side the counselor's thoughts and theory (Worell & Remer, 1992). Much like in collaborative therapy (see Chapter 12), the feminist counseling process is a *mutual exploration* of how best to resolve clients' issues in which counselors recognize clients' expertise in their own lives.

In addition, feminist counselors use *self-disclosure* to increase the sense of equality in the relationship and help clients develop hope and courage in their own lives. Counselors' egalitarian self-disclosure also involves admitting when they are wrong, being open to correction, and acknowledging personal defensiveness rather than assuming that relational disruptions are solely clients' faults. Instead, the counseling relationship is—in good times and bad—a two-way street where the counselor is equally responsible for bumpy roads and misunderstandings.

Mutual Empathy and Growth

A unique feminist concept, *mutual empathy* refers to two-way empathy in which each person—counselor and client—is able to see, know, and feel the inner experience of the other as well as experience *responsiveness* from the other. Mutual empathy involves *both persons impacting the other*, caring for the other, and responding to the other. This experience of mutuality repairs empathetic failures in early, formative childhood relationships, and recent research indicates that there is active brain resonance between people experiencing empathy and that this alters the functioning of the brain in positive ways (Schore, 1994). The counselor allows clients to see that what they say touches and moves the counselor in a personal and human way. These exchanges help clients to feel more connected, reducing their sense of isolation from others and increasing their capacity for relationships that foster growth (see "Growth Fostering Relationships and the Five Good Things" in "The Juice"). In addition, the counselor is authentically and personally touched in the process, enhancing the counselor's growth also.

Counseling relationships built on mutuality should not be misunderstood as sappy, saccharin-sweet relationships in which there is not conflict, disagreement, or confrontation. In fact, these relationships demand high levels of honesty and authenticity, which inherently bring differences and conflicts to the surface. However, because of the relational context, these differences can lead to "good conflict," in which each person's unique experiences, beliefs, and feelings are heard and *responded to*, allowing for each member to learn and grow (Jordan, 2010). In good conflict, even though there is a difference, each person fundamentally feels safe and trusts that the relationship is not threatened. Thus, the counselor cannot retreat into a position of power but instead maintains an egalitarian, human presence and respectfully works through the differences with clients. In fact, moments of conflict and disconnection provide the most fertile opportunities for growth, for it is precisely in these moments when counselors can stay present and responsive and help clients have a *corrective relational experience*, enabling clients to develop new relational patterns (Jordan, 2010). Clients first learn to do this with the counselor and then transfer this to relationships outside the counseling process.

Authenticity

Feminist counselors cultivate *authenticity* in their relationships with clients. "Authenticity" in the counseling context does not mean that the counselor expresses any old emotion, thought, or reaction that spontaneously arises but instead implies a genuine *responsiveness* that keeps the well-being and needs of the client in mind. Clinical judgment and ethics always guide the counselors' expressions of authenticity (Jordan, 2010). In determining which authentic expressions are appropriate with a given client, feminists ask themselves, "*Will this* [information, action, expression, etc.] *facilitate the client's growth? Will this further healing? Will this strengthen the relationship?*" Errors can occur, and when they do, the counselor needs to be ready to apologize and correct the relational disconnection, remaining responsive and open to hearing the client's response.

Feminist Code of Ethics

Feminists at the Feminist Therapy Institute (2000) have developed a *Feminist Code of Ethics*, which counselors use to guide their work and relationships with clients *in addition to* other professional codes. This ethical code describes a commitment to recognizing the impact of dominant cultural norms, acknowledging power differentials in relationships, managing overlapping relationships to avoid abuse, establishing counselor accountability, and promoting social change:

> Feminists believe the personal is political. Basic tenets of feminism include a belief in the equal worth of all human beings, a recognition that each individual's personal experiences and situations are reflective of and an influence on society's institutionalized attitudes and values, and a commitment to political and social change that equalizes power among people. Feminists are committed to recognizing and reducing the pervasive influences and insidious effects of oppressive societal attitudes and society. (p. 1)

Men and Feminist Counseling

Can men be feminist counselors? Do feminist counselors work with men? Yes and yes. Although many of the seminal ideas originate in feminist literature, the applications and values behind them are universal. Contemporary feminist approaches, such as relational-cultural therapy, emphasize diversity and relational responsiveness more than simply women's issues. The values that define feminist approaches—ending oppression, equality, and mutuality—have validity for men and women and have the potential to help both sexes live more authentically and with greater social connection.

Ironically, in the future, feminist approaches may have increased relevance for men. Twenty-first-century economic, political, and social changes are rapidly redefining the role of men in society, and men have—as a group—had more difficulty adapting to these changes than women had in the 20th century as their social roles were redefined (Rosin, 2010). For example, in 2010, for the first time, more American women worked then men. At the same time, 60% of college graduates were female. Many men are struggling to define themselves in a postindustrial economy, where flexibility, relationships, and collaboration matter more than physical strength and size. Additionally, male socialization pushes many men into disconnection from themselves and emotions in boyhood, leaving them searching for ways to connect in adulthood (Shepherd, 2005). In the years ahead, feminist counselors may find they are surprisingly well equipped to help men struggling to find meaning, identity, and connection as their social roles are dramatically and rapidly redefined.

The Viewing: Case Conceptualization
The Personal Is Political; the Political Is Personal

One of the foundational assumptions of feminist counseling is that *the personal is political*, meaning that a person's internal reality—and therefore pathology—is inherently interconnected with political issues from the broader social context (Brown, 2006; Remer, 2008). This is true for men as well as women, heterosexuals as well as those with alternative sexual orientations, and persons of all cultural and ethnic backgrounds. The reverse is also true: the political is also personal (Brown, 2006), meaning that what happens at the societal level affects people in a very personal way. Thus, when developing a case conceptualization, feminist counselors help clients separate internal and external sources of problems by *raising awareness* of oppression, privilege, and societal impact on individual experience. For example, a professional Hispanic mother who is feeling depressed would be encouraged to look at the numerous and contradictory expectations society maintains for the roles of "mother" and "professional" as well as the American stereotypes of Hispanic women as well as the Hispanic community's expectations of her. Similarly, a working-class African American father struggling with substance abuse would be encouraged to examine social roles associated with his class, race, and gender in relation to his problems. In the case study at the end of this chapter, the counselor helps Jayla examine the political effects of being a professional African American woman in an emotionally abusive relationship, considering multiple, interlocking layers of marginalization.

The Politics of DSM-IV Diagnosis

Like other postmodernists feminists have long challenged, as an oppressive practice, the diagnoses outlined in the *Diagnostic and Statistical Manual of Mental Disorders* (4th ed., text revision [*DSM-IV*]). Long from over, this critique is more alive than ever:

> I would submit that feminist critiques of the diagnostic process exemplified by the *DSM* remain fresh and will be even more necessary in the future as increasing numbers of people receive one of these labels during the course of their lives. What does it mean that almost half of the U.S. population qualifies for a formal diagnosis, according to recent news reports? Feminist critique demands a complex analysis and synthesis of the emerging data about the biology of various forms of distress, on the one hand calling into question assumptions about the hard-wired, evolutionarily immutable nature of some phenomena, and on the other calling attention to the profound changes made to neuro-anatomy by exposure to traumatic stress. Feminist theory requires that we conceptualize our clients' distress/ [using] a range of factors that include the parameters of distress and dysfunction as currently subjectively experienced by our clients. (Brown, 2006, p. 19)

As you may have surmised, feminist counselors are in no rush to find a *DSM-IV* label to slap on clients. Instead, they carefully develop a thoughtful case conceptualization that includes the impact of social norms, cultural differences, gender politics, trauma, and clients' subjective experience and understanding of their situations (Brown, 2010). Most feminists would agree that in some cases, a diagnostic label can be helpful and even liberating. For example, women who have been sexually abused often feel quite relieved to hear that flashbacks, nightmares, and hypervigilance are quite normal responses to trauma. In every case, feminist counselors are keenly aware of the political impact that diagnosis has in relationships (e.g., how friends, partners, and family see the person), in medical treatment (e.g., services and fees by insurance companies), and, most important, on how clients see and understand themselves.

Gender Roles

One of the primary areas of assessment, feminist counselors carefully explore clients' *gender role expectations* and how these relate to the presenting problem and clients' lives more broadly (Miler, 1986). Feminists note that "gender is commonly the first identity that people experience, coming before other identity markers such as culture, ethnicity, or social class, because gender, as a sex-derived social construct, is frequently the variable of greatest importance to the human world into which a child is born" (Brown, 2010, p. 52). Counselors explore how the client has internalized social messages about gender and how an individual's social class, cultural background, profession, and sexual orientation shape the clients' understanding of gender roles. For example, many women who report feeling depressed strongly maintain gendered expectations that women put the needs of others before their own, physically, emotionally, and professionally. Not surprisingly, the National Institute of Mental Health (2010) reports that women are more likely than men to be diagnosed with major depressive disorder as well as any mental health disorder. The social pressure for women to be nice, not make waves, and care for others takes a personal toll and sets the stage for depression (Kaplan, 1991). Feminist counselors explore the interaction of gender role and the development of psychological distress.

Self-in-Relation

One of the original theories at the Stone Center, *self-in-relation* theory refers to an alternative model for conceptualizing women's development (Surrey, 1991). In contrast to traditional developmental theories, "self-in-relation involves the recognition that, for women, the primary experience of self is relational, that is, the self is organized and developed in the context of important relationships" (p. 52). Thus, rather than follow the Ericksonian developmental model that emphasizes autonomy, self-reliance, self-actualization, and other forms of separation, feminists describe women as developing their sense of self *in and through relationships*. Thus, when developing case conceptualizations with clients, the counselor views women's development through a relational lens, exploring the evolution and development of self through significant relationships in the woman's life.

Marginalization and Oppression

Contemporary feminist counselors have far more on their agenda than women's issues. They are aware that in addition to gender, people can be marginalized because of culture, race, sexual orientation, age, ability, economic class, religion, and numerous other factors. All of these contribute to a person feeling *disconnected* and marginalized from the dominant group, rejected for one's "otherness." Chronically having to hide parts of the self to be accepted leads to psychological symptoms and pathology (Jordan, 2010). Thus, feminist counselors consider *social oppression* and isolation to be the root cause of clients' problems (Brown, 2010). By identifying these sources of marginalization in the case conceptualization process, counselors identify where and how to help clients build the connections they need to live full, authentic lives.

Relational Images

Relational-cultural counselors assess clients' *relational images*, internal constructs and expectations of relationship based on early life experience, and carefully trace how these affect present-day relationships (Jordan, 2010). People who experience chronic disconnection and relational trauma develop negative relational images that diminish their ability to fully participate in growth-fostering relationships and restrict their ability to experience authenticity. Such negative images are projected onto to other relationships, repeating a painful life pattern. Thus, the case conceptualization process involves identifying these patterns, which are both verbally described and often reenacted in the counseling relationship. In particular, counselors pay attention to *controlling images* that result in *shame* and *disempowerment*, defining what is acceptable and who the client is. These controlling images are often experienced as immutable by clients, resulting in *internal oppression*, where the client rejects parts of the self, thus becoming disconnected from the self as well as others. The counseling relationship is used as a forum for clients to modify their relational images so that they can experience more satisfying relationships, referred to as *correctional relational experiences* (similar to *corrective emotional experiences* described in Chapter 4). In the case study at the end of this chapter, the counselor assesses Jayla's early relational images with her mother, who was the sole caretaker of her and her sister.

Relational Resilience and Courage

A critical quality for healing, *relational resilience* refers to the ability to move back into relationship following disconnection and empathetic failures as well as the ability to ask for help when needed (Jordan, 2010). Counselors don't force or push clients to work through disconnections either in session or in their personal lives but instead create a context in which it is safe to do so, modeling that the well-being of the relationship has priority over making a point and being right. Developing relational resilience requires courage but not the form of heroic legend, which glorifies individual accomplishment and typically domination of another. Instead, *relational courage* is far quieter and scarier: it requires vulnerability and the willingness to open up to another. The counselor's role is to help "en-courage" clients so that they are willing to take the risks that intimacy and relationship demand.

"Mattering" and Connection

When assessing, feminist counselors pay particular attention to the growth-fostering relationships and other contexts in which clients feel that they "matter," that they are valued and cherished by another (Jordan, 2010). This sense of "mattering" to someone—either in a personal relationship or in broader social communities—is considered vital to mental and relational health and well-being; recent research has shown that this is particularly important for persons diagnosed with severe mental illness (Davidson, Tondora, Lawless, O'Connell, & Rowe, 2008). Counselors listen for both areas of strength—relationships where clients feel they matter to someone—and areas where a sense of connection needs to be built and use these to identify goals and build on strengths.

Disconnection Strategies and the Central Relational Paradox

In addition to identifying sources of connection, feminist counselors also identify the strategies clients use to disconnect from others when they feel vulnerable. Counselors use several questions to guide their assessment of disconnection:

Assessment of Disconnection

1. What strategies are used to disconnect from others: family, partner, friends, colleagues, children, and so on?
2. Where were these methods first learned and used?
3. Does shame or disempowerment fuel the need for disconnection?
4. How useful are these strategies in current relationships?
5. Does the client know how and when to reconnect?

One way that people cope with repeated disconnection is to alter the self to fit the wishes of others at the expense of personal authenticity; this is referred to as the *central relational paradox* because it describes how, in response to disconnection, a person seeks connection by avoiding authentic connection. This paradoxical attempt to connect without connecting must change in order for clients to experience grow-fostering relationships that promote wellness.

Targeting Change: Goal Setting
Sociopolitical Awareness and Empowerment

Feminist counselors strive to increase a person's *sociopolitical awareness* of how their individual identity is interconnected with one's broader place in society and *empower* clients to define themselves by alternative standards. Feminists strive to have all clients become more aware of how their *gender, ethnicity, social class, sexual orientation, physical characteristics,* and *physical abilities* significantly affect a person's identity and sense of self-worth (Worell & Johnson, 2001). Thus, one of the goals is to help clients develop greater awareness of how these sociocultural variables inform their identity, critically evaluate their effects, and ultimately develop their identity by crafting their sense of identity with full awareness using personal values and the values from communities that have personal significance.

Connection

The overarching goal of feminist counseling, specifically relational-cultural counseling, is to build *connection*, specifically *growth-fostering relationships* (Jordan, 2010). When clients are able to establish such relationships, they create contexts in which they can authentically experience themselves while feeling a zest for life, valuing the self, being productive, and learning more about who they are: quite simply, a recipe for a lifelong process of evolving into one's best self.

The Doing: Interventions and Ways of Promoting Change

Introduction to Feminist Techniques

The emphasis of feminist counseling is on case conceptualization and the quality of the counseling relationship more so than intervening. In fact, interventions from other approach may be used *if adapted* to in a gender and culturally sensitive manner (Enns, 1992; Worell & Remer, 1992). The techniques below are some of the more unique ones used in feminist counseling.

Gender Role Analysis

A hallmark and defining intervention, *gender role analysis* involves encouraging clients to exam how cultural rules about male and female behavior affect the client's current distress, including multiple cultural rules from the different contexts of a client's life, such as religious, work, family, and ethnic traditions (Enns, 2000; Worell & Remer, 1992). Used with both men and women, gender role analysis helps clients better identify the often unacknowledged pressures and beliefs that support the problem. In the case study at the end of this chapter, the counselor helps Jayla to increase her awareness of how her gender role interacts with being a professional and African American and her tolerance of inappropriate behavior from her boyfriend.

Questions to Facilitate Gender Role Analysis

- What beliefs do you have about being a "good woman" (or man) that might be related to the presenting problem?
- In what ways do you see gender stereotyping affecting you at work, at home, in your family, with friends, with your children, in your religious community, in your ethnic community, and so on?
- What did you learn from your parents about what it means to be a girl/boy or man/woman? Which of these still affect you today?
- What do you believe is a woman's (or man's) role in work? In a relationship? In a family? Regarding finances? Regarding health?
- What are your relationships like with men, women, heterosexuals, and persons who identify as gay/lesbian/bisexuals/transgendered?
- (If in a heterosexual relationship) How do you see gender roles playing out in your relationship? Do you like these effects?
- (If in same-sex relationship) How do you see gender stereotypes and gay/lesbian stereotypes playing out in your relationships?
- What is your philosophy on gender relations and cultural issues?
- How have gender, culture, sexual orientation, class, ability, and other diversity variables affected how you see yourself?

Assertiveness Training

Perhaps, *Assertiveness training*, a classic cognitive-behavioral technique, is adapted by feminists for helping empower clients, most notably women, who have been socialized to put the needs of others before their own (Worell & Remer, 1992). Assertiveness training involves teaching clients the difference between assertive, passive, and aggressive behaviors:

- *Assertive:* Able to balance the needs of self and others
- *Passive:* Attends only to the needs of others
- *Aggressive:* Attends only to the needs of self

Using a psychoeducational approach, clients are taught in role plays and real-world experiments how to advocate for their needs while honoring the needs of others in difficult interpersonal situations.

Self-Esteem Training

Proposed as an alternative to assertiveness training for women with very low self-esteem and/or constricted by rigid gender role stereotypes, self-esteem training emphasizes increasing a client's self-awareness and confidence, which ultimately enables her to assert her needs in interpersonal relationships (Stere, 1985). Self-esteem training involves developing four areas of personal skills:

1. *Accepting feelings as rational and valid:* Validating feelings of guilt and resentment related to sociocultural inequities; trusting feeling reactions; expressing feelings
2. *Being able to please self:* Knowing what one wants; feeling worthy; taking action and making requests on one's own behalf
3. *Identifying personal strengths:* Valuing feminine qualities; feeling courage to be successful; making positive self statements
4. *Being gentle with self and accepting personal "imperfections":* Developing realistic expectations for self; feeling calm when criticized; stating what shortcomings are

Corrective Relational Experiences

Relational-cultural theory describes how the mutuality of counseling relationship provides numerous opportunities for *corrective relational experiences*, experiences in which old relational images are reworked by the counselor providing an alternative, connecting response in a situation where the client had experienced only disconnect in other relationships (Jordan, 2010). For example, clients who had highly critical parents often experience extreme, painful disconnection with even the slightest negative comment. When counselors are able to stay connected and empathetic with clients who feel criticized or as if they have failed in some way, the counselor provides a *corrective relational experience* by not disengaging when clients have come to expect the other to abandon them. By maintaining an empathetic and mutual engaged relationship, counselors help clients work through various corrective relational experiences, first in session and ultimately in relationships outside of the counseling context. For example, in the case study at the end of this chapter, the counselor uses in-session corrective relational experiences to help Jayla learn how to better relate to her boyfriend.

Self-Empathy

Relational-cultural approaches emphasize the importance of developing *self-empathy* in clients, the ability to bring empathetic awareness and a gentle presence to one's own experience (Jordan, 2010). Rather than judging or rejecting, clients learn how to stay with their feelings and experience empathy for how they came about. Clients first experience empathy from without, from the counselor, but are then encouraged to use this same kind of empathy in their inner dialogues. Counselors promote self-empathy by questioning their negative self statements, such as "I shouldn't feel this way" or "I was a fool to do X." Such statements are countered with questions, such as "You are so accepting of others, but you do not accept the same qualities (actions, feelings, etc.) in yourself." If a client is particularly self-loathing, the counselor may ask the client to imagine it was a friend who was experiencing the situation and to have the client identify how she would see the situation in that case.

Social Activism and Social Justice

The feminist counseling is not a solitary process. Clients cannot meaningfully redefine their gender and personal identity stories or seek connection in a vacuum or even in the dyad of the counseling relationship. By definition, changing one's gender identity and building connection happens in relationship and community. Thus, for clients to change, their relationships and social connections must also change. One way this is commonly achieved is through *social activism* and *social justice work* of various forms, activities that clients often spontaneously seek in the closing phase of treatment. This can involve something as stereotypical as becoming involved in activist groups but more often takes far subtler forms, such as getting a group of mothers or fathers together from work or taking a stand on body issues in a circle of friends. Sometimes clients ask counselors where they can make a difference in the community with certain groups, such as children who have been sexually abused or immigrants needing assistance, and counselors should be ready and able to help them connect with appropriate community resources. Often, helping others who have experienced similar painful situations can be a transformative experience in which a client shifts from feeling like a victim to full recovery.

In addition, feminist counselors themselves are committed to social justice causes, using both professional and personal venues to effect societal change. This may take the form of advocating for clients in obtaining mental health or other services, in court situations, or in other contexts related to the client. Additionally, feminist counselors typically are involved in broader social movements, women's movements, clients' rights groups, children's advocacy, political campaigns, and similar efforts to promote social change.

Putting It All Together: Feminist Treatment Plan Template

Use this treatment plan template for developing a plan for clients with depressive, anxious, or compulsive types of presenting problems. Depending on the specific client, presenting problem, and clinical context, the goals and interventions in this template may need to be modified only slightly or significantly; you are encouraged to significantly revise the plan as needed. For the plan to be useful, goals and techniques should be written to target specific beliefs, behaviors, and emotions that the client is experiencing. The more specific, the more useful it will be to you.

Treatment Plan

Initial Phase of Treatment (First One to Three Sessions)
Initial Counseling Task

1. *Develop working counseling relationship. Diversity note:* Adapt style of connection for ethnicity, gender, age, and so on.
   Relationship building intervention:
   a. Develop **growth-fostering relationship** using **mutual empathy** and **authenticity**.

2. *Assess individual, systemic, and broader cultural dynamics. Diversity note:* Attend to relational and conflict management preferences based on gender, ethnicity, and other diversity factors.
   Assessment Strategies:
   a. Identify **gender role expectations** and the affects of the **political on the personal**, including sources of **marginalization** and **oppression**.
   b. Assess sources of "**mattering**," **relational resilience**, and **disconnection strategies**.

Initial Phase Client Goal *(One to Two Goals):* Manage crisis issues and/or reduce most distressing symptoms

1. *Increase* **empowerment** and feelings of "**mattering**" to reduce [specific crisis symptoms].
   Interventions:
   a. Identify sources of **marginalization**, **oppression**, and **disconnection** that fuel sense of crisis.
   b. Identify **relationships and communities** that provide support and connection when needed to manage feelings that lead to crisis.

(continued)

Working Phase of Treatment (Two + Sessions)
Working Phase Counseling Task

1. *Monitor quality of the working alliance. Diversity note:* Attend to issues of power and client's sense of **empowerment** to provide honest feedback to counselor. *Assessment Intervention:*
   a. Look for evidence of and ask about client experiencing **five good things** in counseling relationship; use Session Rating Scale.

Working Phase Client Goals *(Two to Three Goals).* Target individual and relational dynamics using theoretical language (e.g., decrease avoidance of intimacy, increase awareness of emotion, increase agency)

1. *Increase* awareness of the effects of **politics-as-personal, gender roles,** and **marginalization** to reduce [specific symptoms: depression, anxiety, etc.].
   Interventions:
   a. **Gender role analysis** and **analysis of sociopolitical influences** and how they affect the problem.
   b. Connect with friends, groups, and causes that create a sense of **empowerment** in relation to the problem issue.

2. *Increase* ability to relate to people and situations from an **assertive** position of respect for self and other to reduce [specific symptoms: depression, anxiety, etc.].
   Interventions:
   a. **Assertiveness training** to learn how to balance asserting one's needs while respecting those of others.
   b. **Self-esteem training** to develop a greater sense of self-acceptance.

3. *Increase* number and quality of **mutual growth-fostering relationships** to reduce [specific symptoms: depression, anxiety, etc.].
   Interventions:
   a. **Corrective emotional experiences** to learn how to relate more authentically.
   b. Learn to identify **disconnection strategies** and ways to repair the disconnection.

Closing Phase of Treatment (Last Four or More Sessions)
Closing Phase Counseling Tasks

1. *Develop aftercare plan and maintain gains. Diversity note:* Include relational and community resources to support client after counseling ends.
   Intervention:
   a. Identify **relational** and **sociopolitical** forces that are likely to generate problems in the future, prevention, and potential assertive responses.

Closing Phase Client Goals *(One to Two Goals):* Determined by theory's definition of health and normalcy

1. *Increase* client's sense of **relational resilience, "mattering,"** and **empowerment** to reduce feelings of disconnection [*or* anxiety, fear, etc.]
   Interventions:
   a. Apply learning from **corrective emotional experiences** in session to relationships outside.
   b. Empower client to advocate for **relational resilience** and **marginalized others** in relationships.

2. *Increase* **advocacy** and **social justice** efforts for self and/or marginalized others to reduce sense of disempowerment [*or* depressive, anxious, compulsive behaviors, etc.].
   Interventions:
   a. Identify contexts and relationships for **advocacy efforts** that enhance client's sense of self-esteem.
   b. Identity relationships and organizations that foster client's ongoing **growth** and **resilience.**

Snapshot: Research and the Evidence Base

Quick Summary: Similar to other narrative and collaborative counseling, feminists have conducted relatively little empirical research on their specific approach; however, they draw from the common factors and attachment research to support their work (Brown, 2010).

Similar to humanists, feminists cite the common factors evidence that indicates that a supportive, nonjudgmental counseling relationship is consistently correlated with positive outcomes to support their models that emphasize an egalitarian relationship (Brown, 2006). In addition, recent neurological research provides support for the premise that humans are "hardwired" for relational connection and, in fact, that the human brain needs human relationship to develop and function properly (Jordan, 2010). These streams of research, although not on feminist theory directly, do support many of the core premises of the approach. Some research has been conducted on training counselors to become aware of feminism and power issues. For example, Keeling, Butler, Green, Kraus, and Palit (2010) demonstrated that the Gender Discourse in Therapy Questionnaire was effective in helping counselors better identify gender issues in counseling. More research needs to be conducted on the effectiveness of the feminist model as well as on training counselors working from all perspectives on how to identify gender issues in session.

Snapshot: Working With Diverse Populations

Quick Summary: Designed for addressing cultural and gender issues, feminist approaches are well suited for diverse populations; however, feminist counselors need to be careful not to force values or political agendas on clients.

In addition to narrative, feminist counseling approaches is one of the few mental health theories that places societal issues of oppression at the heart of treatment, and most feminist practitioners believe that advocacy and social justice in the general community is part of their roles as counselors (Brown, 2006). Feminists believe in equality in relationships, equality between the sexes, self-determination, and the primacy of relationships and connection. Although many clients also embrace these values, feminist counselors need to be aware that these values are not shared by all people, some of these values contracting religious beliefs and some traditional cultural values. Thus, even though these approaches are designed to reduce oppression, because they include specific values, it is possible for clients to feel misunderstood if the approach is not adapted for their personal beliefs and values. In particular, some men feel immediately unsafe when they hear their counselor identifies as a "feminist." Thus, feminist counselors should make extra efforts to develop solid, respectful relationships when working with clients who are likely to have different religious, political, and/or cultural beliefs and values.

Feminist Case Study and Treatment Plan

A 43-year-old corporate attorney, Jayla has come to counseling because she says that she believes her current relationship has eroded her self-esteem and she is feeling more and more depressed. She has been with Mark for over 10 years and says that she feels lucky to be with a man who is not intimated by her successful career. As she makes more than he does, she pays for many of their living expenses and their lavish vacations. She says they argue often because "I am not going to keep my mouth shut just to keep the peace; I am a lawyer after all." In their arguments, Mark often makes comments that question her competence and intelligence, and over the years Jayla believes she is beginning to believe him. He also tries to control what she wears, as he can be jealous and often puts down her choice of friends; she denies that he has ever hit or thrown things at her. She describes being raised by her mother, "who was an amazing woman of faith and strength"; she worked two jobs to raise her and her sister and ensured that both girls did well in school and stayed out of trouble. Her mother, who was the only parent she knew, died 2 years ago from breast cancer, and Jayla takes pride in trying to be strong in her memory. She and her sister remain very close and have helped each other through the loss of their mother. Jayla has no kids but wonders if it is not too late to change that.

Feminist Case Conceptualization

This case conceptualization was developed by selecting key concepts from "The Viewing: Case Conceptualization" section of this chapter. You can use any of the concepts in that section to develop a case conceptualization for this or other cases.

The Personal Is Political; the Political Is Personal

As a successful African American woman, AF (adult female) is experiencing two forms of oppression in her relationship: stigma as a successful woman and as an African American woman. Her boyfriend is emotionally abusive, which in part may be triggered by his insecurity with their reversed roles with her being the primary breadwinner. His need to control and be superior are likely informed by his socially reinforced definition of what it means to be a man.

The Politics of DSM-IV Diagnosis

Given that AF's situation is clearly related to gender and race politics, *DSM-IV* diagnoses, which focus on individual pathology, are not the best explanation for her situation. Describing her situation in terms of the gender and race politics is more likely to help her successfully cope and manage.

Gender Roles

Gender role expectations are at the heart of AF's situation. She learned a very independent model for being a woman and has flourished as professional in a competitive field. In contrast, her boyfriend is using a more traditional definition of male–female roles in which the man has the right to make decisions about how a woman conducts herself. On the one hand, AF believes that she is asserting herself by standing up to him and arguing; on the other, she says that over the years she feels as though these arguments and constant questioning are causing her to slowly lose her confidence. She has begun to question herself more and more, leading to a sense of depression.

Self-in-Relation

AF reports developing a confident self-in-relation to her mother and sister, both of whom were strong, independent women who were/are supportive of her. Unfortunately, her current relationship with her boyfriend has increasingly not been a place where her true self feels safe and can flourish, and instead she feels she must fight to defend herself.

Marginalization and Oppression

Undoubtedly, AF has experienced numerous forms of marginalization and oppression as an African American woman in a highly competitive, male-dominated profession. These experiences are likely replicated in her current relationship. Her response has been to fight and stand up for herself in the face of oppression, but the negative comments still affect her self-esteem and confidence.

Relational Images

Although AF's mother worked long hours, AF still reports feeling connected to her mother and her sister. These growth-fostering relationships still sustain her today and are informing her uneasiness with her current romantic relationship, where she is not feeling safe and supported.

Relational Resilience and Courage

AF has demonstrated relational resilience and courage in that she continues to work on her relationship with her boyfriend, even though she has not made significant progress. This tendency to try to work through the relationship may actually be keeping her stuck.

"Mattering" and Connection

AF feels less and less like she matters in her relationship with her boyfriend; however, she still feels a sense of connection and mattering with her sister.

Disconnection Strategies and the Central Relational Paradox

When feeling disconnected, AF tries to reconnect by debating the point with the other and trying to convince the other to see her perspective. Debating and arguing draws on her professional strengths but is not working in her current relationship to reestablish connection.

Feminist

Initial Phase of Treatment (First One to Three Sessions)
Initial Phase Counseling Tasks

1. *Develop working counseling relationship. Diversity note:* Adapt communication style based on AF's level of education, professional background, and ethnic background. *Relationship building intervention:*
   a. Develop **growth-fostering relationship** with AF using **mutual empathy** and **authenticity**.

2. *Assess individual, systemic, and broader cultural dynamics. Diversity note:* Adapt assessment to consider AF's level of education, professional background, and ethnic background.
   Assessment Strategies:
   a. Identify **gender role expectations** and the effects of the **political on the personal**, including sources of **marginalization** and **oppression** that relate to her gender, race, and professional position.
   b. Assess sources of "**mattering**," **relational resilience**, and **disconnection strategies** in current and past relationships.

Initial Phase Client Goal

1. *Increase* **empowerment** and feelings of "**mattering**" to reduce feelings of depression.
   Interventions:
   a. Analyze sources of **marginalization, oppression,** and **disconnection** that fuel sense of crisis, namely, her current relationship and any similar professional dynamics.
   b. Identify **relationships and communities,** such as her sister, that provide support and connection when needed to manage feelings that lead to crisis.

Working Phase of Treatment (Three or More Sessions)
Working Phase Counseling Tasks

1. *Monitor quality of the working alliance. Diversity note:* Attend to issues of power and client's sense of **empowerment** to provide honest feedback to counselor.
   Assessment Intervention:
   a. Monitor for evidence of and ask about client experiencing **five good things** in counseling relationship; use Session Rating Scale.

Working Phase Client Goals

1. *Increase* awareness of the effects of **politics-as-personal, gender roles,** and **marginalization** and how they play out in current relationship to reduce depression and increase self-esteem.

(continued)

Interventions:
   a. **Gender role analysis** and **analysis of sociopolitical influences** in relationship and in career.
   b. Connect with friends, sister, religious groups, and causes that create a sense of **empowerment** as a successful African American woman.

2. *Increase* ability to relate to boyfriend from an **assertive** position of respect for self and other to reduce loss of confidence and self-esteem.
    Interventions:
    a. **Assertiveness training** to learn how to balance asserting her needs while respecting those of her boyfriend.
    b. **Self-esteem training** to develop a greater sense of self-acceptance in the relationship and in professional settings.

3. *Increase* number and quality of **mutual growth-fostering relationships** to reduce loss of confidence.
    Interventions:
    a. **Corrective emotional experiences** in session to learn how to relate more authentically.
    b. Learn to identify **disconnection strategies** used in relationship and find ways to repair the disconnection.

Closing Phase of Treatment (Last Four or More Sessions)
Closing Phase Counseling Tasks

1. *Develop aftercare plan and maintain gains. Diversity note:* Include relational and community resources to support client after counseling ends.
    Intervention:
    a. Identify **relational** and **sociopolitical** forces that are likely to generate problems in the future, prevention, and potential assertive responses.

Closing Phase Client Goals

1. *Increase* client's sense of **relational resilience**, "**mattering**," and **empowerment** in intimate relationships to reduce feelings of inferiority and depression.
    Interventions:
    a. Apply learning from **corrective emotional experiences** in session to romantic relationships.
    b. Empower client to advocate for **relational resilience** in relationships.

2. *Increase* **advocacy** and **social justice** efforts for self and marginalized others to reduce sense of disempowerment.
    Interventions:
    a. Identify contexts and relationships for **advocacy efforts** that enhance other African American women's sense of self-esteem.
    b. Identity relationships and organizations that foster personal ongoing **growth** and **resilience**.

ONLINE RESOURCES

Associations

Feminist Therapy Institute
www.feminist-therapy-institute.org

Feminist Therapy Code of Ethics
www.feminist-therapy-institute.org/ethics.htm

Stone Center at Wellesley College
www.wellesley.edu/Counseling/index.html

References

*Asterisk indicates recommended introductory readings.

Brown, L. (1994). *Subversive dialogues: Theory in feminist therapy*. New York: Basic Books.

*Brown, L. (2006). Still subversive after all these years: The relevance of feminist therapy in the age of evidence-based practice. *Psychology of Women Quarterly, 30*(1), 15–24. doi:10.1111/j.1471-6402.2006.00258.x

*Brown, L. (2010). *Feminist therapy*. Washington, DC: American Psychological Association.

Comstock, D. (Ed.). (2005). *Diversity and development: Critical contexts that shape our lives and relationships*. Pacific Grove, CA: Brooks/Cole.

Davidson, L., Tondora, J., Lawless, M. S., O'Connell, M. J., & Rowe. M. (2008). *A practical guide to recovery-oriented practice: Tools for transforming mental health care*. New York: Oxford University Press.

Enns, C. Z. (1992). Toward integrating feminist psychotherapy and feminist philosophy. *Professional Psychology: Research and Practice, 23*, 453–466.

Enns, C. Z. (2000). Gender issues in counseling. In S. D. Brown, & R. W. Rice (Eds.), *Handbook of counseling psychology* (3rd ed., pp. 601–669). New York: Wiley.

Enns, C. (2004). *Feminist theories and feminist psychotherapies: Origins, themes, and diversity* (2nd ed.). New York: Haworth.

Enns, C., Sinacore, A., Ancis, J., & Phillips, J. (2004). Toward Integrating feminist and multicultural pedagogies. *Journal of Multicultural Counseling and Development, 32*(extra), 414–427.

Feminist Therapy Institute. (2000). *Feminist code of ethics*. Georgetown, ME: Author.

Gilligan, C. (1993). *In a different voice: Psychological theory and women's development*. Cambridge, MA: Harvard University Press.

Jordan, J. (1997). *Women's growth in diversity*. New York: Guilford.

Jordan, J. (2010). *Relational-cultural therapy*. Washington, DC: American Psychological Association.

Jordan, J., Kaplan, A., Miller, J., Stiver, I., & Surrey, J. (1991). *Women's growth in connection: Writings from the Stone Center*. New York: Guilford.

Kaplan, A. G. (1991). The self-in-relation: A theory of women's development. In J. Jordan, A. G. Kaplan, J. B. Miller, I. P. Stiver, & J. L. Surrey (Eds.), *Women's growth in connection: Writings from the Stone Center* (pp. 206–222). New York: Guilford.

Keeling, M. L., Butler, J., Green, N., Kraus, V., & Palit, M. (2010). The Gender Discourse in Therapy Questionnaire: A tool for training in feminist-informed therapy. *Journal of Feminist Family Therapy: An International Forum, 22*(2), 153–169. doi:10.1080/08952831003787883

Miller, J. B. (1986). *Toward a new psychology of women* (2nd ed.). Boston: Beacon.

Miller, J. B., & Stiver, I. (1997). *The healing connection: How women form relationships in therapy and in life*. Boston: Beacon.

National Institute of Mental Health (2010). *Depression statistics*. Retrieved from http://www.nimh.nih.gov/statistics/1MDD_ADULT.shtml

Remer, P. (2008). *Feminist therapy*. In J. Frew & M. D. Spiegler (Eds.), *Contemporary psychotherapies for a diverse world* (pp. 397–441). Boston: Lahaska Press.

Rosin, H. (2010, July/August). The end of men. *The Atlantic*.

Schore, A. (1994). *Affect regulation and the origins of the self: The neurobiology of emotional development*. Hillsdale, NJ: Lawrence Erlbaum Associates.

Shepherd, D. (2005). Male development and the journey toward disconnection. In D. Comstock (Ed.), *Diversity and development: Critical contexts that shape our lives and relationships* (pp. 133–157). Pacific Grove, CA: Brooks/Cole.

Stere, L. K. (1985). Feminist assertiveness training: Self-esteem groups as skill training for women. In L. B. Rosewater & L. E. A. Walker (Eds.), *Handbook of feminist therapy: Women's issues in psychotherapy* (pp. 51–61). New York: Springer.

Surrey, J. L. (1991). The self-in-relation: A theory of women's development. In J. Jordan, A. G. Kaplan, J. B. Miller, I. P. Stiver, & J. L. Surrey (Eds.), *Women's growth in connection: Writings from the Stone Center* (pp. 51–66). New York: Guilford.

Worell, J., & Johnson, D. (2001). Therapy with women: Feminist frameworks. In R. K. Unger (Ed.), *Handbook of the psychology of women and gender* (pp. 317–329). New York: Wiley.

Worell, J., & Remer, P. (1992). *Feminist perspectives in therapy: An empowerment model for women*. New York: Wiley.

Section III

Theoretical Integration and Case Conceptualization

Theoretical Integration

And Now for the Exciting Conclusion

As you may (or may not) recall, in the cliffhanger Chapter 2, I refused to tell you more about integration and eclecticism and instead encouraged you to read through Chapters 4 through 13 with a curious and open mind. Now that you are done with the grand tour of theories, you are probably still wondering, "Do I really have to choose?" The answer is, of course, a frustrating yes *and* no. To unravel the multiple layers of this question, let's begin exploring what integration and eclecticism entail in the daily work of counseling.

As discussed in Chapter 2, the common factors movement coincides with a more general movement in counseling and psychotherapy toward theoretical *integration* and *eclecticism* (Miller, Duncan, & Hubble, 1997). Just as it sounds, "integration" refers to combining two or more theories into a coherent approach, while "eclecticism" implies a process of borrowing from more than one theory. At first, integration and eclecticism sound like you can have your cake and eat it too—almost too good to be true. Well, it's not that simple.

Doing integration or eclecticism poorly is easy enough. However, doing it well is far more challenging. It's like putting together a gourmet meal at a salad bar. It's possible; you have all of the right ingredients. But you are more likely to put together a hodge-podge of a meal that is unpleasant for your dinner companions to look at and leaves you feeling bloated. In fact, it takes a trained and restrained person with chef-like instincts to create something of value from the rich and diverse offerings of a salad bar. Similarly, it takes more effort and discipline to do integrative therapy well than it does to work from a single approach, which has been put together and field-tested for you by a gourmet of the psychotherapy world. Thus, choosing to work from a single theory is more like eating at a five-star restaurant: the menu is shorter, but you can be sure that everything on it will be excellent. At the salad bar, you need to put a lot more thought and energy into creating an equal rival. Thus, I generally do not recommend that new counselors start with an integrative or eclectic approach because it is far more difficult to do well. That said, as new counselors become more skilled and experienced, they are likely to move in the direction of integration.

Integration Options

The term "integration" is used a lot in the field, but rarely it seems that folks are using the same definition. This perhaps accounts for why there is so much debate. So the next time you find yourself arguing with a colleague about "integration," you might just want to clarify which variety of integration is being discussed:

- Common factors
- Theoretical integration
- Assimilative integration
- Technical integration
- Systematic treatment selection
- Syncretism and sloppy thinking

Common Factors Approach

As described in Chapter 2, counselors who use the *common factors approach* for integration conceptualize treatment using a common factors model, which identifies the core ingredients of counseling models, such as counseling alliance, client resources, and hope. Counselors who use this approach can then integrate concepts from various approaches using the common factors model. For example, a counselor may use the core conditions from person-centered counseling (see Chapter 6) to build the counseling relationship and solution-generating questions from solution-focused counseling (see Chapter 11) to generate hope. These practices are then incorporated and coherently connected using the common factors theory.

Theoretical Integration

As the name implies, counselors who use *theoretical integration* combine two or more theories into a single coherent theoretical model with the intention to improve or expand the potentials of either alone. Most evidence-based treatments (manualized treatments for a specific population; vaguely remember Chapter 2) are examples of theoretical integration. Emotionally focused therapy is an example of how systems theory, humanistic theory, and attachment theory have been combined to treat couples with better-than-average results (Johnson, 2004). Similarly, the now well-established cognitive-behavioral approaches (see Chapter 9) are an example of integrating behavioral and cognitive theories. Furthermore, many of the family counseling and therapy approaches are also examples of theoretical integration. Early pioneers, such as Virginia Satir (1972) and Carl Whitaker (Whitaker & Keith, 1981), integrated humanistic-existential and systemic approaches to develop their unique family models. In addition to these more formalized integrative models, individual clinicians also develop their unique integrative approaches, which are distinguished from technical eclecticism (see below) by the clear and thought-out combining of two or more theories.

Assimilative Integration

Closely related to theoretical integration, "assimilative integration" refers to having a firm theoretical grounding in one approach while selectively integrating practices from other approaches to allow for a broader range of intervention possibilities (Norcross & Beutler, 2008). In this approach, for example, a counselor may integrate solution-based scaling into a humanistic approach to identify goals and progress. After years of practice, the vast majority of counselors who identify with a single school of counseling most likely also practice some form of assimilative integration.

Technical Eclecticism

Counselors using *technical eclecticism* draw freely from techniques of various theories without significant concern about the theoretical underpinnings. Instead, the primary focus is identifying interventions that are likely to work for a specific client with a specific concern (Norcross & Beutler, 2008). Eclectics put little emphasis on the philosophical and theoretical principles underlying a technique and instead focus on trying to achieve desired outcomes from a specific theory. Increasingly, counselors are able to include evidence-based practice (using a literature review of research studies to identify potential treatments; see Chapter 2) to more precisely inform the choice of treatment.

Systematic Treatment Section

Systematic treatment selection models, such as Norcross and Beutler's (2008), provide an organized template for integrating theories that incorporates evidence-based practice (see Chapter 2). These approaches are designed to identify appropriate treatments and therapeutic relationships for a specific client. In Norcross and Beutler's approach, they (a) use evidence-based practices to identify what the research has shown to be an effective treatment for a particular client or problem, (b) draw from multiple systems of counseling to address client issues, (c) use five diagnostic and nondiagnostic dimensions to develop a case conceptualization, and (d) adapt treatment methods *and* the counseling relationship to best meet client needs. The five areas used to develop a case conceptualization include the following:

- *Mental health diagnosis:* The client is diagnosed using standard medical diagnoses in the *Diagnostic and Statistical Manual of Mental Disorders* (American Psychiatric Association, 2000).
- *Stages of change:* The client's readiness for change is described in one of four stages: contemplation, preparation, action, or maintenance.
- *Coping style:* The client's coping style is generally described as *internalizing* (e.g., depressed, self-critical, inhibited) or *externalizing* (e.g., aggressive, impulsive, stimulation-seeking).
- *Resistance level:* A client's resistance level refers to his or her willingness to take direct intervention from the counselor: if the client's resistance level is low, the counselor can use more directive techniques, whereas if the client's resistance is high, nondirective and paradoxical interventions are more appropriate.
- *Patient preferences:* Finally, the counselor considers client's preferences for the type of relationship and treatment; this often serves to accommodate diversity issues as well as the interaction of diversity issue between counselor and client (e.g., gender differences, age differences, ethnicity differences, educational differences).

Syncretism and Sloppy Thinking

As you might imagine, it is quite possible—or even likely—to use the labels "integration" or "eclectic" to simply mask a haphazard approach of doing what you feel like when you feel like it without much understanding of what you are doing or why or if there is any scientific or theoretical reason to do (i.e., "bad therapy"). Norcross and Beutler (2008) refer to this as *syncretism*, which simply refers to combining various philosophies. It can take the form to a less-than-optimal approach to an outright lawyers-will-be-involved harmful approach.

Too often, counselors develop pet theories or techniques because they have not received proper training, often unaware of what is being missed. Unfortunately, this is increasingly common, as intensive post-degree training in specific treatment approaches or areas of specialty are less common in the United States because of the increasing costs and drop in reimbursement rates over the years. Perhaps the best way to ensure you don't slip into sloppy, syncretic thinking is to seek intensive training in at least one approach. In addition, understanding philosophical differences between schools of counseling will also help prevent the mass confusion that leads to less-than-effective forms of syncretism.

Integration With Integrity

The key to integrating with integrity is understanding the difference between *philosophy* and *theory*. Each theoretical model is built on basic philosophical assumptions, such as what counts as "truth," what counts as "real," what it means to be human, and how humans change. Each theoretical model defines certain practices based on these assumptions. In most cases, skillful integration involves grounding yourself clearly in *one* set of philosophical assumptions and then *integrating* practices from other models and modifying them as necessary to *fit largely within a single set of philosophical principles*.

When counselors fail to work from a single, consistent set of philosophical assumptions, their clients are likely to become confused. For example, if one week the counselor focuses on emotional expression (based on the assumption that their internal, subjective reality is the focus of treatment), then the next week focuses on observable behaviors (based on the assumption that treatment should focus on externally validated behavior), and then later moves to an exploration of multiple, contradictory realities (based on the view that reality is constructed), the client is likely to be as confused as first-semester counseling student taking a comprehensive theory exam without reading the textbook. In contrast, if counselors ground their approach in a single philosophical approach, such as humanistic, they can then draw on techniques from diverse phenomenological models—person centered, Gestalt, and existential—and techniques from other models to support the general phenomenological process, such as analyzing a person's defense mechanisms (psychodynamic therapy) or schemas (cognitive therapy) to identify how they impede the client's process of self-actualization.

Overview of Philosophical Schools

	Modernist	Phenomenological	Systemic	Postmodern
Truth	Objective truth	Subjective truth	Contextual truth	Multiple, coexisting truths
Reality	Objective; observable	Subjective; individually accessible	Contextual; emerges through systemic interactions; no one person has unilateral control	Coconstructed through language and social interaction; occurs at individual, relational, societal levels
Counseling relationship	Expert; hierarchical	Empathetic other	Participant in counseling system	Nonexpert; coconstructor of meaning
Counselor's role in change process	Teaching and guide clients in better ways of being, interacting	Creating context that supports natural self-actualization process	"Perturb" system, allowing system to reorganize itself; no direct control of system	Facilitate a dialogue in which client constructs new meanings and interpretations
Associated schools	Psychodynamic; cognitive-behavioral	Person centered; existential; Gestalt; Adler	Systemic	Solution focused; narrative; collaborative; feminist; multicultural

Modernism

Modernism is founded on logical-positivist assumptions of an external, knowable "truth." In modernist approaches, the counselor assumes a role as expert, as in common in cognitive-behavioral and traditional psychodynamic therapies. The work of counselors who ground their approach in modernist philosophy are generally characterized by the following:

Common Modernist Assumptions

- The counselor is an expert who assumes the primary responsibility for identifying pathology, problems, and goals, often assuming the role of teacher or mentor.
- The counselor uses theory and research as the primary source of identifying problems and diagnosing.
- The counselor uses theory and research to select treatment approaches; clients are expected to adapt to selected treatment.

Although broadly grounded in modernistic assumptions about knowledge, traditional psychodynamic and cognitive-behavioral theories have their own unique stance on the primary source of truth, the means through which it is best identified, and how best to define the counseling relationship.

	Psychodynamic	Cognitive-Behavioral Therapies
Primary source of objective truth	Counselor's analysis of client dynamics based on theory	Measurable, external variables
Truth identified through …	"Reality check"; comparing client experience against external perceptions, events, etc.	Scientific experimentation; counselor definition of "reality" and/or social norms (identified through research)
Counseling relationship	Hierarchical; counselor indirectly leads client toward goals	Educator; counselor straightforward in directing client towards goals

Phenomenology: Humanistic-Existential

Phenomenological therapies are founded on a philosophy that prioritizes the individual's subjective truth and include Carl Rogers's (1951) person-centered therapy, Fritz Perls's Gestalt therapy (Parsons, 1975), and existential therapy (Frankl, 1963). In addition, although Adler's theory is generally considered a "dynamic" theory, its *philosophical foundations* are best classified as a phenomenological approach because the operating assumptions are closer to the humanistic-existential approaches (Sweeney, 2009); this an excellent example of why understanding the philosophical assumptions is critical to understanding the theory.

Most phenomenological theories share the following assumptions:

Common Phenomenological Assumptions

- All people naturally tend toward growth and strive for self-actualization, a process of becoming authentically human.
- The primary focus of treatment is the subjective, internal world of clients.
- Counseling interventions target emotions with the goal of promoting catharsis, the release of repressed emotions.
- A supportive, nurturing environment promotes counseling change.

Although based on similar philosophical traditions, person-centered, Gestalt, existential, and Adlerian approaches have different styles and assumptions, including differences related to the preferred ways to address self-actualization, change, confrontation, and counselor use-of-self.

	Person Centered	Gestalt	Existential	Adler
Self-actualization best promoted through …	Emotionally safe and nurturing environment	Counselor being "fully human"; warmth and confrontational	Directing reflecting on existential issues, such as death, alienation, etc.	Social interest and relational connection
Change promoted through …	Nondirective, process-oriented reflections	Affective confrontation of phony layers of self	Encouraging exploration of existential anxiety, fear of death, loss, etc.	Psychoeducation; tasks; challenging private logic

(*continued*)

Style of confrontation	Gentle, supportive	Direct and harsh when needed to break through denial	Intellectual; stark; "reality" focused	Educational direction
"Authentic" use of self-of-counselor defined as …	Genuine caring for the client	Showing full range of human emotions within counseling relationship	Acknowledging shared human experiences	Encouragement; egalitarian relationship

Systemic

Rather than a formal philosophical school, systemic therapies are grounded in *general systems theory*, which highlights that living systems are open systems, connected with and embedded within other systems (von Bertalanffy, 1968), and *cybernetic systems theory*, which emphasizes a system's ability to self-correct in order to maintain homeostasis (Bateson, 1972), the latter being more influential in development of specific counseling models, such as the brief therapy approach of the Mental Research Institute (MRI) (Watzlawick, Weakland, & Fisch, 1974), strategic therapy (Haley, 1976; Madanes, 1981), and the Milan team's systemic approach (Boscolo, Cecchin, Hoffman, & Penn, 1987). Systems theories emphasize *contextual* truth, truth generated through repeated interpersonal interactions that set a norm and rules for behavior. General tenets shared by systemic counselors are the following:

Common Systemic Assumptions

- One cannot *not* communicate; all behavior is a form of communication.
- An individual's behavior and symptoms always make sense in the person's broader relational contexts.
- All behaviors, including unwanted symptoms, serve a purpose within the system, allowing the system to maintain or regain its homeostasis or feeling of "normalcy."
- No one individual unilaterally controls behavior in a system; thus, no one person can be blamed for problems in a couple or family relationship. Instead, problematic behavior is viewed as emerging from the interaction patterns between members of the system.
- Counseling change involves alternating the interaction patterns within the system.

Within the field of systemic family therapy, Bateson's (1972) distinction between *first-order* and *second-order cybernetics* had a significant impact on how counselors worked with families. "First-order cybernetics" refers to describing systemic functioning as if the counselor is an objective, neutral observer describing the counselor an outsider. *Second-order cybernetic* theory applies the rules of first-order cybernetics on itself, positing that the counselor cannot be an objective, outside observer but instead creates a new system with the family: the observer–observed or counselor–family system. This second-order system is subject to the same dynamics as the first, including the drive to maintain homeostasis and rules for relating that are mutually reinforced. Second-order cybernetic theory maintains that whatever the counselor observes in the family reveals more about the *counselor's* values and priorities than the family's because any description exposes what the counselor pays attention to and what the counselor ignores or misses. Second-order cybernetics laid the foundation for transition to postmodern therapy, specifically constructivism in the MRI and Milan schools (Watzlawick, 1984).

In general, all systems counselors are influenced by both first- and second-order cybernetic theory. In practice, counselors will generally emphasize one level of systems analysis or another. Broadly speaking, strategic therapy worked more at the first-order approach with the MRI and Milan approaches gravitating toward second-order and later constructivist approaches:

- *First-order cybernetic approaches* lean toward modernist tendency to find a more objective form of truth. Counselors who practice systemic therapies using a first-order orientation use more assessment instruments of family functioning and rely heavily on the counselor's perception of the system to guide practice.
- *Second-order cybernetic approaches* lean more toward a postmodern approach to truth (see below). Their focus is on how the counselor and client coconstruct a second-order system, which has its own unique set of rules for establishing truth.

	First-Order Cybernetics	Second-Order Cybernetics
Level(s) of analysis	Family system	Family system (level 1) and counselor–family system (level 2)
Interventions target	Correcting interactional sequences	"Perturbing" or interrupting interactional sequences
Counselor role	Tends to appear as a knowledge-able expert	Cocreator of counseling system
Assessment focuses on ...	Behavioral sequences	Meaning-making systems (epistemology)

Postmodern

Postmodern therapies are based on the premise that objective truth can never be fully known because it must always pass through a person's subjective and intersubjective filters, which always affects what is seen. Postmodern counselors share several common assumptions:

Common Postmodern Assumptions

- The human mind does not have access to an outside reality independent of human interpretation; objectivity is not humanly possible.
- All knowledge and truth is culturally, historically, and relationally bound and therefore intersubjective, constructed between people.
- What a person experiences as "real" and believes to be "true" is shaped primarily through language and relationships.
- Language and the words used to describe one's experiences significantly affect how one's identity is shaped and experienced.
- The identification of a "problem" is a social process that occurs through language both at the immediate local level and at the broader societal level.
- Therapy is a process of coconstructing new realities related to the client's personal identity and relationship with the problem.

Within counseling, there are three philosophical schools of postmodernism that are particularly influential (Anderson, 1997; Hoffman, 2002; Watzlawick, 1984):

- *Constructivism:* Constructivists focus on the construction of meaning within the individual organism, thus focusing on how information is received and interpreted.
- *Social constructionism:* Social constructionists focus on how people cocreate meaning in relationships. They emphasize how truth is generated at the local (immediate) relational level.
- *Structuralism/poststructuralism:* Structuralists and poststructuralists focus on the analysis of how meanings are produced and reproduced within a culture through various practices and discourses.

Postmodern Philosophical Schools

	Constructivism	Social Constructionism	Structuralism/ Poststructuralism
Level of reality construction	Individual organism	Local relationship	Societal, political
Associated theories	Later MRI and Milan theories; contemporary Gestalt*; contemporary cognitive-behavioral therapy*	Collaborative therapy; reflecting teams; relational and intersubjectivity theories*	Narrative therapy; feminist and culturally informed therapies
Focus of interventions	Recasting interpretations with new language	Dialogues that highlight multiple meanings and interpretations	Deconstruction and questioning of dominant discourses (popular knowledge)
Counselor role	Facilitate alternative interpretations	Noninterventive; facilitate dialogical process	Help identify social and historical influences

*Several contemporary versions of Gestalt, cognitive-behavioral, and psychodynamic relational and intersubjectivity theories actually have strong postmodern elements.

Wrapping Up Integration

Hopefully, you now know that skillfully using an integrative approach is not a carefree cop-out for someone who doesn't want to feel "tied down" to any one theory. To be done well, it requires *more skill* and *more discipline* than using a single theoretical model, especially if you are going to be able to answer questions about the evidence base to support your work. That said, it should not automatically be avoided and is perhaps an appropriate long-term goal for your professional development, especially if it helps address unique client needs. Similar to cooking, when starting out, it is generally easiest to begin by following tried-and-true recipes than it is to forge out your own to create a new fusion of flavors. By trying to implement a single model at first, you develop a certain set of skills. Once that is mastered, you can determine what else might be useful to enhance that skills set and slowly build up a repertoire that works for you and those you serve.

ONLINE RESOURCES

Associations

Center for Clinical Excellence: Common Factors
www.centerforclinicalexcellence.com

Heart and Soul of Change
http://heartandsoulofchange.com

Society for the Exploration of Psychotherapy Integration
www.cyberpsych.org/sepi

Systematic Treatment Selection
www.systematictreatmentselction.com

Transtheoretical Model
www.uri.edu/research/cprc

References

American Psychiatric Association. (2000). *Diagnostic and statistical manual of mental disorders* (4th ed., text revision). Washington, DC: Author.

Anderson, H. (1997). *Conversations, language, and possibilities: A postmodern approach to therapy.* New York: Basic Books.

Bateson, G. (1972). *Steps to an ecology of mind.* San Francisco: Chandler.

Boscolo, L., Cecchin, G., Hoffman, L., & Penn, P. (1987). *Milan systemic family therapy.* New York: Basic Books.

Frankl, V. (1963). *Man's search for meaning.* Boston: Beacon.

Haley, J. (1976). *Problem-solving therapy: New strategies for effective family therapy.* San Francisco: Jossey-Bass.

Hoffman, L. (2002). *Family therapy: An intimate history.* New York: Norton.

Johnson, S. M. (2004). *The practice of emotionally focused marital therapy: Creating connection* (2nd ed.). New York: Brunner-Routledge.

Madanes, C. (1981). *Strategic family therapy.* San Francisco: Jossey-Bass.

Miller, S. D., Duncan, B. L., & Hubble, M. (1997). *Escape from Babel: Toward a unifying language for psychotherapy practice.* New York: Norton.

Norcross, J. C., & Beutler, L. E. (2008). Integrative psychotherapies. In R. J. Corsini & D. Wedding (Eds.), *Current psychotherapies* (8th ed., pp. 481–511). Pacific Grove, CA: Brooks/Cole.

Parsons, W. R. (1975). *Gestalt therapies in counseling.* New York: Holt, Rinehart and Winston.

Rogers, C. (1951). *Client-centered therapy.* Boston: Houghton Mifflin.

Satir, V. (1972). *Peoplemaking.* Palo Alto, CA: Science and Behavior Books.

Sweeney, T. J. (2009). *Adlerian counseling and psychotherapy: A practitioner's approach* (5th ed.). New York: Routledge/Taylor & Francis Group.

von Bertalanffy, L. (1968). *General system theory: Foundations, development, applications* (Rev.). New York: George Braziller.

Watzlawick, P. (1984). *The invented reality: How do we know what we believe we know? Contributions to constructivism.* New York: Norton.

Watzlawick, P., Weakland, J., & Fisch, R. (1974). *Change: Principles of problem formation and problem resolution.* New York: Norton.

Whitaker, C. A., & Keith, D. V. (1981). Symbolic-experiential family therapy. In A. S. Gurman & D. P. Kniskern (Eds.), *Handbook of family therapy* (pp. 187–224). New York: Brunner/Mazel.

15

Integrative Case Conceptualization

Case Conceptualization and Great Counseling

As already discussed, one thing (besides hourly fees) separates a great counselor from a friend, bartender, or hairdresser: what each does with the information that is shared by clients. After hearing a heartfelt story of struggle, friends, bartenders, and hairdressers tend to do one of two things: give advice or offer sympathy. Counselors and therapists do something very different. They use what they have heard to develop a deeper understanding of clients, often a more sensible and compassionate story than clients tell themselves. When counselors listen to clients, they take the information that they are hearing to develop a map of the person's experience and inner world. This map is called case conceptualization, and it is the key to skillful, competent counseling. In fact, it is the primary reason we need counseling theories at all: once you have a clear conceptualization of what is going on, "what to do" is generally plainly evident. Thus, if you can develop a clear and meaningful case conceptualization, the counseling journey is relatively quick and smooth. If you miss the boat with this first step, you won't get very far.

Counseling theories provide counselors with unique lenses through which to view the problems that clients bring to them. Much like a detailed map, theories allow counselors to view clients and their problems in a broader and more comprehensive context. This broad view allows counselors to see how the pieces fit together in a client's life and provides clues as to the best path out of a sticky situation. In each of the earlier theory chapters (Chapters 4 through 13), you read about case conceptualization using a single model. In this chapter, you will learn about a comprehensive case conceptualization approach that helps you consider a single case from multiple theoretical perspectives, which is ideal for learning about each theory and the interconnections across theories and provides an excellent tool for thinking more broadly about cases.

Realistic Expectations

After forming a strong working relationship with clients, case conceptualization is the second most important skill in counseling. However—and I will tell this to you without high-calorie sugarcoating—case conceptualization is the hardest skill to learn. In short, a comprehensive, integrative case conceptualization requires that you understand and apply most of what is in this book. That said, case conceptualization is also the most empowering and liberating counseling competency—because once you can do this, you will know how to handle almost every situation. So, roll up your sleeves and get ready for intense work.

In most cases, the first time you complete the case conceptualization in this text, it will take 10 or more hours over the course of a week (this is one assignment you cannot cram for the night before it is due unless you live on a planet that spins slower than the earth). However, each time you do another one, you will find that you can complete it more quickly and easily because you are learning how to integrate and use the theoretical concepts. By doing this once, you learn what to listen for and ask about in session with clients (or pay attention to in a video or vignette if doing this for a class assignment). The next time you do it, you begin to better understand how dynamics in one section correlate with dynamics in another. After you do 10 to 20 of these, your ability to conceptualize will significantly increase your counseling abilities both in in-session interventions and in out-of-session communications with your supervisor and other professionals.

Elements of Case Conceptualization

As counselors become more experienced, case conceptualization takes place primarily in their heads—while clients are talking. It happens so fast that often they have a hard time tracing their steps. However, new counselors need to take things more slowly. Similar to learning a new dance step, the new move needs to be broken down into small pieces with specific instructions for where the hands and feet go; with practice, the dancer is able to put the pieces together more quickly and smoothly until it becomes "natural" to him or her. That is what we are going to do here with case conceptualization. So, let's start with identifying the components of a counseling case conceptualization for working with an individual (a similar format of case conceptualization for working with couples and families is presented in the related text *Mastering Competencies in Family Therapy*):

1. *Introduction of client:* Define who the client is (individual, couple, or family) and identify most salient demographics (e.g., age, ethnicity, language, job, grade).
2. *Presenting concern:* Specify how all parties involved are defining the problem: client, family, friends, school, work, legal system, society, and so on.
3. *Background information:* Summarize recent changes, including precipitating events, as well as related historical background.
4. *Strengths and diversity:* Identify personal, relational, and spiritual strengths as well as resources and limitations related to diversity issues.
5. *Theoretical case conceptualization(s):* Use one or more of the following to develop an initial theoretical understanding of the client's personal and relational dynamics:
   - *Psychodynamic/Adlerian conceptualization:* Includes defense mechanisms, object relation patterns, Erickson's psychosocial development stages, and Adlerian style of life and basic mistakes
   - *Humanistic-existential conceptualization:* Expression of authentic self, existential analysis, and Gestalt contact boundary disturbances
   - *Cognitive-behavioral conceptualization:* Behavioral baseline, A-B-C analysis, and schema analysis
   - *Family systemic:* Family life cycle stage, boundaries, triangles, hierarchy, complementarity, and intergenerational patterns
   - *Solution-based and cultural discourse conceptualization:* Previous solution, unique outcomes, miracle question, dominant discourses, identity narratives, and preferred discourses

Alternatively, you can use the "The Viewing: Case Conceptualization" section of your preferred theory to develop a shorter, theory-specific case conceptualization for your client. The complete form for case conceptualization is at the end of this chapter and is also available on the publisher's and book's websites (www.cengage.com and www.masteringcompetencies.com). Below you will find basic instructions for completing each section; you will find the concepts in the "Theoretical Conceptualization" sections described in more depth in the corresponding theory chapter later in this book.

Examples of how to complete a case conceptualization are found at the end of each of the theoretical chapters of this text.

Introduction to Client

I. Introduction to Client and Significant Others

❏ AF   ❏ AM   ❏ CF   ❏ CM   *Age:* _____   *Ethnicity/Language:* _____

Occupation/Grade in School: _____

Relational/Family Status: _____

Case conceptualization starts by identifying the most salient demographic features that relate to treatment. Common demographic information includes the following:

- Gender
- Age
- Ethnicity
- Current occupation/work status or grade in school
- Family status, sexual orientation, and so on.

This initial introduction provides the reader with a basic sketch of the client that will be elaborated on as the case conceptualization unfolds:

Symbols:

AF = adult female   CF = child female

AM = adult male   CM = child male

Presenting Concern

II. Presenting Concern(s)

Client Description of Problem(s): _____

_____

_____

Significant Other/Family Description(s) of Problems: _____

_____

_____

Broader System Problem Descriptions: Description of problem from referring party, teachers, relatives, legal system, and so on:

_____:_____

_____:_____

Often, new and even experienced counselors assume that the "presenting concern" is a straightforward and clear-cut matter. Once in a while it is, but most of the time it is surprisingly complex. Anderson and Goolishian (Anderson, 1997; Anderson & Gehart, 2007) developed a unique means of conceptualizing the presenting problem in their collaborative language systems approach, also referred to as collaborative therapy (see Chapter 12).

This postmodern approach maintains that each person who is talking about the problem is part of the *problem-generating system*, the set of relationships that generated the perspective or idea that there is a problem. Each person who is talking about the problem has a different definition of the problem; sometimes the difference is slight and sometimes stark. For example, when parents bring a child to counseling, the mother, father, siblings, grandparents, teachers, school counselors, doctors, and friends have different ideas as to what the problem *really* is. The mother may think it is a medical problem, such as attention-deficit/hyperactivity disorder (ADHD); the father may believe it is related to his wife's permissiveness; the teacher may say it is poor parenting; and the child may think there really is not a problem at all.

Historically, counselors move rapidly to define the problem in a way that fits with their theoretical worldview: either a formal diagnosis (ADHD, depression, etc.) or another mental health category (such as parenting style, defense mechanism, family dynamics, etc.) with little reflection on the contradictory opinions and descriptions of the problem by the various people involved. Having a single problem definition helps focus the treatment. However, if adhered to too rigidly, having a single problem definition can quickly become a liability rather than an asset. The more a counselor can remain open to the alternative descriptions of the problem, the more maneuverability, adaptability, and creativity can be infused in treatment. In addition, remaining cognizant of the variability of understanding throughout treatment allows the counselor to maintain stronger rapport with each person involved because each person's perspective is honored and referred to throughout the treatment.

A description of the presenting problem should include the following:

1. The reason(s) each client states he or she is seeking counseling or has been referred
2. Any information from the referring agent (teacher, doctor, psychiatrist, etc.) and his or her description of the problem
3. A brief history of the problem and family (if applicable)
4. Descriptions of the attempted solutions and the outcome of these attempts
5. Perspectives from significant persons and institutions in the client's broader social network, including professional associates, religious organizations, close friends, and so on

Background Information

> ### III. Background Information
>
> *Trauma/Abuse History* (recent and past): _____
>
> _____
>
> *Substance Use/Abuse* (current and past; self, family of origin, significant others): _____
>
> _____
>
> _____
>
> *Precipitating Events* (recent life changes, first symptoms, stressors, etc.): _____
>
> _____
>
> _____
>
> _____
>
> *Related Historical Background* (family history, related issues, previous counseling, medical/mental health history, etc.): _____
>
> _____
>
> _____

Obtaining background information about the problem is the next step. Traditionally, counselors include information such as the following:

- History of childhood and adulthood abuse and trauma, including childhood abuse, rape, domestic violence, natural disasters, war, witnessing violence, and so on
- History of substance abuse by client, client's family, and significant others
- Precipitating events that are associated with the onset of the problem, such as recent life changes, breakups, losses, developmental milestones, career moves, and so on
- Related historical background, including history of mental disorders, previous counseling, significant health concerns, and so on

Often, this background information is considered the "facts" of the case. However, as counselors have historically cautioned, how we language the facts makes all the difference (Anderson, 1997; O'Hanlon & Weiner-Davis, 1989; Watzlawick, Weakland, & Fisch, 1974). For example, whether you begin by saying that the client "recently won a state level academic decathlon" or whether you begin with "her mother recently divorced her alcoholic father" paints two very different pictures of the same client for both you and anyone else who reads the assessment. Therefore, although this may seem like the "factual" part of the report where you as a professional are not imposing your bias, in fact, you impose bias by the subtle choice of words, ordering of information, and emphasis on particular details.

Based on research about the importance of the counseling relationship and of hope (Lambert & Ogles, 2004; Miller, Duncan, & Hubble, 1997), I recommend that counselors write the background section in such a way that the counselor and anyone reading the report, including potentially the client, would have a positive impression of and hope for the client because these two factors have an effect on the outcome of treatment.

Assessment of Strengths and Diversity

Everything up to this point has been an introduction that provides a context and framework for understanding the actual assessment elements of the case conceptualization. In the following areas of assessment, counselors assess their clients using theoretical constructs from the major counseling theories to paint a multidimensional picture of clients and their life situation.

Client Strengths

IV. Client Strengths

Personal: _____

_____

Relational/Social: _____

_____

Spiritual: _____

_____

Client strengths and resources should be the first thing assessed. This is a lesson I learned the hard way. When I began teaching case conceptualization, I put the client strength section at the end because it is more clearly associated with solution-based and postmodern approaches (see Chapters 11 and 12; Anderson, 1997; de Shazer, 1988; White & Epston, 1990), which were developed later historically. What I discovered is that after reading about the presenting problem, history, and problematic family dynamics, I was often feeling quite hopeless about the case. However, often on reading the strengths section at the end, I would immediately perk up and find myself having hope, deep respect, and even excitement about the clients and their future. I have since decided to *start* by assessing strengths and believe it puts the counselor in a more resourceful mind-set.

Emerging research supports the importance of identifying client strengths and resources. Researchers who developed the *common factors model* (as you may remember from Chapter 2; Lambert & Ogles, 2004; Miller et al., 1997) estimate that 40% of outcome variance can be attributed to client factors, such as severity of symptoms, access to resources, support system, and so on; the remaining factors include the quality of the counseling relationship (30%), counseling interventions and treatment models (15%), and the client's sense of hope (15%). Counselors can leverage client factors best by assessing for resources. Furthermore, assessing for strengths also strengthens the counseling relationship (30%) and can be done in such a way as to instill hope (15%), thus drawing on three of the four common factors. The potential impact of assessing strengths is hard to overestimate.

To conceptualize a full spectrum of client strengths and resources, counselors can include strengths at several levels:

- Personal/individual strengths
- Relational/social strengths and resources
- Spiritual resources

Personal/Individual Strengths

When assessing for personal/individual strengths and resources, you can begin by reviewing two general categories of strengths: abilities and personal qualities.

- *Abilities:* Where and how are clients functioning in daily life? How do they get to session? Are they able to maintain a job, a hobby, or a relationship? Are there any special talents, either now or in the past? If you look, you will always find a wide range of abilities with even the most "dysfunctional" of clients, especially if you consider the past as well as present and future.

  Naming the abilities can increase clients' sense of hope and confidence to address the problem at hand. I find this especially helpful with children. If a child is having academic problems at school, the family, teachers, and child may not notice how the child is excelling in an extracurricular activity, such as karate, soccer, or piano. Often noticing these areas of accomplishment makes it easier for all involved to find hope for improving the situation.

  Identifying the abilities may give clients or counselors creative ideas about how to solve a current problem. For example, I worked with a recovering alcoholic who hated the idea of writing but spoke often of how music inspired her. By drawing on this strength, we developed the idea of creating a special "sobriety mix" of favorite songs to help maintain sobriety and prevent relapse, an activity that had deep significance and inspiration for her.

- *Personal qualities:* Another area where counselors can identify client strengths is personal qualities. Ironically, the best place to find these is embedded within the presenting problem or complaint. Usually, the thing that brings them to see a counselor is the flip side of another strength. For example, if a person complains about worrying a lot, that person is equally likely to be a diligent and productive worker. Persons who argue with a spouse or child are more likely to speak up for themselves and are generally invested in the relationship in which they are arguing. In virtually all cases, the knife cuts both ways: each liability contains within it a strength in another context. Conversely, a strength in one context is often a problem in another. Here is a list of common problems and the strengths that may be found in clients with the presenting problems.

Problem	Possible Associated "Shadow Strengths"
Depression	• Awareness of what others think and feel • Connected to others and/or desires connection • Has dreams and hopes • Has had the courage to take action to realize dreams • Realistic assessment of self/others (according to recent research; Seligman, 2002)
Anxiety	• Pays attention to details • Desires to perform well • Careful and thoughtful about actions • Able to plan for future and anticipate potential obstacles
Arguing	• Stands up for self and/or beliefs • Fights injustice • Wants the relationship to work • Has hope for better things for others/self
Anger	• In touch with feelings and thoughts • Stands up against injustice • Believes in fairness • Able to sense their boundaries and when they are crossed
Overwhelmed	• Concerned about others' needs • Thoughtful • Able to see the big picture • Sets goals and pursues them

As you can see, identifying strengths relies heavily on the counselor's viewing skills. A skilled counselor is able to "see" the strengths that are the flip side of the presenting problem while remaining aware of the problem tendencies that are the inverse of a particular strength.

Relational/Social Strengths and Resources

* *Social support network:* Family, friends, professionals, teachers, coworkers, bosses, neighbors, church members, salespeople, as well as numerous others in a person's life can be part of a network of social support that help the client in physical, emotional, and spiritual ways.
    * *Physical forms of support* include people who may help with errands, picking up the children, or doing tasks around the house.
    * *Emotional support* may take the form of listening or helping resolve relational problems.
    * *Community support* includes friendships and acceptance provided by any community and is almost always there in some form with a person who may be feeling marginalized because of culture, sexual orientation, language, religion, or similar factors. These communities are critical for coping with the inherent stress of marginalization.

Simply naming, recognizing, and appreciating that there is support can immediately increase a client's sense of hope and reduce feelings of loneliness.

Spiritual Resources

* *Spiritual:* Increasingly, counselors are increasing their awareness of how clients' spiritual resources can be used to address the problems they bring to counseling (Morgan, 2006; Sperry, 2001; Walsh, 2003). Counselors should become familiar with the major religious traditions in their community, such as Protestantism, Catholicism, Judaism, Islam, New Age religions, Native American practices, and so on.

Drawing on the epistemological foundations of Bateson (1972, 2002) and more recent postmodern philosophies (Gergen, 1999), I have developed a definition of spirituality that I find particularly helpful for work as a counselor:

> **Spirituality:** How a person conceptualizes his or her relationship to the universe or God (or however he or she constructs that which is larger than the self). In short, how a person relates to life (in the largest sense of the word).

Using this definition, everyone has some form of spirituality, which ultimately relates to how a person believes the universe operates. The rules of "how life should go" inevitably inform (a) what the person perceives to be a problem, (b) how a person feels about it, and (c) what that person believes can "realistically" be done about it, all of which a counselor wants to know about to help develop an effective treatment plan.

Questions to Assess Spirituality

A counselor can use some of the following questions to assess a client's spirituality, whether traditional or nontraditional:

- Do you believe there is a God or some form of intelligence that organizes the universe? If so, what types of things does that being/force have control over?
- If there is not a God, by what rules does the universe operate? Why do things happen? Or is life entirely random?
- What is the purpose and/or meaning of human existence? How does this inform how a person should approach life?
- Is there any reason to be kind to others? To oneself?
- What is the ideal versus realistic way to approach life?
- Why do "bad" things happen to "good" people?
- Do you believe things happen for a reason? If so, what reason?
- Does the person belong to a religious community or spiritual circle of friends that provides spiritual support, inspiration, and/or guidance in some way?

With the answers to these questions, counselors can create a map of the client's world that can then be used to develop conversations and interventions that are deeply meaningful and a good "fit" for the client. An accurate understanding of a client's "map of the life" reveals what logic and actions will motivate the client to make changes, providing counselors with invaluable resources for changes. For example, I have often found that many clients from traditional religious backgrounds as well as more New Age groups believe that "things happen for a reason." I have had numerous clients use this one belief to radically and quickly transform how they feel, think, and respond to difficult situations.

Diversity

Related to strengths, diversity issues refer to characteristics such as age, gender, sexual orientation, cultural background, immigration status, socioeconomic status, religion, regional community, language, family background, family configuration, or ability. Much like strengths and symptoms, in most cases, each form of diversity brings with it both unique resources and limitations. For many, traumatic and oppressive experiences related to being a minority or simply "different" are at the core of their problematic situation, if not an exacerbating factor. Some counseling theories, such as feminist theory, narrative, and collaborative, consider these at the heart of the case conceptualization process (see Chapters 12 and 13). But in all cases, counselors need to take time to think about how the client's situation is affected by limitations created by diversity issues, such as living in poverty or being an immigrant, and consider these when conceptualizing the client's situation. As silly as it may sound to new counselors, it is *very* easy to not adjust the conceptualization assessment on the basis of theory. For example, how to adjust what a secure attachment looks like in a

Japanese versus an Italian family? What happens when you consider generation of immigration and socioeconomic status? What is normal then? Quickly, things become murky.

Furthermore, in most cases, each limitation that arises from being different has a correlating resource. For example, gays and lesbians are marginalized in numerous ways in our society and are often targeted for abuse, resulting in various levels of trauma; these experiences add significantly to their overall level of psychological stress. However, because of this marginalization, they tend to develop unusually strong social and friendship networks that help them to not only cope but also thrive. Similarly, many cultural and ethnic groups are marginalized in dominant society, but they also tend to have stronger-than-average social and religious networks that provide them a sense of belonging and support.

Theoretical Conceptualizations

The remainder of this form includes five potential areas of conceptualization using the major schools of theory covered in this book:

- Psychodynamic/Adlerian
- Humanistic-existential
- Cognitive-behavioral
- Family systemic
- Postmodern and feminist

Using one or more these allows for a slightly more integrative approach. Alternatively, you can use the "The Viewing: Case Conceptualization" section of a single theory to develop a theory-specific conceptualization.

Psychodynamic and Adlerian Conceptualization
Psychodynamic Defense Mechanisms

V. Psychodynamic Defense Mechanisms

❑ Acting out: *Describe:* _____

❑ Denial: *Describe:* _____

❑ Displacement: *Describe:* _____

❑ Help-rejecting complaining: *Describe:* _____

❑ Humor: *Describe:* _____

❑ Passive aggression: *Describe:* _____

❑ Projection: *Describe:* _____

❑ Projective identification: *Describe:* _____

❑ Rationalization: *Describe:* _____

❑ Reaction formation: *Describe:* _____

❑ Repression: *Describe:* _____

❑ Splitting: *Describe:* _____

❑ Sublimation: *Describe:* _____

❑ Suppression: *Describe:* _____

❑ Other: _____

Psychodynamic defense mechanisms refer to automatic psychological processes that a person uses to ward off anxiety and external stressors and thus describe strategies the person frequently uses to handle problems. A person may be conscious or unconscious about using a defense mechanism; generally, the more aware one is of using a defense mechanism, the more functional he or she is. In addition, certain defense mechanisms are considered more functional than others. For example, humor, sublimation, and suppression are considered more functional than mechanisms that require image distortion or disavowal, such as idealization, denial, and projection.

Originally described in early psychoanalytic writing, these defense mechanisms are widely recognized by counselors practicing from a variety of theoretical perspectives. An assessment of *defensive functioning* has been recommended for inclusion in the next edition of the *Diagnostic and Statistical Manual of Mental Disorders* and a comprehensive list is included in the present edition (American Psychiatric Association, 2000). The current recommendation is to identify up to seven defense mechanisms that the client uses in session or describes using outside of session.

The purpose of identifying defense mechanisms is to better understand the client's internal dynamics, particularly those that are contributing to the presenting problem. That said, not all defenses are bad, and, in fact, they can be quite helpful at times. For example, at the beginning of Chapter 2, I share how my career in writing began as a type of sublimation. Similarly, I encourage new counselors to master the art of suppression: putting difficult ideas out of one's mind. Sublimation is an important skill that enables them to continue to focus on their clients during work hours even when they are dealing with difficult matters in their personal lives (disappointing side note: life still happens to professional counselors and therapists). Thus, you should carefully reflect on what defense mechanisms your clients use, considering how they may be helpful in certain contexts.

The more common defense mechanisms are listed below; additional defense mechanisms are listed in the appendices of the *Diagnostic and Statistical Manual of Mental Disorders* (4th ed., text revision).

Acting Out

A common term that has trickled into the vernacular, the technical meaning of acting out as a defense mechanism refers to dealing with inner emotional conflict through action rather than reflecting on feelings. These actions may or may not translate to "bad behavior" but rather to a pattern of engaging in a behavior (e.g., physically fighting, starting verbal fights) to deal with inner conflict.

Denial

One of the more famous defense mechanisms ("Denial is not just a river in Egypt") and one of the more difficult to assess initially (because your client probably won't mention it), denial refers to refusing to acknowledge a painful reality that is readily apparent to others. Denial is commonly seen in families with substance and alcohol abuse as well as people in dead-end jobs and relationships.

Displacement

Most frequently observed in family dynamics, displacement refers to transferring feelings about one person (or situation) to another, less threatening substitute object. For example, if a person is angry at a spouse but afraid to raise the issue, it is usually easier to displace this anger onto one's young children, with whom a person is more likely to win an argument.

Help-Rejecting Complaining

Commonly observed in counseling sessions, help-rejecting complaining is just like it sounds: a person deals with stress by complaining but invariably rejects suggestions, advice, or help that others offer. I'd offer an example here, but I am confident you just came up with five examples from your personal list of friends, family, and acquaintances.

Humor

All joking aside, humor can be used as a defense mechanism whereby a person manages emotional conflict by identifying the amusing or ironic qualities of the situation. Humor can be used in a highly adaptive way, and it can also be used so rigidly that it almost becomes a form of denial.

Passive Aggression

Another of the more cited defense mechanisms, passive aggression refers to when a person portrays a facade of cooperation but then covertly resists, resents, or undermines, thus indirectly expressing aggression. Sometimes this is easy to detect, as in a classic case of "backstabbing," and other times it is more subtle, such as endless procrastination or "forgetting."

Projection

Projection refers to falsely attributing one's own unacceptable feelings, impulses, or wishes onto another, typically without being aware of what is going on. In clinical practice, this is often seen in the case where one partner has cheated and then projects these intentions onto the faithful partner; this can happen whether or not the infidelity has been discovered.

Projective Identification

Projective identification takes simple projection to a whole new level. Similar to simple projection, projective identification involves falsely attributing to another one's own unacceptable feelings. However, in this case, the person is aware of having the unacceptable feelings but inappropriately justifies them by claiming that they are reasonable reactions to the other person, which often results in the other person acting in such a way as to confirm the projection, making it difficult to clarify who did what to whom first. The classic example of this is jealousy: a person is jealous of his partner's relationship with other men but claims that is because of her behavior. His jealousy causes her to be more secretive to avoid conflict, which further confirms his hypothesis about her, quickly creating a negative, downward spiral.

Rationalization

A favorite of the educated, rationalization refers to dealing with emotional conflict by concealing true motivations by developing elaborate reassuring but incorrect explanations for thoughts, feelings, and emotions. For example, a person may offer intricate and convoluted explanations for excessive drinking behavior, staying in a bad relationship, or failing to take needed action.

Reaction Formation

Often linked with repression, reaction formation refers to dealing with difficult inner conflict by engaging in actions that are diametrically opposed to the denied thought, feelings, and behaviors. A frequent example of this is someone who becomes a rigid religious adherent to cope with unacceptable sexual or materialistic desires; often this backfires, and the person makes headlines when they are caught in a sex or financial scandal.

Repression

More pathological than suppression, repression refers to eliminating unacceptable desires, thoughts, or experiences from conscious awareness to the extent that the person is unaware of the inner conflict. Often the repression is used to describe how traumatized persons will sometimes repress memories associated with the event as a means of coping; the memory may later be triggered by another event, conversation, or other reminder.

Splitting

A term from object relations theory, splitting refers to the inability to see an individual—self included—as having both positive and negative qualities. Instead, the person swings from seeing people as all good or all bad: idealizing or villainizing. In some cases, they can rapidly alternate between an all-good or an all-bad view of the same person, creating significant chaos in relationships.

Sublimation

One of the more functional defenses, sublimation refers to dealing with internal conflict by channeling potentially inappropriate feelings or impulses into socially acceptable activities, such as challenging aggression through sports or sadness through art. This defense can be developed to help people find creative ways to use difficult emotions, such as sadness, anger, rage, fear, and so on.

Suppression

Unlike repression, suppression is the *intentional* avoidance of difficult inner thoughts, feelings, and desires. When thoughtfully chosen, this defense can be very useful when facing difficult emotions over extended periods of time, such as grief, complicated loss, and so on.

Object Relations and Attachment Patterns

Object Relational Pattern

Describe relationship with early caregivers in past: _____

_____

_____

Was the attachment with the mother (or equivalent) primarily: ❐ Generally secure
❐ Anxious and clingy   ❐ Avoidant and emotionally distant   ❐ Other: _____

Was the attachment with the father (or equivalent) primarily: ❐ Generally secure
❐ Anxious and clingy   ❐ Avoidant and emotionally distant   ❐ Other: _____

Describe present relationship with these caregivers: _____

_____

Describe relational patterns with partner and other current relationships: _____

_____

_____

Object relations theorists examine the client's relationship with early caregivers to understand the dynamics that are creating current difficulties (Bowlby, 1988; Johnson, 2004; St. Clair, 2000). In general, these patterns can be described in three ways:

- *Secure:* Client feels safe in relationships, is comfortable with intimacy, and does not have unreasonable fears of abandonment or losing self in a relationship. Generally, people with secure relationships seek counseling in response to a specific trauma or event.
- *Anxious:* Client unnecessarily worries about abandonment or rejection, often displaying jealousy and feeling insecure with the slightest criticism (or even without significant praise). The anxiety that such a person experiences in relationships frequently brings him or her to counseling for help.
- *Avoidant:* Clients with avoidant relational patterns often fear being swallowed or lost in a relationship and therefore remain emotionally unavailable and distant to help them preserve a sense of self.

These early childhood patterns typically repeat like variations on a theme in adulthood, both with the primary caregiver and in other relationships. By tracing these patterns, counselors can help clients more quickly identify core dynamic patterns that are affecting all areas of life.

Erickson's Psychosocial Developmental Stage

Describe development at each stage up to current stage

Trust versus mistrust (infant stage): _____

Autonomy versus shame and doubt (toddler stage): _____

Initiative versus guilt (preschool age): _____

Industry versus inferiority (school age): _____

Identity versus identity confusion (adolescence): _____

Intimacy versus isolation (young adulthood): _____

Generativity versus stagnation (adulthood): _____

Integrity versus despair (late adulthood): _____

Erickson's eight stages of psychosocial development are one of the more useful developmental theories in applied clinical counseling. These stages provide a template for understanding the larger developmental concerns that may be underlying the problems clients bring to session. When viewed through a developmental lens, client problems often make more sense, and typically this insight informs are more resourceful direction for counseling. For example, if a middle-aged man presents with depressive symptoms, examining these symptoms in the context of the struggle for generativity versus stagnation can help focus counseling at the deeper underlying issues that may be fueling the depression. In this case, rather than simply trying to relieve symptoms, the focus of counseling can be to help him achieve a sense of purpose and contribution.

Chapman (2006) explains that the developmental challenge at each stage of development is to achieve an effective *ratio* between the two counterbalancing dispositions, such as trust and mistrust, rather than maximize one at the expense of the other. Ideally, a person will develop a tendency toward trust yet also know when it is appropriate to distrust; having blind trust in everyone and everything is not adaptive. Thus, a person strives to find a healthy balance between the two propensities at each stage. Development issues arise when a person develops an extreme tendency toward one of the two dispositions, such as being overly trusting *or* overly distrustful. When one tends toward the first, more positive sounding disposition, this is referred to as a maladaptation; if one tends toward the second, this is referred to as a malignancy. Chapman's (2006) table summarizes:

Trust Versus Mistrust: Infant Stage

Maladaptation (overemphasize trust): Unrealistic, spoiled, deluded
Malignancy (overemphasize mistrust): Withdrawal, neurotic, depressive, afraid

Applicable to the first year or two of life, infants in this stage develop a healthy balance of trust or mistrust based on their experiences with early caregivers. A healthy balance of trust translates to a general sense of hope and safety in the world while simultaneously knowing when caution is warranted. Persons who have had traumatic childhoods or whose parents overly protected often have confusion over when, where, and who to trust, resulting in a sense of being either unrealistically entitled or needlessly afraid.

Autonomy Versus Shame and Doubt: Toddler Stage

Maladaption (overemphasis of autonomy): Impulsivity, recklessness, inconsiderate, thoughtless
Malignancy (overemphasis of shame/doubt): Compulsion, constrained, self-limiting

During toddlerhood, children develop a sense of autonomy and having an impact in their lives while also learning the limits of their abilities. If caretakers are either neglectful or overly protective, children become overburdened with a sense of shame and may grow up to have lingering issues that manifest as extreme self-doubt or debilitating shame and/or shyness. Alternatively, if parents do not allow their children to experience shame and self-doubt, these children tend to become impulsive and inconsiderate of others.

Initiative Versus Guilt: Preschool and Kindergarten Age

Maladaptation (overemphasis of initiative): Ruthless, exploitative, uncaring, dispassionate
Malignancy (overemphasis of guilt): Inhibition, risk-aversive, unadventurous

During preschool and kindergarten, child transition through a developmental stage in which they develop a sense of initiative and purpose tempered by guilt when their actions hurt others. Children who have either overly protective or neglectful parents may develop a strong sense of guilt and insecurity about making their own choices, leading to risk avoidance and inhibition. Alternatively, children who have an underdeveloped awareness of guilt and how their actions affect others become overly aggressive and even ruthless.

Industry Versus Inferiority: School Age

Maladaptation (overemphasis of industry): Narrowly virtuous, workaholic, obsessive specialist
Malignancy (overemphasis of inferiority): Inertia, lazy, apathetic, purposeless

In the early years in school, children learn new skills, developing a sense of competence from which they build their sense of self-worth; thus, the task at this stage is to engage in industrious activities to build confidence in their abilities. Children who are frequently criticized or compared to others and found to be lacking develop a pervasive sense of inferiority. Recent research also shows that overly praised children who are protected from experiencing failure and obstacles also develop a sense of inferiority because as they are thwarted from developing a genuine sense of mastery (Seligman, 2002). Thus, contrary to their parents' intentions, children who are constantly sheltered from the feelings of losing a game, getting bad grades, being left out, and similar feelings of inferiority are actually likely to develop a lingering sense of inadequacy as they get older that can manifest as "underachieving" down the road. Alternatively, overly identifying with one's industriousness can result in obsessiveness in their activities.

Identity Versus Identity Confusion: Adolescence

Maladaptation (overemphasis of identity): Fanaticism, self-important, extremist
Malignancy (overemphasis of identity confusion): Repudiation, socially disconnected, cut-off

Few developmental stages are more fabled—or as well researched—as adolescence. Erickson saw this as a time of identity development when a person first begins to answer questions, such as who am I, and how do I fit in? Developmentally, this is a time of exploring possible identities and social roles, which often takes the form of wild outfits, colorful hair, rebellious music, rotating social groups, and other ways to magnificently annoy one's parents. Teens who are not allowed to explore their identity or are made to feel guilty for not pursuing certain life paths may experience role confusion, failing to identify a clear or viable sense of identity. Alternatively, role confusion can also take the form of failing to adopt viable social role and instead developing a reactive identity that is based on a rebellious need to "not be" what someone wants, often taking the form of drug use, a radical social group, gang membership, or dropping out of high school. In such cases, teens are not able to conceive of themselves as productive members of one's family or society.

Intimacy Versus Isolation: Young Adulthood

Maladaptation (overemphasis of intimacy): Promiscuous, needy, vulnerably
Malignancy (overemphasis of isolation): Exclusivity, loner, cold, self-contained

In recent generations, young adulthood has become much longer than in years prior as more people seek higher education and views of marriage and "settling down" change. During this time, people establish intimate relationships in their personal, social, and work lives, developing their own families and social networks. People who struggle with this stage can become either overly focused on their relationships, possibly becoming sexually promiscuous or overly identified with being in a relationship, or increasingly socially isolated.

Generativity Versus Stagnation: Adulthood

Maladaptation (overemphasis of generativity): Overextension, do-gooder, busy-body, meddling
Malignancy (overemphasis of stagnation): Rejecting, disinterested, cynical

The developmental tasks of adulthood focus on feeling as though one meaningfully contributes to society and the succeeding generations and is often measured by whether one is satisfied with life accomplishments. A midlife crisis refers to feeling that one's life is stagnant, off course, and/or in need of fixing, which some pursue by trying to make radical life changes—sometimes these help, and at other times these get a person even more off course. Often, the consequences of developmental deficiencies from prior stages come to a head during this time and can now be worked through and more readily addressed. Additionally, developmental issues at this stage can take the form of being overly involved and extended in one's social or work world or, alternatively, becoming cynical and disconnected.

Integrity Versus Despair: Late Adulthood

Maladaptation (overemphasis of integrity): Presumption, conceited, pompous, arrogant
Malignancy (overemphasis of despair): Disdain, miserable, unfulfilled, blaming

The final developmental stage is an increasingly important one for counselors to understand as more elderly are receiving professional services. During this stage, people balance a sense of integrity with a sense of despair as they look back over their lives and face the inevitability of death. Those who are able to face the end of life with a greater sense of integrity and wisdom are able to integrate the experiences of their life to make meaning and accept what and who they have been. In contrast, others struggle to make peace with their lives and with life more generally and experience inconsolable sadness and loss or, alternatively, develop a false sense of self-importance that is conveyed as arrogance and self-righteousness.

Adlerian Style of Life Theme

Style of Life Theme
❏ Control: _____
❏ Superiority: _____
❏ Pleasing: _____
❏ Comfort: _____
Basic Mistake Misperceptions: _____
_____
_____

When working with clients, one of the most important areas that Adlerian counselors assess is a person's *style of life*, which can be described a person's characteristic way of thinking, doing, feeling, living, and striving: one's road map for life. This "style" or map of life both shapes and is shaped by the goals we choose for our lives and becomes the thread that runs through all aspects of our lives. Eckstein (2009) identifies four general patterns that are commonly adopted as a style of life: control, superiority, pleasing, and comfort. Although these are not the only way to assess a client's style of life, they are an easy way to begin. A person may have more than one of these themes in their style of life.

Control

A person whose lifestyle is characterized by control frequently seek to control others, themselves, and/or the situation in order to create a sense of safety and security. However, you have no doubt lived long enough to realize that total control over anyone, including oneself, is not humanly possible. Thus, those whose life theme includes elements of control are frequently frustrated, often perceiving others as being resistant or difficult. These people tend to often be drawn into power struggles and distancing themselves from people and situations over which they have no control. Counseling can help people with a controlling lifestyle accept what they cannot change and develop greater tolerance for others.

Superiority

Those whose life theme is characterized by superiority, not be confused with control, are commonly referred to as "perfectionists." They need to be better than others as well as "right," useful, and competent. However, underneath an outer layer of what appears to be superiority, they tend to have an ongoing inner doubt about whether they are "good enough." Inside they tend to be hard on themselves, often taking on more than they can reasonably handle. Sometimes this standard of superiority gets projected onto others, especially children, and the person becomes impossible to please. Counselors can help those with superiority life themes develop more realistic expectations for themselves and others.

Pleasing

Those whose life theme involves pleasing, one of the easiest to work with and most commonly seen in counseling settings, focus their energies on understanding the needs of others and finding ways to meet them. They often need everyone else to be happy before they can be happy, thus making their happiness dependent on how they are treated by others. Typically, a person with a pleasing lifestyle gives and gives and gives and then at a certain point becomes resentful. In some cases, others take advantage of them or abuse them; in other cases, those around them are unaware of the sacrifices they are making. Their fear of rejection and habit of pleasing others at the expense of their own integrity can cause significant hardship in their lives. In counseling, they can learn to set healthy boundaries and find ways to assert their needs in relationships while still respecting those of others.

Comfort

Those whose life theme involves comfort seek comfort at the expense of taking the risks involved with pursuing life goals and achievement. They tend to avoid the stress of responsibility and delayed reward often due to a sense of inadequacy or fear of failure. In moderation, seeking comfort leads to underachieving, while in its extreme, it may take the form of addiction. Counselors can help those with this theme to take small steps toward their goals, emphasizing small successes along the way.

Basic Mistake Perceptions

Each person's style of life reveals his or her *private logic* about how life and the world work. Children begin developing their personal maps of the universe—their private logic— from their earliest experiences. Thus, virtually everyone ends up with a system of private logic that has some *basic mistakes*, perceptions about the world that are inaccurate. Basic mistakes are similar to what cognitive counselors call *irrational beliefs* but refer to the core and most general irrational beliefs that inform one's view of life, self, and others. Adlerian counseling involves helping people identify these often unconscious or semiconscious erroneous assumptions about life to enable a person to develop a system of private logic that supports him or her in pursuing life goals.

Basic mistakes are individual and unique. Thus, assessing them requires carefully listening to what clients say and asking about their thinking process in situations related to the presenting problem: "What did you find so offensive in what your husband said?" or "What motivated you to take such a desperate action?" With careful listening, astute observations, and probing questions, counselors can help clients identify basic mistake misperceptions that contribute to their current concerns. Examples include the following:

- *Overgeneralizations:* "People cannot be trusted"; "No one cares about me."
- *Unrealistic expectations:* "I should always be happy"; "Life should be easy."
- *Unsustainable goals:* "Everyone must be happy for me to be happy"; "I must always be the best at what I do."
- *Misperceptions about life/God:* "Life should be fair"; "God will give me what I want."
- *Denying one's worth:* "I will never be good enough."; "I am not worth loving."
- *Problematic values:* "I must get to the top at any cost."; "I do not apologize for my actions."

Humanistic-Existential Conceptualization

Expression of Authentic Self

Humanistic Assessment: Expression of Authentic Self

Problems: Are problems perceived as internal or external (caused by others, circumstance, etc.)?   ❏ Predominantly internal   ❏ Mixed   ❏ Predominantly external

Agency and responsibility: Is self or other discussed as agent of story? Does client take clear responsibility for situation?   ❏ Strong sense of agency and responsibility   ❏ Agency in some areas   ❏ Little agency; frequently blames others/situation   ❏ Often feels victimized

Recognition and expression of feelings: Are feelings readily recognized, owned, and experienced?   ❏ Easily expresses feelings   ❏ Identifies with prompting   ❏ Difficulty recognizing feelings

Here-and-now experiencing: Is the client able to experience full range of feelings as they are happening in the present moment?   ❏ Easily experiences emotions in present moment   ❏ Experiences some present emotions with assistance   ❏ Difficulty with present moment experiencing

Personal constructs and facades: Is the client able to recognize and go beyond roles? Is identity rigid or tentatively held?   ❏ Tentatively held; able to critique and question   ❏ Some awareness of facades and construction of identity   ❏ Identity rigidly defined; seems like "fact"

Complexity and contradictions: Are internal contradictions owned and explored? Is client able to fully engage the complexity of identity and life?   ❏ Aware of and resolves contradictions   ❏ Some recognition of contradictions   ❏ Unaware of internal contradictions

"Shoulds": Is client able to question socially imposed "shoulds" and "oughts"? Can client balance desire to please others and desire to be authentic?   ❏ Able to balance authenticity with social obligation   ❏ Identifies tension between social expectations and personal desires   ❏ Primarily focuses on external "shoulds"

(continued)

> *Acceptance of others: Is client able to accept others and modify expectations of others to be more realistic?* ❑ Readily accepts others as they are   ❑ Recognizes expectations of others are unrealistic but still strong emotional reaction to expectations not being met   ❑ Difficulty accepting others as is; always wanting others to change to meet expectations
>
> *Trust of self: Is client able to trust self as process (rather than a stabile object)?* ❑ Able to trust and express authentic self   ❑ Trust of self in certain contexts   ❑ Difficulty trusting self in most contexts

In humanistic approaches to counseling, such as person centered and Gestalt, assessment focuses on the person's ability to experience and express one's authentic self. As you can imagine, this is a subtle process that is difficult to assess. Carl Rogers (1961) identifies several telltale signs of authenticity. These are discussed in the following sections.

Problems

Rogers noticed that as people move toward greater authenticity, they begin to see problems and solutions to problems primarily as an internal rather than an external matter. People early in the growth process tend to see problems as caused by others or attributable to external circumstances, such as someone not doing what he or she wants or an unfortunate event. In contrast, as people move toward greater authenticity, they begin to describe problems as their needing to take some action or respond differently to a situation; they no longer see others or situations as the problem; rather, the problem is that they need to change their role in the situation.

Agency and Responsibility

When listening to clients with an attuned ear, it is often easy to discern whether they see themselves as the agent of their lives and therefore take responsibility for their actions as well as the situations. Early in the growth process, clients tend to blame others or their circumstances or report feeling like a victim. They describe events happening *to them*, with others serving as the agents in the story. In contrast, as they begin to become more self-actualized, the same circumstances are described with the client as the agent or protagonist of the story, and they take responsibility for the situation and their response.

Recognition and Expression of Feelings

Humanistic counselors carefully observe a person's ability to recognize, own, express, and experience their emotions. As people become more self-actualized, they more readily access and manage emotions. When some clients begin counseling, they have extreme difficulty identifying their emotions: when asked what they are feeling, they can only describe what they are thinking. Through the counseling process, they learn to identify and more fully experience their emotions. Finally, the counselor helps them to "own" them (take responsibility) and respectfully express them in appropriate contexts with appropriate people.

Here-and-Now Experiencing

Once a counselor has helped a client to more readily identify emotions, the next step is to be able to experience and express emotions as they arise in the present moment. Typically, clients are first able to do this in a safe environment in session with their counselor and then in less controlled, real-life situations. Clients who learn how to experience emotions in the here and now can feel emotions as they arise, are consciously aware of feeling these emotions, and can do so without overreacting to them.

For example, if a client gets disappointing news about not getting a job or promotion, he can feel the disappointment and is aware that he is feeling the disappointment yet does not overreact by getting angry, depressed, or self-harming (drinking, etc.).

Personal Constructs and Facades

Carl Rogers paid careful attention to the social roles and facades his clients played. His counseling approach aimed to get people to move beyond these limiting personal constructs—rigid definitions of self—to move toward a more fluid form of identity that was constantly evolving and expanding. The more rigid one holds to a personal construct—"I am a hard worker" or "I am beautiful"—the more limited one's life becomes because so much energy must go toward maintaining this identity. Thus, humanistic counselors look for more tentatively held ideas of self and personhood as a sign of living more authentically.

Complexity and Contradictions

News flash: You are a hypocrite. I am a hypocrite. We are all riddled with contradictions, complexities, and confusions. As a person becomes more self-aware, the better able one is to see these contradictions and accept them as part of what it means to be human.

"Shoulds"

Also targeted by Gestalt and cognitive counselors, "shoulds" and "oughts" are socially imposed rules about how one should think, feel, and behave. Every culture has these "shoulds"; in fact, in essence, each culture is a list of "shoulds." Thus, it is impossible to live with other humans and not have a list of socially defined "shoulds." The key is how one relates to these. If a person swallows them whole and contorts themselves to fit into these "shoulds," the authentic self has little room for expression. Instead, the ideal is to thoughtfully balance one's need for authentic self-expression with the socially imposed "shoulds," sometimes having to forgo social acceptance to maintain one's integrity. That said, someone who flaunts going against cultural norms is not expressing the authentic self but rather finding identity by being a reactive rebel who is still defined by socially imposed "shoulds"—just in negative relief.

Acceptance of Others

Relating to other humans is challenging. Even in the best of relationships, at a certain point a fundamental difference or failure occurs that leaves one or both feeling betrayed, hurt, or angry. Accepting imperfection in others tends to occur when one begins to accept that in oneself. Thus, humanistic counselors carefully assess clients' abilities to accept others and to modify their expectations of others to be more realistic. In theory, it would be great if everyone spoke with kind words in a kind tone to everyone. In theory, it would be great if everyone could follow through on their promises and act with integrity in difficult situations. The more you are in relationship with others, the more you realize that such perfection is not possible. That said, it is important to keep striving for these ideals and to balance this realism with realistic expectations for thoughtful and kind behavior.

Trust of Self

Finally, humanistic counselors assess the extent to which clients are able to experience their identity as *process* rather than a stabile object. People who experience their identity as a stabile "thing" are attached to labels, routines, status, objects, and anything else that symbolizes their identities. As a person becomes more self-actualized, these things matter less and less, and a person becomes more comfortable with the idea that identity is fluid and evolving. Important identity factors today—grades, degree, job, relationship, and children—will likely be less important at some point in the future. Self-actualization involves trusting the ongoing unfolding of the self with less and less need to label it, pin it down, or claim it.

Existential Analysis

Existential Analysis

Sources of life meaning (as described or demonstrated by client): _____

_____

_____

General themes: ❏ Personal achievement/work   ❏ Significant other   ❏ Children
❏ Family of origin   ❏ Social cause/contributing to others   ❏ Religion/spirituality
❏ Other:

Satisfaction with and clarity of life direction:

❏ Clear sense of meaning that creates resilience in difficult times
❏ Current problems require making choices related to life direction
❏ Minimally satisfied with current life direction
❏ Has reflected little on life direction up to this point; living according to life plan
   defined by someone/something else
❏ Other: _____

Based on existential logotherapy (Frankl, 1963), existential analysis of a client's life situation involves looking at their life from the highest possible vantage point. It's such a "big-picture" view that it is easy to forget when one is focused on so many other details, such as frequency of symptoms, childhood history, and current relationships. However, this wide-angle view often provides invaluable information about how to expedite the counseling process. Two initial areas for assessment are the following:

- Sources of life meaning: What inspires the client and makes them feel whole and fulfilled?
- Satisfaction with and clarity of life direction: Does the client have a clear sense of purpose and direction for his or her life? Is life on or off track?

The importance of these perennial existential questions has had a boost from science in recent years. In studying happiness and life satisfaction, positive psychologists report a strong correlation between having a sense of meaning and purpose and being happy (Seligman, 2002). Thus, counselors need to understand where clients find meaning and purpose at the outset of counseling in order to effectively guide treatment to help the client achieve greater levels of happiness.

An existential analysis of meaning and purpose is particularly useful when working with certain types of clients. For example, when working with clients who have suicidal feelings, counselors can assess for sources of life meaning and life satisfaction to determine how serious the threat is and how best to motivate a client to value life again. Similarly, clients who struggle with depression have often lost their sense of direction in life and need to have their life dreams reinvigorated. As is developmentally expected, most teens I work with struggle with issues of life meaning and direction and appreciate being able to discuss these personal issues with an open-minded and patient adult. In all cases, knowing where clients draw their inspiration reveals what will ultimately motivate them toward change no matter what the initial presenting concern.

Gestalt Contact Boundary Disturbances

> ## Gestalt Contact Boundary Disturbances
>
> ❑ *Desensitization:* Failing to notice problems
> ❑ *Introjection:* Take in others' views whole and unedited
> ❑ *Projection:* Assign undesired parts of self to others
> ❑ *Retroflection:* Direct action to self rather than other
> ❑ *Deflection:* Avoid direct contact with another or self
> ❑ *Egotism:* Not allowing outside to influence self
> ❑ *Confluence:* Agree with another to extent that boundary blurred
>
> *Describe:* _____
>
> _____

As described in Chapter 8, Gestalt counselors view each moment of lived experience primarily in terms of a form of *contact* between the self (organism) and the outside world (others and environment; Perls, Hefferline, & Goodman,1951; Yontef, 1993). If a person is able to make direct contact and authentically *encounter* the outside world, the person is living a fully and authentic life. However, for a variety of reasons—early life lessons, fears, or social dictates—people avoid genuine contact to protect themselves. These *contact boundary disturbances* refer to distortions in perceptions of self or others.

An encounter involves a continuum of seven phases, beginning with initial perception, moving toward direct encounter, and ending in withdrawal. The human experience involves an endless ebb and flow of making contact with one person/object/idea and then withdrawing, then making contact and withdrawing from another in an endless series of connections and disconnections. A person can avoid contact at any of the seven phases using specific resistance processes at each stage (Woldt & Toman, 2005):

Continuum Phase	Resistance Process	Example of Resistance
1. *Sensation/perception:* Organism perceives input from environment.	*Desensitization:* Failing to notice problems	Ignoring increasing violence by partner in fights
2. *Awareness:* One's lived experience becomes focused on the environmental sensation.	*Introjection:* Take in others' views whole and unedited	Becoming what your parents wanted you to be
3. *Excitement/mobilization:* The organism mobilizes to prepare for contact.	*Projection:* Assign undesired parts of self to others	Rejecting sexual aspects of self and then perceiving others as "oversexed"
4. *Encounter/action:* The organism takes action to engage the other.	*Retroflection:* Direct action to self rather than other	Rather than creating conflict with others, focus criticism on self
5. *Interaction/full contact:* A back-and-forth exchange happens; the self becomes part of "we."	*Deflection:* Avoid direct contact with another or self	Working long hours to avoid spouse or avoiding own emotions

(continued)

| 6. *Assimilation/integration:* The organism takes in and integrates new information, behavior, and so on. | *Egotism:* Not allowing outside to influence self | Claiming to be "in love" but not being open to changing self to meet needs of relationship |
| 7. *Differentiation/withdrawal:* The organism withdraws from contact and returns to its individual state. | *Confluence:* Agree with another to extent that boundary blurred | Agreeing with spouse to extent that one no longer allows self to have a divergent opinion |

When assessing clients, Gestalt counselors look for where their clients are "stuck" in the cycle of making contact and direct their interventions to encourage clients make contact and complete the encounter cycle.

Cognitive-Behavioral Conceptualization

Baseline of Symptomatic Behavior

Baseline Assessment of Symptomatic Behavior

Symptom #1 (behavioral description): _____

Frequency: _____

Duration: _____

Context(s): _____

Events before: _____

Events after: _____

Symptom #2 (behavioral description): _____

Frequency: _____

Duration: _____

Context(s): _____

Events before: _____

Events after: _____

The *Baseline Assessment of Symptomatic Behavior* originated in behavioral counseling (Spiegler & Guevremont, 2003) but is commonly required by insurance companies and other third-party payers whose preferred model is the *medical model*, which focuses on observable symptoms. Therefore, if you like to get paid, it's a good idea to become competent in the art of baseline assessment. Thankfully, compared to everything else in this assessment, it's a snap.

Steps to Baseline Assessment

Step 1. Define the problem behavior in specific, observable behaviors that are easily counted.

Examples: To measure depression, you could measure any of the following:
(a) hours per day with depressed mood; (b) days per week with mild, moderate, or severe depressed mood; or (c) days per week avoiding social contact and/or normal activities.

Step 2: Get a baseline: Create a chart for the client that collects the following data:

- *Frequency of problem behavior:* Measured in minutes, hours, days, or weeks.
- *Duration and/or severity of each episode:* Duration can be in minutes or hours; severity is typically measured as mild, moderate, or severe.
- *Context in which the behavior happened:* Could be place, relationship, timing, or some other potentially contextual trigger for the behavior.
- *Events before each episode:* Used to identify potential triggers (e.g., rain, an argument).
- *Events after each episode:* Used to identify potential reinforcement and/or clarify trigger of the behavior (e.g., when her husband comes home the wife's anxiety diminishes).

Sample of Baseline Assessment Chart

	Frequency	Duration/ Severity	Context	Events Before	Events After
Monday					
Tuesday					
Wednesday					
Thursday					
Friday					
Saturday					
Sunday					

The client then completes the chart for a period of 1 to 4 weeks to get a baseline assessment of the problem behavior. This becomes the measuring point for progress once treatment commences so that progress can be closely measured. Relying on the most objective data available in mental health, baseline assessment is considered one of the best measures of progress. However, for those who have spent some time collecting such data, it becomes quickly apparent that because these data rely heavily on client recall and description, they are less consistent and reliable as one might hope. In fact, often a spouse or parent may be a more reliable source of behavioral information than the client trying to remember their internal states.

A-B-C Analysis of Irrational Beliefs

> ### A-B-C Analysis of Irrational Beliefs
>
> *Activating event ("problem"):* _____
>
> *Consequence (mood, behavior, etc.):* _____
>
> *Mediating beliefs (unhelpful beliefs about event that result in C):*
>
> 1. _____
>
> 2. _____
>
> 3. _____

One of the more common assessment techniques in cognitive-behavior approaches, Albert Ellis's (1999) A-B-C framework is used to identify problematic beliefs that result in undesirable emotions and behaviors. The A-B-C framework works as follows:

A = Activating event ➔ B = Belief ➔ C = Consequence

In this case, A, the activating event, triggers B, a belief, that results in C, a consequence. In theory, this happens with all events all the time. However, when a person has what Ellis terms an irrational belief or what I prefer to call a problematic belief, the consequences are essentially the presenting problem for which the client is seeking help.

Here are some examples:

- A = Fight with boyfriend ➔ B = Our relationship is in trouble; no one will ever love me ➔ C = Feeling depressed; acting desperate; text messaging every 2 minutes; eating a pint of ice cream.
- A = Trip to shopping mall ➔ B = People judge me by the way I look; I am not as good as everyone else; something is wrong with me ➔ C = Feelings of inadequacy; feeling anxious and panicked; afraid to make eye contact; avoiding people; leaving the mall early; overspending online at home.

The role of the counselor is to help identify B, the unhelpful belief, because most clients *experience* the chain of events as A ➔ C and describe it as "I am depressed *because* my boyfriend and I had a fight," not "I am depressed because I believe no one will ever love me." To identify these underlying beliefs, counselors can ask questions such as the following:

Questions for Identifying Unhelpful Beliefs

- When you think about the activating event (helps to name it), why does it make sense to then feel _____ (C) or do _____ (C)?

Example: When you think about going to the mall (A), why does it make sense to feel anxious (C) and leave as soon as possible (C)?

- What beliefs do you have about yourself and/or _____ (A) that may lead you to feel _____ (C) or do _____ (C)?

Example: What beliefs do you have about you or your relationship that may lead you to feel depressed or act impulsively after a fight?

Beck's Schema Analysis

Beck's Schema Analysis

❏ *Arbitrary inference:* _____

❏ *Selective abstraction:* _____

❏ *Overgeneralization:* _____

❏ *Magnification/minimization:* _____

❏ *Personalization:* _____

❏ *Absolutist/dichotomous thinking:* _____

❏ *Mislabeling:* _____

❏ *Mind reading:* _____

Another common cognitive assessment technique is *schema analysis*, pioneered by Aaron Beck (1976). Schema is a technical psychological term that refers to a structured set of beliefs about some aspect of the world, such as one's worth, others' motives, or luck. To connect back up with Ellis's A-B-C framework, Beck's schema analysis can be viewed as a categorization of specific unhelpful beliefs. Assessing unhelpful beliefs using Beck's categorization of schemas can be very helpful in the counseling process by naming the beliefs more concretely and by identifying habitual patterns of thought. Categories of schema include but are not limited to the following:

- *Arbitrary inference:* Drawing conclusions without sufficient or relevant evidence, including pessimism and catastrophizing (e.g., assuming that someone is angry with you just because they do not return a phone call when expected).
- *Selective abstraction:* Making assumptions based on certain facts while ignoring other—usually more positive—facts (e.g., assuming that you will lose a long-term friend because of a minor miscommunication).
- *Overgeneralization:* Holding extreme beliefs based on relatively little data (e.g., because I was not a good soccer player in elementary school, I am terrible at all sports).
- *Magnification and minimization:* Overemphasizing or underemphasizing a particular fact and drawing inaccurate conclusions; in statistical terms, making assumptions that are based on an unrepresentative data set (e.g., believing that no one thinks you are beautiful because of a comment that one person made).
- *Personalization:* Assuming that an external event or someone else's action somehow says something about you (e.g., believing something is wrong with you because a partner cheats on you—hint, hint, *you* didn't make the choice to be unfaithful).
- *Absolutist or dichotomous thinking:* Categorizing things as all-good or all-bad or as either-or extremes (e.g., either she loves me or she doesn't).
- *Mislabeling:* Unfairly characterizing one's entire identity on the basis of limited events (e.g., I am a terrible counselor because one client did not return for a second session).
- *Mind reading:* Believing that you know what another person is thinking without sufficient supporting evidence (e.g., I know he does not like me because of the look on his face when I am at the meetings).

Family Systemic Conceptualization

Stage of Family Life Cycle

❐ Single adult   ❐ Marriage   ❐ Family with young children   ❐ Family with adolescent children   ❐ Launching children   ❐ Later life

Describe struggles with mastering developmental tasks in one of these stages:

Family Boundaries

Typical style for regulating closeness and distance with others: _____

_____

_____

Boundaries with

Parents: ❐ Enmeshed ❐ Clear ❐ Disengaged ❐ NA: *Diversity note:* _____

Siblings: ❐ Enmeshed ❐ Clear ❐ Disengaged ❐ NA: *Diversity note:* _____/_____

Significant other: ❐ Enmeshed ❐ Clear ❐ Disengaged ❐ NA: *Diversity note:* _____

Children: ❐ Enmeshed ❐ Clear ❐ Disengaged ❐ NA: *Diversity note:* _____

Extended family: ❐ Enmeshed ❐ Clear ❐ Disengaged ❐ NA: *Diversity note:* _____

Other: _____: ❐ Enmeshed ❐ Clear ❐ Disengaged ❐ NA: *Diversity note:* _____

(continued)

Triangles/coalitions

    ❏ Coalition in family of origin: *Describe:* _____

    ❏ Coalitions related to significant other: *Describe:* _____

    ❏ Other coalitions: _____

Hierarchy between self and parent/child   ❏ NA

With own children: ❏ Effective   ❏ Rigid   ❏ Permissive

With parents (for child or young adult):   ❏ Effective   ❏ Rigid   ❏ Permissive

Complementary patterns with _____: ❏ Pursuer/distancer   ❏ Over/underfunctioner

❏ Emotional/logical   ❏ Good/bad parent   ❏ Other:_____ Example: _____

_____

Intergenerational patterns

Family strengths: _____

Substance/alcohol abuse: ❏ N/A   ❏ Example: _____

Sexual/physical/emotional abuse: ❏ N/A   ❏ Example: _____

Parent/child relations: ❏ N/A   ❏ Example: _____

Physical/mental disorders: ❏ N/A   ❏ Example: _____

Historical incidents of presenting problem: ❏ N/A   ❏ Example: _____

Stage of Family Life Cycle Development

When assessing families, it is helpful to identify their stage in the life cycle (Carter & McGoldrick, 1999). Each stage is associated with specific developmental tasks; symptoms arise when families are having difficulty mastering these tasks:

- *Leaving home: single adult:* Accepting emotional and financial responsibility for self.
- *Marriage:* Commit to new system; realigning boundaries with family and friends.
- *Families with young children:* Adjust marriage to make space for children; join in child-rearing tasks; realign boundaries with parents/grandparents.
- *Families with adolescent children:* Adjusting parental boundaries to increase freedom and responsibility for adolescents; refocus on marriage and career life.
- *Launching children:* Renegotiating marital subsystem; developing adult-to-adult relationships with children; coping with aging parents.
- *Family in later life:* Accepting the shift of generational roles; coping with loss of abilities; middle generation takes more central role; creating space for wisdom of the elderly.

Interpersonal Boundaries

A family counseling term that has found its way into many self-help books, *boundaries* are the rules for negotiating interpersonal closeness and distance (Minuchin, 1974). These rules are generally unspoken and unfold as two people interact over time, each defining when, where, and how he or she prefers to relate to the other. Structural counselors characterize boundaries in one of three ways—clear, diffuse, or rigid—all of which are strongly influenced by culture.

Clear Boundaries and Cultural Variance

Clear boundaries refer to a range of possible ways couples can negotiate a healthy balance between closeness (we-ness) and separation (individuality). Cultural factors shape how much closeness versus separation is preferred. Collectivist cultures tend toward greater degrees of closeness, whereas individualistic cultures tend to value greater independence. The best way to determine if a couple's boundaries are clear is to determine whether symptoms have developed in the individual, couple, or family. If they have, it is likely that there are problems with the boundaries being too *diffuse* or too *rigid*. Most people who come in for counseling have reached a point where previous boundaries and rules for relating that may have worked in one context are no longer working. For relationships to weather the test of time, couples, families, and even friends must constantly renegotiate their boundaries (rules for relating) to adjust to each person's evolving needs. The more flexible people are in negotiating these rules, the more successful they will be in adjusting to life transitions and setbacks.

Enmeshed/Diffuse Boundaries

When a couple or family begins to overvalue togetherness at the expense of respecting the individuality of each, their boundaries become *diffuse*, and relationship becomes *enmeshed* (note: technically boundaries are not enmeshed; they are diffuse). In these relationships, individuals may feel that they are being suffocated, that they lack freedom, or that they are not cared for enough. Often, in these relationships, people feel threatened whenever the other disagrees or does not affirm them, resulting in an intense tug-of-war to convince the other to agree with them. Couples with diffuse boundaries may also have diffuse boundaries with their children, families of origin, and/or friends, resulting in these outside others becoming overly involved in one or both of the partners' lives (e.g., involving parents, friends, or children in couple's arguments).

Disengaged/Rigid Boundaries

When relationships emphasize independence over togetherness, boundaries can become *rigid* and the relationship *disengaged*. In these relationships, people may not allow others to influence them, often choosing careers over relationship priorities, and frequently have minimal emotional connection. In couple partnerships that are disengaged, one or the other may compensate for distance in the couple relationship by having diffuse boundaries with children, friends, family, or an outside love interest (e.g., an emotional or physical affair). Often difficult to accurately assess, the key indicator of rigid boundaries is whether they are creating problems individually or for the partnership.

Questions for Assessing Boundaries

Here are some sample questions to think about while working with an individual, couple, or family to assess boundaries:

- Does the couple have clear couple boundaries that are distinct from their parenting and family-of-origin relationships?
- Does the couple spend time alone not talking about the children?
- Do family members experience anxiety or frustration when there is a difference of opinion?
- Is one hurt or angry if another has a different opinion or perspective on a problem?
- Do they use "we" or "I" more often when speaking? Is there a balance?
- Does each have a set of personal friends and activities separate from the family and partnership?
- How much energy goes into the family versus career and outside interests?
- What gets priority in their schedules? Children? Work? Personal activities? Couple time?

Triangles/Coalitions: Problem Subsystems and Triangles

Problem systems are identified in most systemic family counseling approaches. Triangles (Kerr & Bowen, 1988), covert coalitions (Minuchin & Fishman, 1981), or cross-generational coalitions (Minuchin & Fishman, 1981) all refer to a similar systemic process: tension between two people is resolved by drawing in a third (or forth, "*tetrad*"; Whitaker & Keith, 1981) person to stabilize the original dyad. Many counselors include inanimate objects or other processes as potential "thirds" in the triangulation process, such as drinking, drug use, work, hobbies, and so on, that are used to help one or both partners sooth their internal stress at the expense of the relationship.

Counselors assess for triangles and problematic subsystems in several ways:

- Clients overtly describe another party as playing a role in their tension; in these cases, the clients are aware at some level of the process going on.
- When clients describe the problem or conflict situation, another person plays the role of confidant or takes the side of one of the partners (e.g., one person has a friend or another family member who takes his or her side against the other).
- After being unable to get a need met in the primary dyad, a person finds what he or she is not getting in another person (e.g., a mother seeks emotional closeness from a child rather than husband).
- When counseling is inexplicably "stuck," there is often a triangle at work that distracts one or both parties from resolving critical issues (e.g., an affair, substance abuse, a friend who undermines agreements made in counseling).

Identifying triangles early in the assessment process enables counselors to intervene more successfully and quickly in a complex set of family dynamics.

Hierarchy Between Child and Parents

A key area in assessing parent and child relationships is the parent–child hierarchy. When assessing parental hierarchy, counselors must ask themselves, Is the parent–child hierarchy developmentally and culturally appropriate? If the hierarchy is appropriate, there are generally minimal problems with the child's behavior. Generally, if the child is exhibiting symptoms or there are problems in the parent–child relationship, there is some problem in the hierarchical structure: either an excessive (authoritarian) or an insufficient (permissive) parental hierarchy given the family's current sociocultural context(s). Immigrant families most always have two different sets of cultural norms for parental hierarchy (the traditional and the current cultural context), resulting in a difficult task of finding a balance between the two.

Assessing hierarchy is critical because it tells the counselor where and how to intervene. Often, inappropriate interventions are used if the counselor assesses only the symptoms. For example, although children with ADHD have similar symptoms—hyperactivity, defiance, failing to follow through on parents' requests, and so on—these same symptoms can occur in two dramatically different family structures: either too much or too little parental hierarchy. In the cases where the parental hierarchy is too rigid, the counselor works with the parents to soften this, develop a stronger personal relationship with the child, and set developmentally and culturally appropriate expectations. On the other hand, if there is not enough parental hierarchy, the counselor works with the parents to increase their consistency with consequences and to increase their attention to setting limits and rules. Thus, the same set of symptoms can require very different interventions.

Complementary Patterns

Complementary patterns characterize most couple relationships to a certain degree and can also characterize sibling relationships, friendships, and other relationships. *Complementary* in this case refers to each person taking on opposite or complementary roles that exist on a range from functional to problematic. For example, a complementary relationship of introvert/extrovert can exist in a balanced and well-functioning relationship as well as an out-of-balance, problematic relationship; the difference is in the rigidity of the pattern. Classic examples of complementary roles that often become problematic include pursuer/

distancer, emotional/logical, overfunctioner/underfunctioner, friendly parent/strict parent, and so on. In fact, Gottman (1999) indicates that the female-purse (demand) and male-withdraw pattern exists to some extent in the majority of marriages he studied. However, in distressed marriages, this becomes exaggerated and begins to be viewed as innate personality traits. Assessing for these patterns can help counselors intervene around these interactional dynamics. In most cases, people readily identify their complementary roles in their complaints about a relationship: "he's too strict with the kids," "she always emotionally overreacts," "I have to do it all the time," "she never wants sex," and so on. These broad, sweeping descriptions of the other denote a likely problematic complementary pattern.

Intergenerational Patterns

Assessing for intergenerational patterns is easiest when using a genogram (McGoldrick, Gerson, & Petry, 2008), which provides a visual map of intergenerational patterns. Counselors can create comprehensive genograms that map numerous intergenerational patterns or problem-specific genograms that focus on patterns related to the presenting problem and how family members have dealt with similar problems across generations (e.g., how other couples have dealt with marital tension). Patterns that frequently included in genograms are the following:

- Substance and alcohol abuse and dependence
- Sexual, physical, and emotional abuse
- Personal qualities and/or family roles; complementary roles (e.g., black sheep, rebellious one, overachiever/underachiever)
- Physical and mental health issues (e.g., diabetes, cancer, depression, psychosis)
- Historical incidents of the presenting problem, either with the same people or how other generations and family members have managed this problem.

Postmodern-Feminist Conceptualization

Solutions and Unique Outcomes

Solutions and Unique Outcomes

Attempted solutions that did not *work:* _____

_____

Exceptions and unique outcomes (times, places, relationships, contexts, etc. when problem is less of a problem; behaviors that seem to make things even slightly better): _____

_____

_____

Miracle question: If the problem were to be resolved overnight, what would client be doing differently the next day? (Describe in terms of doing X rather than not doing Y.)

1. _____

2. _____

3. _____

Attempted Solutions That Did Not *Work*

When assessing solutions, counselors need to assess two kinds: those that have worked and those that have not. The Mental Research Institute group (Watzlawick et al., 1974) and cognitive-behavioral therapy counselors (Baucom & Epstein, 1990) are best known for assessing what has not worked, although they use these in different ways when they intervene. With most clients, it is generally easy to assess failed previous solutions.

Questions for Assessing Solutions That Did Not Work

- *What have you tried to solve this problem?*

Most clients respond with a list of things that have not worked. If they need more prompting, counselors may ask the following:

- *I am guessing you have tried to solve this problem (address this issue) on your own and that some things were not as successful as you had hoped. What have you tried that did not work?*

Previous Solutions That Did Work/Unique Outcomes

Assessing previous solutions that helped is much harder because most clients are less aware of when the problem is not a problem and how they have kept things from getting worse. Solution-focused (de Shazer, 1988; O'Hanlon & Weiner-Davis, 1989) and narrative counselors (Freedman & Combs, 1996; White & Epston, 1990) have developed most of the assessment strategies for assessing what has worked.

Questions for Assessing Solutions and Unique Outcomes

- *What keeps this problem from being worse than it is right now?*
- *Is there any solution you have tried that worked for a while? Or made things slightly better?*
- *Are there times or places when the problem is less of a problem or when the problem is not a problem?*
- *Have you ever been able to respond to the problem so that it is less of a problem or less severe?*
- *Does this problem occur in all places with all people, or is it better in certain contexts?*

These questions generally require more thought and reflection on the part of the client and often require more follow-up questions on the part of the counselor. The answers to these questions often provide invaluable clues to how best to proceed and intervene in counseling.

Miracle Question

The original solution-generating question, the *miracle question* serves to both (a) conceptualize and assess and (b) set goals in solution-based counseling. The question goes as follows:

Miracle question: Imagine that you go home tonight, and during the middle of the night a miracle happens: *all the problems you came here to resolve* are miraculously resolved. However, when you wake up, you have no idea a miracle has occurred. What are some of the first things you would notice that would be different? How would you know that the problems that brought you here were resolved?

The key to successfully using this question to conceptualize the case involves (a) emphasizing that the miracle isn't just any old miracle but specifically resolves *problems that brought you here* today disappear and (b) to get specific, behavioral descriptions of what is different (not what the client wouldn't be doing or feeling). When delivered well, this single intervention can generate just about all of your client goals for treatment. For example, when working with a client who reports feeling depressed, a properly delivered miracle question would uncover goal-informing information, such as he would (a) wake up excited about the day, (b) go for a run, (c) hug and kiss his wife, (d) read a passage from his favorite Rumi book, and (e) arrive at work on time and warmly greet coworkers.

Narrative, Dominant Discourses, and Diversity

Narrative, Dominant Discourses, and Diversity

Dominant discourses informing definition of problem:

- *Cultural, ethnic, socioeconomic status, religious, etc.:* _____

  _____

- *Gender, sexual orientation, etc.:* _____

  _____

- *Contextual, family, and other social discourses:* _____

  _____

Identity narratives: How has having the problem shaped client's identity? _____

  _____

Local or preferred discourses: What is the client's preferred identity narrative and/or narrative about the problem? Are there local (alternative) discourses about the problem that are preferred? _____

  _____

  _____

Assessing dominant social discourses in which a client's problems are embedded often creates a broader and new perspective on a client's situation (Freedman & Combs, 1996; White & Epston, 1990). I frequently find that this broader perspective helps me to feel more freedom and possibility, increasing my emotional attunement to clients and allowing me to be more creative in my work. For example, when I view a client's reported "anxiety" as part of a larger discourse in which the client feels powerless, such as being a sexual minority, I begin to see the anxiety as part of this larger social dance. I also see how it is possible for this person to put less "faith," weight, or credence to the dominant discourse and generate new stories about what is "normal" sexual behavior and what is not. By discussing the difficulty in concretely defining what is "normal" sexual behavior and what is not, the client and I can begin to explore the truths that this person has experienced. We join in an exploratory process that offers new ways for the client to understand the anxiety as well as his or her identity.

Common dominant discourses or broader narratives that inform clients' lives include the following:

- Culture, race, ethnicity, and immigration
- Gender, sexual orientation, and sexual preferences
- Family of origin experiences, such as alcoholism, sexual abuse, adoption, and so on
- Stories of divorce, death, and loss of significant relationships
- Wealth, poverty, power, and fame
- Small-town, urban, and regional discourses
- Health, illness, body image, and so on

Identity Narratives

When a client comes for counseling, the problem discourse has most always become a significant part of one or more person's *identity narrative*, the story people tell themselves as to who they are. For example, a child having problems in school may begin to think, "I am stupid," while his mother may also be feeling like, "I have failed as a mother" because of her child's academic performance. Obviously, these negative sweeping judgments of a person's value or ability need to be addressed in counseling. Assessing these early in the process is useful to understand how to engage and motivate each person.

Local and Preferred Discourses

Local discourses are the stories that occur at the "local" (as opposed to dominant societal) level (Anderson, 1997). These narratives often are built on personal beliefs and unique interpretations and often contradict or significantly modify dominant discourses. Although it is theoretically possible for local discourses to contribute to the problem (e.g., having more oppressive versions of dominant discourses), they are most often a significant source of motivation, energy, and hope addressing problems. Most often, local discourses are a person's "personal truth" that they have been hiding or are ashamed of because of anticipated disapproval from others. Local discourses can address common subculture values, such as valuing certain religious or sexual practices, or highly unique to an individual, such as wanting to sell everything and travel the world. Local discourses are often the source of *preferred discourses* in narrative counseling (Freedman & Combs, 1996), which are the preferred version of one's life and identity that serve as the goal in narrative counseling.

Case Conceptualization, Diversity, and Sameness

Just in case you were beginning to feel like you finally understood something about case conceptualization, let me throw a wrench or two into the mix: diversity and sameness. The problem with case conceptualization and assessments in general (this applies to prior chapters as well) is that there are no objective standards against which a person can be measured for "healthy boundaries," "logical thinking," or "clear communication." Healthy, emotionally engaged boundaries look quite different in a Mexican American family and an Asian American family. In fact, problematic boundaries in a Mexican American family (e.g., cool, disengaged) may look *more like* healthy (e.g., quietly respectful) than problem boundaries (e.g., overly involved) in an Asian American family. Thus, counselors cannot rely simply on objective descriptions of behavior in assessment. Instead, counselor must consider the broader culture norms, which may include *more than one* set of ethnic norms as well as local neighborhood culture, school contexts, sexual orientation subculture, religious communities, and so on. Although you will undoubtedly take a course on cultural issues that will go into more depth on this topic and will read that professional codes of ethics require respecting diversity, it takes working with a diverse range of individuals and families and a willingness to learn from them to cultivate a meaningful sense of cultural sensitivity. I believe this to be a lifelong journey.

Ironically, I have found that new counselors in training today sometimes have the most difficulty accepting diversity in clients from *within* their culture of origin or who are in some ways similar to the counselor. The more similar clients are to us, the more we expect them to share our values and behavioral norms, making us more likely to have a low threshold for differentness. For example, middle-class Caucasian counselors often expect middle-class Caucasian clients to have particular values toward emotional expression, marital arrangements, extended family, and parent–child relationships and may be quick to encourage particular systems of values, namely, their own. Thus, whether working with someone very similar or very different than yourself, counselors need to *slowly* assess and evaluate, always considering clients' broader sociocultural context and norms. Counselors who excel in conceptualization and assessment approach these tasks with profound humility and a continual willingness to learn.

This End Is Just the Beginning

You have just traversed the bridge across the Grand Canyon of counseling. I hope you have that exhausted but exhilarating feeling that comes with great travel adventures. Not only have you been on a grand tour of the major counseling and psychotherapy theories, which is a lot in itself, but you have also learned perhaps the most critical of documentation skills: case conceptualization and treatment planning. If you are new to the field, by embarking on this admittedly challenging expedition early in your career, you have greatly accelerated your journey to becoming a competent counselor by establishing a solid foundation and framework from which to build as you move forward. For those who are more established, I am hoping that many pieces have fallen into place that help to take your practice to the next level.

In any case, I hope this is not the only time you read this book. Although this book is part textbook, it is more importantly a reference and hopefully a career-long companion for you. Each theory covered in this book is rich with insights into the human experience and how counselors can help people meet the challenges in their lives with grace and courage and prevent further crises from arising. For better or worse, counselors and psychotherapists are never done learning as new theories are developed each year and theories from over a hundred years ago still can assist us in our work. Each time you reread a section on one of these theories, I assure you that you will have new aha moments that make a client's situation, your own life, or the counseling profession make more sense. In fact, this book gets better and better each time you read it because you are able to conceptualize the material at deeper and more profound levels because of your practice in between. Thus, this is not an ending but rather the beginning of the next stage of the journey to becoming a competent counselor.

ONLINE RESOURCES

Associations

Family History Maker: U.S. Department of Health and Human Services
www.hhs.gov/familyhistory

References

American Psychiatric Association. (2000). *Diagnostic and statistical manual of mental disorders* (4th ed., text revision). Washington, DC: Author.

Anderson, H. (1997). *Conversations, language, and possibilities.* New York: Basic Books.

Anderson, H., &, Gehart, D. R. (Eds.). (2007). *Collaborative therapy: Relationships and conversations that make a difference.* New York: Brunner-Routledge.

Bateson, G. (1972). *Steps to an ecology of mind.* New York: Ballantine.

Bateson, G. (2002). *Mind and nature: A necessary unity.* Cresskill, NJ: Hampton.

Baucom, D. H., & Epstein, N. (1990). *Cognitive-behavioral marital therapy.* New York: Brunner/Mazel.

Beck, A. (1976). *Cognitive therapy and emotional disorders.* New York: International University Press.

Bowlby, J. (1988). *A secure base: Parent-child attachment and healthy human development.* London: Routledge.

Carter, B., & McGoldrick, M. (1999). *The expanded family life cycle: Individuals, families, and social perspectives* (3rd ed.). New York: Allyn and Bacon.

Chapman, A. (2006). *Erickson's psychosocial development theory.* Available: http://www.businessballs.com/erik_erikson_psychosocial_theory.htm de Shazer, S. (1988). *Clues: Investigating solutions in brief therapy.* New York: Norton.

Eckstein, D. (2009). *An understanding of each person's personal preferences.* Available: http://www.santafecoach.com/DRC/drcpp-test%20theory.htm#comfortpar

Ellis, A. (1999). *Reason and emotion in psychotherapy* (Rev. ed.). New York: Kensington.

Frankl, V. (1963). *Man's search for meaning.* Boston: Beacon.

Freedman, J., & Combs, G. (1996). *Narrative therapy: The social contruction of preferred realities.* New York: Norton.

Gergen, K. J. (1999). *An invitation to social construction.* Thousand Oaks, CA: Sage.

Gottman, J. M. (1999). *The marriage clinic: A scientifically based marital therapy.* New York: Norton.

Johnson, S. M. (2004). *The practice of emotionally focused marital therapy: Creating connection* (2nd ed.). New York: Brunner-Routledge.

Kerr, M., & Bowen, M. (1988). *Family evaluation.* New York: Norton.

Lambert, M. J., & Ogles, B. M. (2004). The efficacy and effectiveness of psychotherapy. In M. J. Lambert (Ed.), *Bergin and Garfield's handbook of psychotherapy and behavior change* (5th ed., pp. 139–193). New York: Wiley.

McGoldrick, M., Gerson, R., & Petry, S. (2008). *Genograms: Assessment and intervention* (3rd ed.). New York: Norton.

Miller, S. D., Duncan, B. L., & Hubble, M. (1997). *Escape from Babel: Toward a unifying language for psychotherapy practice.* New York: Norton.

Minuchin, S. (1974). *Families and family therapy.* Cambridge, MA: Harvard University Press.

Minuchin, S., & Fishman, H.C. (1981). *Family therapy techniques.* Cambridge, MA: Harvard University Press.

Morgan, O. (2006). *Counseling and spirituality: Views from the profession.* Pacific Grove, CA: Wadsworth.

O'Hanlon, W. H., & Weiner-Davis, M. (1989). *In search of solutions: A new direction in psychotherapy.* New York: Norton.

Perls, F., Hefferline, R. F., & Goodman, P. (1951). *Gestalt therapy: Excitement and growth in the human personality*. New York: Julian Press.

Rogers, C. (1961). *On becoming a person: A counselor's view of psychocounseling*. London: Constable.

Seligman, M. (2002). *Authentic happiness: Using the new positive psychology to realize your potential for lasting fulfillment*. New York: Free Press.

Sperry, L. (2001). *Spirituality in clinical practice: Incorporating the spiritual dimention in psychotherapy and counseling*. New York: Routledge.

Spiegler, M. D., & Guevremont, D. C. (2003). *Contemporary behavior therapy* (4th ed.). Pacific Grove, CA: Brooks/Cole.

St. Clair, M. (2000). *Object relations and self psychology: An introduction*. Belmont, CA: Brooks/Cole.

Walsh, F. (Ed.). (2003). *Spiritual resources in family therapy*. New York: Guilford.

Watzlawick, P., Weakland, J., & Fisch, R. (1974). *Change: Principles of problem formation and problem resolution*. New York: Norton.

Whitaker, C. A., & Keith, D. V. (1981). Symbolic-experiential family therapy. In A. S. Gurman, & D. P. Kniskern (Eds.), *Handbook of family therapy* (pp. 187–224). New York: Brunner/Mazel.

White, M., & Epston, D. (1990). *Narrative means to therapeutic ends*. New York: Norton.

Woldt, A. L., & Toman, S. M. (Eds.). (2005). *Gestalt therapy: History, theory, and practice*. Thousand Oaks, CA: Sage.

Yontef, G. (1993). *Awareness dialogue and process: Essays on Gestalt therapy*. Highland, NY: Gestalt Journal Press.

Case Conceptualization Form

COPIES OF THIS FORM ARE AVAILABLE ON THE TEXTBOOK WEBSITE

Counseling Case Conceptualization

Clinical Mental Health

Counselor: _____ Client/Case #: _____ Date: _____

I. Introduction to Client & Significant Others

❏ AF ❏ AM ❏ CF ❏ CM   *Age:* _____   *Ethnicity/Language:* _____

Occupation/Grade in School: _____

Relational/Family Status: _____

II. Presenting Concern(s)

Client Description of Problem(s): _____

_____

_____

Significant Other/Family Description(s) of Problems: _____

_____

_____

Broader System Problem Descriptions: Description of problem from referring party, teachers, relatives, legal system, etc.:

_____ : _____

_____ : _____

III. Background Information

Trauma/Abuse History (recent and past): _____

_____

Substance Use/Abuse (current and past; self, family of origin, significant others): _____

_____

_____

Precipitating Events (recent life changes, first symptoms, stressors, etc.): _____

_____

_____

_____

(continued)

Related Historical Background (family history, related issues, previous counseling, medical/mental health history, etc.): _____

_____

_____

IV. Client Strengths and Diversity

Client Strengths

Personal: _____

_____

Relational/Social: _____

_____

Spiritual: _____

_____

Diversity: Resources and Limitations

Identify potential resources and limitations available to clients based on their age, gender, sexual orientation, cultural background, socioeconomic status, religion, regional community, language, family background, family configuration, abilities, etc.

Unique Resources: _____

_____

Potential Limitations: _____

_____

COMPLETE ONE OR MORE OF THE FOLLOWING SECTIONS (V–IX) BASED ON THE THEORY(IES) YOU PLAN TO USE FOR YOUR TREATMENT PLAN

V. Psychodynamic Conceptualization

Psychodynamic Defense Mechanisms

❏ Acting out: *Describe:* _____

❏ Denial: *Describe:* _____

❏ Displacement: *Describe:* _____

❏ Help-rejecting complaining: *Describe:* _____

❏ Humor: *Describe:* _____

❏ Passive aggression: *Describe:* _____

❏ Projection: *Describe:* _____

❏ Projective identification: *Describe:* _____

❏ Rationalization: *Describe:* _____

❏ Reaction formation: *Describe:* _____

(continued)

❏ Repression: *Describe:* _____

❏ Splitting: *Describe:* _____

❏ Sublimation: *Describe:* _____

❏ Suppression: *Describe:* _____

❏ Other: _____

Object Relational Patterns

Describe relationship with early caregivers in past: _____

_____

_____

Was the attachment with the mother (or equivalent) primarily: ❏ Generally secure
❏ Anxious and clingy   ❏ Avoidant and emotionally distant   ❏ Other: _____

Was the attachment with the father (or equivalent) primarily: ❏ Generally secure
❏ Anxious and clingy   ❏ Avoidant and emotionally distant   ❏ Other: _____

Describe present relationship with these caregivers: _____

_____

Describe relational patterns with partner and other current relationships: _____

_____

_____

Erickson's Psychosocial Developmental Stage

Describe development at each stage up to current stage

Trust versus mistrust (infant stage): _____

Autonomy versus shame and doubt (toddler stage): _____

Initiative versus guilt (preschool stage): _____

Industry versus inferiority (school stage): _____

Identity versus role confusion (adolescence): _____

Intimacy versus isolation (young adulthood): _____

Generativity versus stagnation (adulthood): _____

Ego integrity versus despair (late adulthood): _____

Adlerian Style of Life Theme

❏ Control: _____

❏ Superiority: _____

❏ Pleasing: _____

❏ Comfort: _____

Basic Mistake Misperceptions: _____

(continued)

VI. Humanistic-Existential Conceptualization

Expression of Authentic Self

Problems: Are problems perceived as internal or external (caused by others, circumstance, etc.)?
❏ Predominantly internal ❏ Mixed ❏ Predominantly external

Agency and responsibility: Is self or other discussed as agent of story? Does client take clear responsibility for situation? ❏ Strong sense of agency and responsibility ❏ Agency in some areas
❏ Little agency; frequently blames others/situation ❏ Often feels victimized

Recognition and expression of feelings: Are feelings readily recognized, owned, and experienced?
❏ Easily expresses feelings ❏ Identifies with prompting ❏ Difficulty recognizing feelings

Here-and-now experiencing: Is the client able to experience full range of feelings as they are happening in the present moment? ❏ Easily experiences emotions in present moment ❏ Experiences some present emotions with assistance ❏ Difficulty with present moment experiencing

Personal constructs and facades: Is the client able to recognize and go beyond roles? Is identity rigid or tentatively held? ❏ Tentatively held; able to critique and question ❏ Some awareness of facades and construction of identity ❏ Identity rigidly defined; seems like "fact"

Complexity and contradictions: Are internal contradictions owned and explored? Is client able to fully engage the complexity of identity and life? ❏ Aware of and resolves contradictions ❏ Some recognition of contradictions ❏ Unaware of internal contradictions

"Shoulds": Is client able to question socially imposed "shoulds" and "oughts"? Can client balance desire to please others and desire to be authentic? ❏ Able to balance authenticity with social obligation
❏ Identifies tension between social expectations and personal desires ❏ Primarily focuses on external shoulds

List "shoulds": _____

Acceptance of others: Is client able to accept others and modify expectations of others to be more realistic?
❏ Readily accepts others as they are ❏ Recognizes expectations of others are unrealistic but still strong emotional reaction to expectations not being met ❏ Difficulty accepting others as is; always wanting others to change to meet expectations

Trust of self: Is client able to trust self as process (rather than a stable object)? ❏ Able to trust and express authentic self ❏ Trust of self in certain contexts ❏ Difficulty trusting self in most contexts

Existential Analysis

Sources of life meaning (as described or demonstrated by client): _____

_____

_____

General themes: ❏ Personal achievement/work ❏ Significant other ❏ Children ❏ Family of origin ❏ Social cause/contributing to others ❏ Religion/spirituality ❏ Other: _____

Satisfaction with and clarity on life direction:

❏ Clear sense of meaning that creates resilience in difficult times

❏ Current problems require making choices related to life direction

❏ Minimally satisfied with current life direction; wants more from life

(continued)

❐ Has reflected little on life direction up to this point; living according to life plan defined by someone/ something else

❐ Other: _____

Gestalt Contact Boundary Disturbances

❐ *Desensitization:* Failing to notice problems

❐ *Introjection:* Take in others' views whole and unedited

❐ *Projection:* Assign undesired parts of self to others

❐ *Retroflection:* Direct action to self rather than other

❐ *Deflection:* Avoid direct contact with another or self

❐ *Egotism:* Not allowing outside to influence self

❐ *Confluence:* Agree with another to an extent that boundary blurred

❐ *Describe:* _____

_____

VII. Cognitive-Behavioral Conceptualization

Baseline of Symptomatic Behavior

Symptom #1 (behavioral description): _____

Frequency: _____

Duration: _____

Context(s): _____

Events before: _____

Events after: _____

Symptom #2 (behavioral description): _____

Frequency: _____

Duration: _____

Context(s): _____

Events before: _____

Events after: _____

A-B-C Analysis of Irrational Beliefs

Activating Event (problem): _____

Consequence (mood, behavior, etc.): _____

Mediating Beliefs (unhelpful beliefs about event that result in C): _____

(continued)

1. _____

2. _____

3. _____

Beck's Schema Analysis

Identify frequently used cognitive schemas:

❏ *Arbitrary inference:* _____

❏ *Selective abstraction:* _____

❏ *Overgeneralization:* _____

❏ *Magnification/minimization:* _____

❏ *Personalization:* _____

❏ *Absolutist/dichotomous thinking:* _____

❏ *Mislabeling:* _____

❏ *Mind reading:* _____

VIII. Family Systems Conceptualization

Family Life Cycle Stage

❏ Single adult ❏ Marriage ❏ Family with young children ❏ Family with adolescent children ❏ Launching children ❏ Later life

Describe struggles with mastering developmental tasks in one of these stages: _____

_____

Typical style for regulating closeness and distance with others: _____

_____

_____

Boundaries with

    Parents: Enmeshed Clear Disengaged NA: *Diversity note:* _____

    Siblings: Enmeshed Clear Disengaged NA: *Diversity note:* _____

    Significant other: Enmeshed Clear Disengaged NA: *Diversity note:* _____

    Children: Enmeshed Clear Disengaged NA: *Diversity note:* _____

    Extended family: Enmeshed Clear Disengaged NA: *Diversity note:* _____

    Other: _____: Enmeshed Clear Disengaged NA: *Diversity note:* _____

Triangles/Coalitions

    ❏ Coalition in family of origin: *Describe:* _____

    ❏ Coalitions related to significant other: *Describe:* _____

    ❏ Other coalitions: _____

(continued)

Hierarchy between self and parent/child ❐ NA

   With own children: ❐ Effective ❐ Rigid ❐ Permissive

   With parents (for child or young adult): ❐ Effective ❐ Rigid ❐ Permissive

Complementary patterns with _____ : ❐ Pursuer/distancer ❐ Over/underfunctioner ❐ Emotional/logical
   ❐ Good/bad parent ❐ Other: _____ Example: _____

Intergenerational Patterns

   Family strengths: _____

   Substance/alcohol abuse: ❐ N/A ❐ Example: _____

   Sexual/physical/emotional abuse: ❐ N/A ❐ Example: _____

   Parent/child relations: ❐ N/A ❐ Example: _____

   Physical/mental disorders: ❐ N/A ❐ Example: _____

   Historical incidents of presenting problem: ❐ N/A ❐ Example: _____

IX. Solution-Based and Cultural Discourse Conceptualization (Postmodern)

Solutions and Unique Outcomes

Attempted solutions that did not *work*: _____

_____

Exceptions and unique outcomes (times, places, relationships, contexts, etc. when problem is less of a problem; behaviors that seem to make things even slightly better): _____

_____

_____

Miracle question answer: If the problem were to be resolved overnight, what would client be doing differently the next day? (Describe in terms of doing X rather than not doing Y.)

1. _____

2. _____

3. _____

X. Narrative, Dominant Discourses, and Diversity

Dominant discourses informing definition of problem:

• *Cultural, ethnic, socioeconomic status, religious etc.:* _____

_____

• *Gender, sexual orientation, etc.:* _____

_____

- *Contextual, family, and other social discourses:* _____

_____

Identity/self narratives: How has the problem shaped client's identity? _____

Local or preferred discourses: What is the client's preferred identity narrative and/or narrative about the problem? Are there local (alternative) discourses about the problem that are preferred? _____

_____

A

Treatment Plan Rubric

Note: The sample rubric below is correlated to the CACREP Clinical Mental Health Counseling competencies. On the textbook websites at www.Cengage.com and the www.masteringcompetencies.com, instructors and students will find additional rubrics correlated to all the major mental health competencies, including the following:

- Each of the 2009 CACREP areas of specialty: addictions, career, clinical mental health, marriage, couple, and family, school, and student affairs and college counseling.
- The marriage and family therapy (AAMFT) Core Competencies
- The social work (CSWE) competencies
- 2011 psychology competency benchmarks

Date: _____

Student: _____

Evaluator: _____

Level of Clinical Training:
- ☐ Pre-clinical training; coursework only
- ☐ 0–12 months
- ☐ 12–24 months
- ☐ 2+ years

Rating Scale

5 = Exceptional: Skills and understanding significantly beyond developmental level

4 = Outstanding: Strong mastery of skills and thorough understanding of concepts

3 = Mastered Basic Skills at Developmental Level: Understanding of concepts/skills evident

2 = Developing: Minor conceptual and skill errors; in process of developing

1 = Deficits: Significant remediation needed; deficits in knowledge/skills

NA = Not Applicable: Unable to measure with given data (do not use to indicate deficit)

	5	4	3	2	1	Comp	Score
Theory-Specific Case Conceptualization (Optional)	Sophisticated and subtle case conceptualization narrative using theory-specific elements; integrates diversity, trauma, and substance abuse, and diversity issues; unique and specific.	Thoughtful and specific case conceptualization narrative that includes discussion of major theory-specific elements; addresses diversity and unique client needs.	Case conceptualization narrative uses theory-specific concepts to address salient client issues.	Inconsistent or incorrect use of theory-specific conceptualization elements. Ignores subtle diversity issues.	Significant problems with case conceptualization, such as misunderstanding key theoretical concepts, mixing theories, missing significant diversity issues, etc.	A5 C8 D1 D2 D5 E1 E2 G1	☐ NA
Choice of Theory (if applicable)	Choice of theory demonstrates sophisticated understanding of the evidence base and best approaches for presenting problem; adapts choice for age, culture, ability, trauma, values, etc.	Choice of theory demonstrates thoughtful understanding of presenting problem; good choice for age, culture, ability, values, trauma, etc.	Choice of theory is appropriate for presenting problem.	Minor problem with chosen theory for client; no particular attention to age, culture, ability, values, etc.	Inappropriate choice of theory given problem, research, age, culture, ability, values, etc.	A1 A5 C8 E3 I3 J1 K2	☐ NA
Initial Phase Task: Relationship	Sophisticated application of theory's specific form of counseling relationship; relates directly to specifics of case and diversity issues.	Identifies at least one theory-specific technique for forming relationship and uniquely applies to client needs/diversity issues; more detailed than template in the book.	Identifies an effective technique from theory for forming a counseling relationship.	Minor theoretical inconsistencies related to counseling relationship and/or no specific application to case.	Significant problems or theoretical inconsistencies addressing counseling relationship.	A5	☐ NA

Task						Codes	
Initial Phase Task: Assessment	Sophisticated use of theory-specific assessment; uniquely applied to case; adapts for age, culture, education, service context.	At least one theory-specific assessment; proposed assessments appropriate for age, culture, education, etc.; more detailed than template in the book.	Theoretically consistent assessment techniques that are appropriate for case.	Minor problems or theoretical inconsistencies with proposed assessments.	Significant problems with proposed assessment; does not address critical diversity issues, such as age, culture, education, language, etc.	C7 D1 H1 H4	❑ NA
Initial Phase Client Goal	Sophisticated, well-chosen initial goal that address specific, immediate client needs or crisis; goals clearly prioritized based on research, treatment model, diversity issues, and client needs.	Well-chosen initial goal that address immediate client needs; more detailed than template in the book.	Appropriate initial goal that address immediate client needs.	Minor problems with initial goal; may not be prioritized correctly or specific enough.	Initial goal inappropriate; misses immediate and/or crisis issues.	A5 D1 D2 J2	❑ NA
Initial Phase Interventions	Sophisticated choice of interventions appropriate for initial stage of counseling; theory-specific and tailored to client and diversity needs.	Thoughtful choice of interventions; theory-specific; more detailed than template in the book.	Appropriate choice of interventions for goal that generally fit with theory.	Minor problems or vague interventions; may not be a good fit for theory.	Significant problems with initial interventions; theoretically inappropriate or poor fit for client.	A5 C1 F3	❑ NA
Working Phase Task: Monitor Alliance	Theory-specific handling of diversity issues and client needs for monitoring alliance; specific and realistic.	Meaningful attention to diversity and client needs for monitoring the alliance; more detailed than template in the book.	Identifies appropriate intervention for monitoring alliance.	Minor problems with plans for monitoring alliance.	Does not provide appropriate and/or any means for monitoring alliance.	D1 I3	❑ NA
Working Phase Client Goals	2-3 easily measured and theory-specific goals that skillfully address all issues identified in case conceptualization by identifying client's core issues; goals are unique, specific, and tailored to client situation and diversity needs.	2-3 measurable goals that target assessed issues in case conceptualization; goals consistent with chosen theory; attention to diversity; more detailed than template in the book.	2-3 goals that target major assessed problems; reflect basic understanding of content vs. process; appropriate for client.	Vague goals and/or theoretically inconsistent yet appropriate goals. No clear distinction between content and process.	Inappropriate goals and/or unclear goals; goals outside scope of competence or practice.	A5 D1 D2 J2	❑ NA

	5	4	3	2	1	Comp	Score
Working Phase Interventions	Carefully crafted interventions that support goal achievement; theory-specific and tailored to client; clear and realistic plan of how to achieve goal; interventions include specific examples (e.g., quotes, etc.).	2 detailed interventions for each goal; theory-specific and applied to client; more detailed than template in the book.	1-2 appropriate interventions for each goal that are generally consistent with theory.	Suggested interventions do not support stated goal; theoretically inconsistent.	Poor choice of intervention given stated goals. Poor description of intervention.	A5 C1 F3	☐ NA
Closing Phase Task: Aftercare Plan	Sophisticated and detailed approach to termination and aftercare plans; theory specific and tailored to fit unique client needs/diversity.	Thoughtful approach to termination and aftercare plans that fit with theory; more detailed than template in the book.	Appropriate termination and aftercare plans; broadly reflects theory and client needs.	Minor problems with closing plan; unrealistic or inappropriately adapted for client.	Significant problems with closing plan; unrealistic or inappropriately adapted for client.	C5 D3	☐ NA
Closing Phase Client Goals	Targets theory's long-term goals if appropriate (i.e., definition of health) and client's goals; detailed, clear and specific; promotes overall personal and relational wellness; addresses diversity/client specific.	1-2 goals appropriate for theory in late phase that are specific to client; promotes long-term wellness; more detailed than template in the book.	1-2 goals that address long-term goals related to client's presenting concerns.	Minor problems with closing goals; does not attend to theory's model of health.	Significant problems with closing goals; inappropriate or unrealistic.	A5 D1 D2 D3 J2	☐ NA
Closing Phase Interventions	Sophisticated interventions that support sustained gains; theory-specific and tailored to client; clear and realistic interventions for long-term wellness; interventions include specific examples.	2 interventions that support goal achievement; specific and unique; theory-specific; more detailed than template in the book.	Appropriate interventions that support goal; consistent with theory.	Suggested interventions do not support stated goal; theoretically inconsistent; vague examples of specific interventions.	Poor choice of intervention given stated goals. Poor description of intervention.	A5 C1 F3	☐ NA
Overall Understanding of Theory and Technique	Sophisticated understanding of theory and techniques; plan highly consistent with theory yet uniquely adapted for cultural/context factors; demonstrates original thinking.	Clear understanding of theory and techniques; interventions consistent with theory and appropriate for cultural/context factors; goes beyond template in the book.	Solid understanding of theories and techniques; closely follows template; interventions generally consistent with theory and cultural/context factors.	Some problems with understanding of theory and techniques; interventions often not consistent with theory.	Significant problems with understanding of theories and techniques; interventions generally not consistent with theory.	A5 D2 F3	☐ NA

Overall Plan	Sophisticated plan that reveals depth of understanding of theory and ability to creatively meet client and diversity needs and goals. Extensive detail with some specific examples of interventions (e.g., quotes, etc.).	Thoughtful plan that goes beyond template in the book to reveal unique application of theory; plan addresses most areas related to presenting problem using theory.	Theory-specific plan that closely models template; effectively addresses client's presenting problem.	Minor problems with plan, such as not all aspects fitting with theory, not addressing presenting problems, etc.	Significant problems with plan, such as numerous theoretical inconsistencies, missing key aspects of presenting problem, etc.	C8 D7 G1	❑ NA
Comments:							

B

Comprehensive Case Conceptualization Rubric

> **Note:** The sample rubric below is correlated to the CACREP Clinical Mental Health Counseling competencies. On the textbook websites at www.Cengage.com and the www.masteringcompetencies.com, instructors and students will find additional rubrics correlated to all the major mental health competencies, including the following:
>
> • Each of the 2009 CACREP areas of specialty: addictions, career, clinical mental health, marriage, couple, and family, school, and student affairs and college counseling.
> • The marriage and family therapy (AAMFT) Core Competencies
> • The social work (CSWE) competencies
> • 2011 psychology competency benchmarks

Date: _____

Student: _____

Evaluator: _____

Level of Clinical Training:
☐ Pre-clinical training; coursework only
☐ 0–12 months
☐ 12–24 months
☐ 2+ years

Rating Scale

5 = Exceptional: Skills and understanding significantly beyond developmental level

4 = Outstanding: Strong mastery of skills and thorough understanding of concepts

3 = Mastered Basic Skills at Developmental Level: Understanding of concepts/skills evident

2 = Developing: Minor conceptual and skill errors; in process of developing

1 = Deficits: Significant remediation needed; deficits in knowledge/skills

NA = Not Applicable: Unable to measure with given data (do not use to indicate deficit)

	5	4	3	2	1	Comp	Score
Introduction	Detailed yet succinct intro that identifies client, age, ethnicity, occupation, grade, etc. Descriptions clearly set context for understanding problem.	Complete intro that identifies client, age, ethnicity, occupation, grade, etc.	Basic information related to age, ethnicity, occupation, grade, etc. included.	Missing 1-2 identifiers.	Missing, incorrect or significant problem with identifiers and/or significant involved parties.	C7 H2	☐ NA
Presenting Concern	Description of problem provides sophisticated depiction of all stakeholders' views; word choice conveys empathy with each perspective; descriptions clearly contribute to coherent conceptualization.	Description of problem provides useful description of all stakeholders' views; word choice conveys respect for perspectives.	Includes description of problem for each person and key stakeholders.	Minor problems or lack of clarity with problem descriptions; missing stakeholders.	Significant problems with problem descriptions; missing key perspectives; incorrect characterization.	C7 H2	☐ NA
Background Information	Includes detailed yet succinct description of recent and past events and traumas. Selected information helps develop coherent conceptualization.	Includes useful summary of recent and past events and traumas with time frames.	Includes summary of key recent and past events and traumas.	Insufficient, minimal or missing background information.	Significant information missing; unable to identify significant events.	A9 H2 H4	☐ NA

					Code	NA
Client Strengths & Diversity	Insightful identification of strengths; able to identify subtle diversity resources and limitations and how these may impact counseling process.	Clear articulation of useful strengths; able to identify several key resources and limitations related to diversity, oppression, and marginalization.	Identifies several strengths as well as significant resources and limitations related to diversity.	Underdeveloped description of strengths. Missed one or more significant diversity limitation.	Significant problems identifying clinically relevant strengths and/or diversity issues.	D2 D3 E1 E2	❑ NA
Psycho-dynamic and Adlerian	Sophisticated analysis that coherently and succinctly relates defense mechanisms, object relation patterns, developmental stages and style of life themes. Clear sense of core dynamics emerges.	Thoughtful and coherent descriptions of defense mechanisms, object relation patterns, developmental stages and style of life themes.	Identifies key issues in defense mechanisms, object relation patterns, developmental stages and style of life themes.	Minor errors or inconsistencies in descriptions of defense mechanisms, object relation patterns, developmental stages and/or style of life themes.	Incorrect, poor characterization of defense mechanisms, object relation patterns, developmental stages and style of life themes.	A5	❑ NA
Humanistic-Existential	Sophisticated analysis that coherently and succinctly relates expressions of self, existential issues, and boundary disturbances. Clear sense of core issues developed.	Thoughtful and coherent descriptions of expressions of self, existential issues, and boundary disturbances.	Identifies key issues in expressions of self, existential issues, and boundary disturbances.	Minor errors or inconsistencies in descriptions of expressions of self, existential issues, and boundary disturbances.	Significant problems with expressions of self, existential issues, and boundary disturbances; misidentified issues.	A5	❑ NA
Cognitive-Behavioral	Sophisticated analysis that coherently and succinctly relates behavioral analysis, ABC analysis, and schemas. Clear sense of core themes emerges.	Thoughtful and coherent descriptions of behavioral analysis, ABC analysis, and schemas.	Identifies key issues in behavioral analysis, ABC analysis, and schemas.	Minor problems conceptualizing behavioral analysis, ABC analysis, and schemas.	Significant problems identifying behavioral analysis, ABC analysis, and schemas.	A5	❑ NA
Family Systems	Sophisticated analysis that coherently and succinctly relates assessment of family life cycle, family structure, and intergenerational patterns. Clear depiction of how family patterns relate to problem.	Thoughtful and coherent descriptions of family life cycle, family structure, and intergenerational patterns.	Identifies key issues in family life cycle, family structure, and intergenerational patterns.	Misses minor issues in family life cycle, family structure, and intergenerational patterns.	Misses significant issues related to family life cycle, family structure, and intergenerational patterns.	A5 C8	❑ NA

	5	4	3	2	1	Comp	Score
Solution-Focused	Sophisticated analysis that reveals creativity in identifying solutions that did and did not work; behavioral, positively stated, and easily implementable answers to miracle question.	Able to identified several useful exceptions to the problem; answers to miracle question behavioral and positively stated.	Provides examples of solutions that did and did not work; behavioral answers to miracle question.	Solutions and miracle question not approached from a strengths perspective; lack usefulness and practicality.	Significant problems with assessment of strengths and/or does not demonstrate understanding of miracle question.	A5	❏ NA
Narrative, Dominant Discourses, and Diversity	Thoughtfully identifies effect of dominant discourses in client's life; able to meaningfully identify several cultural, SES, gender, and larger social discourse issues and outline how these intersect. Addresses oppression and marginalization.	Detailed description of the effect of dominant discourses in client's life; able to meaningfully identify at least two cultural, SES, gender, and larger social discourse issues.	Clear description of key diversity issues and broader social discourses affecting client and experience of problem.	Minor issues with identification of social and dominant discourses.	Misses one or more significant diversity issue and/or unable to usefully identify its effect on the client's life.	A5 D2 E1 E2 E5	❏ NA
Overall Conceptualization	All elements of case conceptualization clearly fit to create a unified understanding to guide counseling process. Sophisticated conceptualization that identifies subtle issues.	Well developed conceptualization that enables reader to a have a clear sense of client and core issues.	Provides a useful description of key issues for developing treatment plan. Few if any inconsistencies.	Several minor inconsistencies that are not clearly reconciled.	Significant problems with conceptualization, such as irreconcilable discrepancies or missing key issues.	A5 C7 D7 F3 H1	❏ NA

Comments:

Name Index

Subject Index